Whiplash and Other Useful Illnesses

Whiplash and
Other Useful Illnesses

Andrew Malleson

McGill-Queen's University Press
Montreal & Kingston • London • Ithaca

© McGill-Queen's University Press 2002
ISBN 0-7735-2333-2
Legal deposit second quarter 2002
Bibliothèque nationale du Québec

Printed in Canada on acid-free paper.

Publication of this book has been made possible by a
grant from the Psychiatry Department, University of
Toronto, and the Board of Humane Medicine.

McGill-Queen's University Press acknowledges the
financial support of the Government of Canada
through the Book Publishing Industry Development
Program (BPIDP) for its publishing activities. We also
acknowledge the support of the Canada Council for
the Arts for our publishing program.

National Library of Canada Cataloguing in Publication Data

Malleson, Andrew
    Whiplash and other useful illnesses

    Includes bibliographical references and index.
    ISBN 0-7735-2333-2

    1. Medical jurisprudence—Canada.   2. Whiplash injuries—
    Treatment—Canada.   3. Personal injuries—Canada.
    4. Medical care, Cost of—Canada.   I. Title.

    RA1170.B33M34 2002   614'.1   C2001-903341-9

Typeset in 10/12 Baskerville by True to Type

I dedicate this book to all the chimpanzees, monkeys,
and other animals that died miserable deaths
in vain attempts to prove that whiplashed people are not
"just neurotic" but have been truly injured.

I also dedicate it to the everlastingly patient librarians
at the University Health Network hospitals, Toronto,
who were not driven neurotic by my demands
for inaccessible publications.

Contents

Acknowledgments

Many friends and colleagues have helped with the ideas and information in this book. Some read individual chapters and some the whole manuscript. They all gave useful advice for which I am most grateful. In particular, I wish to thank Dr Cornelia Baines, Dr Joanna Barnes, Dr Richard Earle, Dr June Engel, Dr J.F. Ross Fleming, Dr John Frank, Mr Brian Leck, Dr Michael Livingston, Dr Jon Poole, Dr John Rutka, Dr Ashok Sajani, Dr John Senders, Dr Ann Taylor, Ms Elizabeth Till, and my niece and my nephews: Drs Kate, Peter and Steven Malleson; and my wife, Dr Donna Stewart. I especially want to thank Sherry Stein, who has an eagle eye for typos, spelling mistakes, and solecisms; and also, Jane McWhinney, editor for McGill-Queen's University Press, who patiently and with great competence made sure that I wrote what I meant to write, and that I did so with decorum and without "too many" words.

I would like in addition to acknowledge with much gratitude grants from the Department of Psychiatry at the University of Toronto, and from Dr Dimitri Oreopoulos and other members of the Board of Humane Medicine, whose exceptional generosity made the publication of this book possible.

Andrew Malleson
MB, BS, DPM, MRCP, MRCPsych, FRCP(C)

Preface

AN APOLOGY TO READERS OF BOTH SEXES

The customary use of a masculine pronoun to include both male and female indicates much that is wrong in our gender relationships. It certainly offends many women. The use of the duplicated pronoun – he/she – is offensive to the English language. Writing about whiplash compounds an author's pronoun problems, since twice as many women suffer from whiplash as do men.

Referring to a whiplashed person as him, when he is more likely to be a her is logically reprehensible. The consistent use of her, while being more accurate, conveys the impression that only women suffer whiplash, and, since I clearly regard whiplash as a questionable condition, such a use of the female pronoun would undoubtedly be most offensive. I have therefore decided to stick to the customary masculine pronoun. It should, however, be remembered that statistically the hes and hims are more likely to be shes and hers. I mean neither gender offence.

Whiplash and
Other Useful Illnesses

Magnificent in its simplicity and how it seizes the imagination of patients, doctors and lawyers. It is so easy to picture the occurrence of a whiplash injury that, as we think about it, we can almost feel the resulting pain in the neck.

– James Hodge[1]

We are not the only dishonest species, but we are surely the most dishonest, if only because we do the most talking.

– Robert Wright, *The Moral Animal*[2]

Absolute power corrupts but lack of power corrupts absolutely.

– Adlai Stevenson

A society that spends so much on healthcare that it cannot spend adequately on other health-enhancing activities may actually be reducing the health of its population.

– R.G. Evans and G.L. Stoddart[3]

Healthcare Entrepreneurs in Search of Work

Healthcare systems are in trouble. Although more and more public and private money is being poured into healthcare, it is never enough. Medicine has had some astounding successes, and histories of medicine paint glowing pictures of its victories over ignorance and disease. The shadier side of medicine is usually quietly forgotten.

Healthcare is now the world's largest industry. Just as the lumber industry depends upon trees for its existence, so the healthcare industry depends upon illness. The lumber industry worries about a shortage of trees, but the healthcare industry is confronted by an even greater problem. Never before, at least in the developed world, have we lived such healthy lives or inhabited such a healthy environment, and never before have there been so many healthcare practitioners in search of work. Doctors, other healthcare professionals, and the many lawyers and businessmen who depend upon the health industry for their livelihoods are entrepreneurs. They make their own work. When illnesses are in short supply, they create new ones. Increasingly expensive investigational techniques are deployed in the unending search for illnesses to treat.

I grew up in the depression years in Maida Vale, a red-light district of London, in a row of dilapidated Victorian houses owned by the Church of England. From our house, my mother and two women colleagues ran a busy medical practice. Watching patients come and go, I learned that, while people have courage in adversity, they are also quite capable of putting illness to good use; patients get attention. My father was a character actor and from him I learned also that people are not always what they seem to be. Perhaps because of these early impressions of the world, I have always had a particular interest in the uses and abuses of illness, especially illnesses that are intentionally or unconsciously feigned.

For the last fifteen years, as a sideline to my psychiatry practice, I have assessed medico-legal patients, many of whom claimed disability from alleged injuries caused by small motor vehicle accidents. About three-quarters of all auto injury claims are for whiplash sprain, and, in keeping with this statistic, most of my medico-legal referrals are whiplash claimants.[1]

As an actual injury, whiplash offers little of interest. If there is any injury at all, it is usually a sprain of the neck and, like sprains in other parts of the body, it heals within a few days or weeks and any associated discomfort disappears. Medico-legal whiplash is a different matter. Up to 10 per cent of "whiplash victims" are reported as "permanently disabled."

First described in 1953 in the United States, whiplash rapidly achieved notoriety. Within ten years it had become a subject heading in the Cumulated Index Medicus (the huge database of medical journal articles) and, as a term for a neck injury, it had made it into a Webster's dictionary. Whiplash quickly became a worldwide epidemic and a multibillion-dollar industry.

The average whiplash claimant submits a request for a few thousand dollars. Some claims are genuine, most are greatly exaggerated, and some are totally bogus. Insurance companies, finding it neither economically feasible nor worth the public's disgruntlement to challenge these claims, meekly pay up. Such claimants seldom come my way. I see claimants who dismiss such paltry compensation. They usually arrive in my office five or more years after their accident, determined to be big winners in the "whiplash lottery."

Of the years between the accident and their arrival at my office, whiplash claimants relate remarkably similar experiences. Their symptoms, instead of abating, have multiplied. They have been examined and sometimes treated by several dozen medical specialists, as well as chiropractors, acupuncturists, and other alternative healthcare practitioners. After the various physical treatments applied by these specialists have failed to work, the claimant is sent to psychologists and psychiatrists. These doctors for the mind attribute the claimant's difficulties to the psychological trauma of the accident and to the stress of the physical pain and suffering that he subsequently endured. The claimant receives psychotherapy, antidepressants, and more tranquilizers. Again, all is in vain, nothing helps!

Typically, regardless of ethnic background, social class, or gender, the claimants report having been exceptionally well and active before the accident; the accident changed everything. They can no longer work, care for their families, have sex, or in any other way enjoy life. Their stories are so similar that when one such claimant failed to keep an appointment with a very established plaintiff lawyer, the lawyer reputedly said to the interpreter, "Well, we don't really need her; we both know what she is going to say anyway."

When acting as the defence psychiatrist (an expert witness for an insurance company) I am usually the last in a long line of expert witnesses to examine the claimant. Along with the claimant comes the medico-legal brief – a collection of binders sometimes more than a foot thick – which contains the claimant's medical reports. Doctors' and lawyers' time is expensive, and medical reports are time-consuming to write and to read. Some briefs contain well over a hundred medical reports and so represent a fortune's worth of professional time.

Since the authors of these reports frequently authenticate the legitimacy of claimants' complaints by referring to articles on whiplash, I became curious about the whiplash literature. A careful examination revealed that, although these articles are often published in reputable medical journals, the extensive literature is filled with scientifically spurious studies. One misleading article after another shows how doctors and lawyers managed to finesse whiplash from a trifling injury into a permanent disability that keeps both doctors and lawyers gainfully employed. One Danish doctor, for example, titled his medical journal article, "With Whiplash, the Future Comes from Behind," and a gloomy future (except for some unmentioned compensation) he painted it to be.[2]

Before whiplash became of medico-legal interest, people in rear-end collisions seem to have lived contentedly with their rear-ended necks. Even today, in the few parts of the developed world where whiplash remains unknown or uncompensated, the rear-ended have no more problems with their necks than do the rest of the population. Iatrogenic, or doctor-made, illnesses are common, but seldom can one follow the steps by which they are created. Whiplash is an exception. It is such an unusually circumscribed condition that it is possible to trace how orthopaedic surgeons, ENT surgeons (laryngologists), ophthalmologists, radiologists, dentists, neurologists, psychiatrists, psychologists, rheumatologists, and physiatrists, not to mention chiropractors and other alternative practitioners, managed to bring whiplash into their own professional domain and raise it from a minor disorder into a major world-wide epidemic.

I have used whiplash along with some other fashionable illnesses to illustrate the ways in which much of medicine and the law actually works. We need this knowledge if we are ever to succeed in creating healthcare services that can hope to meet our needs. Running a healthcare service without knowing how practitioners and patients function is like running a nursery school without knowing how teachers and children interrelate. Whiplash may be a pain in the neck, but I hope, in this respect at least, that it will prove a *genuinely* useful condition.

It is perhaps impossible to write about whiplash and not take sides. I take sides. I believe that minor car collisions seldom cause serious neck injury, and that the routine attribution of ongoing symptoms to whiplash injury is incorrect. Many experienced clinicians believe just the opposite, but in my opinion they are mistaken. I wish to make you sceptical of whiplash, but since I too am handsomely rewarded for my opinions, you should also be sceptical about this book. I aim to provide an overall account of whiplash that is credible, realistic, internally consistent, and sufficiently well referenced to enable any reader with access to library facilities to check out the facts. I have not written this book to obtain more referrals. I am seventy years old; I am tired of whiplash and I hope never to see another case again.

Overall, this book is the story of the shady side of medicine and its insalubrious association with the law. It is the story of mindlessness, folly, deception, exuberant but often self-serving sympathy for patients, and outright greed. It is the story of how illnesses are manufactured and then require endless and remunerative sustenance. It is a story that brims over with medical and legal intrigue.

PART ONE

*Finessing Whiplash
into a Permanent Disability*

1

Making Whiplash Sound Serious: Caveat Lector

If you really believe it, it is not a lie.
– George Costanza in *Seinfeld*

Whiplash has become a major epidemic in Western society.
– Michael Livingston

It is true that some physicians are excellent scientists. During their years at medical school, however, most doctors are not trained in the scientific method; they are apprenticed into the tradition of diagnosing and treating illness. Then, faced with earning a living, they need to recruit patients. To do so, they must provide the services that patients want. Doctors who decide to manage whiplash patients must let potential patients, lawyers, and other doctors know of their interest, and one way to do this is to write an article on whiplash for a medical journal. Although such articles adopt a neutral and seemingly scientific stance by providing both sides of the whiplash problem, they often end up presenting whiplash as a catastrophic injury. These articles both inform other doctors about whiplash and serve as the shop window that displays the doctor's expertise.

I have chosen to model a portion of this chapter on such articles as a way of informing you about medico-legal whiplash. My description of whiplash, like other whiplash articles, uses the customary scientific format, though I hope that, unlike many such articles, it has no factual errors. I correctly report the findings of other authors and appropriately reference their works. On this level, at least, my presentation of whiplash is scientifically sound. As an account of whiplash it is nonsense, however, for the authors I cite either rely upon faulty scientific techniques or quote other authors who have done so.

In presenting whiplash in this way I have given myself a problem. Friends and colleagues whom I asked to read my description of whiplash became so convinced that whiplash is indeed a catastrophic injury that they could see little point in reading a book to show that it is not. I hope their erroneous conviction will have proved useful, for it emphasizes just how easy it is to present whiplash as a severe injury. As you proceed, *remember that you too will be convinced that whiplash is an*

injury requiring much skilled medical attention and generous compensation.
You must also remember that whiplash forms the basis of a multimillion-dollar
industry from which many people make a living. The industry relies upon the
public's acceptance of whiplash as an injury with catastrophic consequences.

WHIPLASH: A CAUSE FOR CONCERN?

Cars and human bodies do not mix well. People in fast-moving hunks
of metal involved in collisions easily get hurt. In the United States,
about 50,000 occupants of vehicles are killed each year, and for each
person killed, many more are injured with varying degrees of severity.[1]
Neck injuries are the most common form of motor vehicle injury.
Indeed, it is claimed that 85 per cent of all neck injuries result from
vehicle collisions, and, of these neck injuries, 85 per cent result
from rear-end collisions.[2]

The true incidence of whiplash injury is unknown. At the low end
the estimate is one million new cases annually, generated by about 12
million motor vehicle accidents.[3] The high-end estimate is that as
many as 5 million Americans sustain a whiplash injury each year, from
which 3 million do not fully recover.[4] In 1994, 2.6 million American
citizens were reported to have chronic pain as a result of whiplash
injury, and in 650,000 cases this pain was reported to be severe and
ongoing.[5] The massive American insurance company State Farm estimates that the annual cost of whiplash in the United States is somewhere between $13 billion and $18 billion.[6]

The term "whiplash" was first used to denote the motion of the head
and neck induced by forces of acceleration or deceleration, though
the term has since come to signify the injuries induced by this motion.
The head is said to be jerked violently backwards or forwards, by forces
sufficiently powerful to cause serious neck and brain injury even in the
absence of any direct blow to the head or body.[7] Delicate nerve cells in
the brain and spinal cord, once destroyed, never recover, so their loss
can have disastrous consequences. Many authors report that whiplash
causes deterioration of cognition, memory, and behaviour.[8]

The literature describes a range of serious whiplash neck injuries:
fracture of vertebrae, rupture of intervertebral discs, painful separation of the intervertebral disc from the vertebral end plate, damage to
the vertebral arteries (two of the four arteries that supply blood to the
brain), acute bilateral internal carotid arterial dissection, and rupture
of the oesophagus to name just a few.[9]

In the huge majority of whiplash cases, however, no such injury can
be demonstrated, and the symptoms are then attributed to "a muscu-
loligamental sprain or strain of the neck." The condition is called

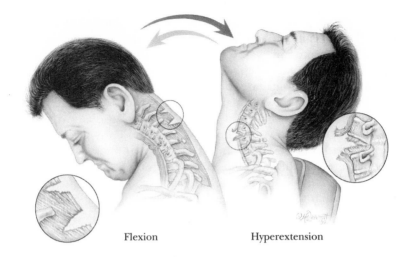

Flexion   Hyperextension

Fig. 1–1   An artist's impression of whiplash neck injury, © Teri J. McDermott 1992

"common whiplash," a condition in which demonstrably serious injuries such as neck fractures and dislocations are, by definition, absent.[10]

A sprain of the neck, as with sprains elsewhere in the body, is painful. The pain either begins immediately or is delayed until a few hours or even days later when the injured tissues have become swollen and stiff. Sprains heal, but sometimes neck pain and stiffness persist or get worse and the complaints continue indefinitely. Despite recent improvements in motor vehicle safety features, whiplash remains a problem, and its symptoms become increasingly disabling and chronic.[11]

By general acceptance, whiplash injury is considered "chronic" when its symptoms persist for more than six months. Chronic whiplash is also referred to as "late whiplash syndrome," "cervical syndrome," "whiplash syndrome" or simply as "whiplash."[12] By whatever name, chronic whiplash is a well-delineated clinical condition remarkably consistent in its presentation: neck pain, headaches, memory and thinking problems, fatigue, anxiety, and depression.[13] (*Dear reader, please remember that this is how whiplash articles are written but is in no way a reflection of reality.*)

Despite intensive modern treatments, the prevalence of chronic whiplash neck complaints remains high. Barnsley, Lord, and Bogduk, Australian whiplash experts, reviewed a number of whiplash disability studies and concluded: "Taken together, the studies indicate that between 14 per cent and 42 per cent of patients with whiplash injuries develop significant chronic neck pain, and that approximately 10 per cent will have constant, severe neck pain for the foreseeable future."[14] Other authors have reported similar findings.[15]

Whiplash symptoms are described as particularly unpleasant. Robert Bingham, a Californian orthopaedic surgeon, discussed the 122 whiplash patients he had treated in the previous two years: "I truly believe that they would rather have almost any accident other than whiplash injury. They suffer from constant pain, day and night. They wake up in the morning with it. It bothers them during their activities all day. It interferes with their sleep at night. And no medicine, other than a general anaesthetic or strong narcotic, will relieve it completely."[16]

As the failure of sprained muscles and ligaments to heal is an unsatisfactory explanation for the persistence of whiplash pain, all sorts of other injuries are suggested as explanations for the ongoing whiplash symptoms. Not surprisingly, the frequent failure of whiplash patients to recover gives whiplash a bad reputation – so bad, in fact, that its very name has become equated with a dire prognosis.

Many authors comment on whiplash headache.[17] Fifty to 80 per cent of patients are reported to have headaches within two months of whiplash injury.[18] Murrey M. Braaf and Samuel Rosner, New York surgeons and early experts on whiplash, reviewed over 1,000 whiplash cases and found headache to be the most common and annoying symptom. In some cases head pain may be so severe as to overshadow any or all other complaints and cannot be relieved by simple analgesics.[19]

Whiplash is reported to damage the sympathetic nervous system, a chain of nerve fibres and cells that extends from the abdomen up into the neck. It is part of the body's self-regulating system, which aids in controlling such physiological functions as blood pressure and digestion. Several authors have reported abnormal eye signs consistent with this injury.[20]

Clinically less obvious damage to the sympathetic nervous system is a cause of Barré syndrome, a perplexing condition consisting of headache, vertigo, ringing in the ears, intermittent loss of voice, hoarseness, fatigue, temperature changes, uncomfortable feelings of the hands and forearms provoked by emotion, temperature, humidity, or noise, and increased muscle tone.[21] Barré syndrome has been reported in 20 per cent of whiplash patients.[22]

Numerous whiplash simulation experiments with animals confirm that the acceleration/deceleration forces of whiplash cause neck injury and severe brain damage.[23] Ophthalmologists report whiplash damage to the eyes.[24] ENT surgeons report whiplash damage of the inner ear that causes distressing and disabling dizziness, buzzing in the ears, and sometimes deafness.[25] Dentists report mandibular whiplash leading to chronic and incapacitating temporomandibular joint disorder.[26] Orthopaedic surgeons report whiplash to be a potent cause of persistent backache and other musculoskeletal pains,[27] and rheumatologists that whiplash victims frequently develop incapacitating fibromyalgia.[28]

Minds can be damaged in accidents as well as bodies. Psychologists and psychiatrists emphasize that the deleterious effects of the frightening experience of the collision cause victims to develop a post-traumatic stress disorder.[29] Recent studies into the psychological effects of motor vehicle accidents demonstrate that close to 40 per cent of accident victims (mostly whiplash victims) seeking treatment for ongoing physical symptoms have signs of post-traumatic stress disorder.[30]

Whiplash-causing accidents often appear trivial, but many authors report that this triviality is misleading, noting both the magnitude of the forces involved even in low-velocity collisions and the particular vulnerability of the human neck and human brain to this type of injury.[31] J.A. McKenzie and J.F. Williams, mechanical engineers from Melbourne, Australia, note that "a struck vehicle acquired a peak acceleration almost equal to the striking vehicle, an acceleration which resulted in the head and shoulders of the occupant attaining acceleration levels almost 2 to 2.5 times greater [than that of the vehicle]."[32]

Henry La Rocca, professor of orthopaedic surgery at Tulane University in New Orleans and editor-in-chief of the prestigious journal *Spine*, in summarizing these studies, comments: "Enormous forces are applied to the head and neck complex, even with low speed impact ... Typical head accelerations of eleven times gravity were recorded resulting in the application of traction forces in excess of one hundred pounds to the head-neck complex ... These data demonstrate conclusively that a low speed rear-end accident is capable of applying a seriously damaging force to the head and neck."[33]

Emil Seletz, an orthopaedic surgeon from Beverly Hills, California, writing in the *Journal of the American Medical Association (JAMA)*, describes these forces:

When a 3,500-lb car travelling at 10 mph strikes the rear of another car, it may transmit to this car a force of 25 tons. The person's body (in the car that is struck) continues to move forward while, being hinged at the neck, the head snaps backward. The average head weighs about 8 lbs, and the cervical vertebrae are very delicate; the force that is pushing the head backward is even greater than believed, since the base of the neck acts as a fulcrum and the leverage is applied near the top of the head. Therefore, the head snaps back with the equivalent of several tons of force – without any support, since the muscular control of the neck is caught off guard.[34]

The magnitude of whiplash force is inimicable to the human body. Bingham, in his study on whiplash injuries, encapsulates the modern human predicament: "The environment of civilized man, over the period of history, has not changed his primitive body, yet we put this same primitive body into a vehicle at any speed over 15 mph, and then subject it to the terrible forces of acceleration and deceleration in a collision. The human body just cannot take this. The cervical spine is the area most likely to be injured in our modern automobile."[35]

Robert Maigne, president of the International Federation of Manual Medicine and head of physical medicine at the Hôtel Dieu Hospital in Paris, whose many publications have been translated into several languages, comments: "The accident need not be severe in order to generate cervical trauma." He notes that even braking suddenly can do it. "The head, which weighs over 5 lbs and is balanced over the cervical spine, being supported by only two small articular surfaces no greater than a thumbnail, is ... thrown backwards pulling the cervical spine with it."[36]

Arthur Croft, a California chiropractor and co-founder of the American College of Forensic Sciences, confirms that the severity of the collision bears little relationship to the severity of the whiplash injury. "The notion that one can calculate or predict the type or extent of soft tissue damage sustained by the occupants of a vehicle merely by calculating the 'g' forces produced in the vehicle by the resultant collision should clearly be laid to rest. The practice of calculating bodily injury to the victim by estimating the cost of auto damage is naïve at best and should be condemned."[37]

Women are more vulnerable to whiplash than men.[38] The female neck measures on average 4 cm less in circumference than the male's, though the average lengths for both are virtually the same. This anatomical difference is deemed to make female necks even more vulnerable to whiplash.[39]

It is easy to see from the above material that whiplash injury has grave consequences for human health. But it is difficult to provide consistent figures for whiplash-induced disability because various observers make their assessments with different measures and at different time intervals after the accident. Also, many whiplash victims are housewives who do not work outside the home, a circumstance that makes the determination of disability status yet more difficult. However, some figures are available.

John Pearce, a neurologist from Hull, England, in a study of 100 British whiplash plaintiffs, found that 21 per cent were still off work one month after the accident, 14 per cent after three months, and 6 per cent after one year.[40] In a huge Swedish study of motor vehicle accidents, Åke Nygren reported a "permanent medical disability rate" of 9.6 per cent following rear-end collisions.[41] John I. Balla, an Australian neurologist and expert on whiplash, found that two-thirds of his whiplash patients showed social disability to the extent that they had either downgraded their jobs or had difficulties performing housework or sports and recreational activities. Ten per cent of the patients had remained off work for over two years.[42]

No definite whiplash disability figures are available for North America, though if even only a small percentage of North Americans who submit insurance claims for acute whiplash progress to disability, the number must be high. Whatever the exact figures, Barnsley, Lord, and Bogduk are correct in commenting: "The costs of whiplash injuries in terms of lost productivity and human suffering too often are underestimated."[43]

BACK TO REALITY

Has all this made you nervous? Are you going to sell the car and walk? We live in a dangerous world and there are lots of sensible things to worry about, but I hope you will soon learn that whiplash is *not* one of them. First, though, to ensure we are all on the same wavelength, I want to clear up the problem of injury severity.

Like other injuries, whiplash comes in many shapes and sizes. It is customary to divide whiplash injuries into mild, moderate, and severe but, as there have been few hard and fast rules on how to pigeonhole whiplash into these three categories and since claimants with no apparent injury at all often refer to their whiplash as severe, the classification is far from precise.

A more useful classification comes from Quebec. Customarily, drivers buy auto insurance from private insurance companies but in Quebec and Saskatchewan the provincial governments provide their citizens with auto insurance coverage. The Quebec government, discomfited by the high cost of whiplash claims, established the Quebec Task Force on Whiplash-Associated Disorders. In 1995, under the leadership of Walter Spitzer, one of Canada's foremost epidemiologists, a group of experienced scientists completed its four-year three-million-dollar international study of whiplash.[44] Their study is by far the largest ever made of whiplash. They divided whiplash-associated disorders (WADs) into the following grades:

0 = No complaints about neck; no physical signs;
I   = Neck complaints of pain, stiffness, or tenderness only. No physical signs;
II = Neck complaints and musculoskeletal signs (limitation of movement and point tenderness);
III = Neck complaints and neurological signs;
IV = Fracture or dislocation.

The task force evaluated only grades I to III, that is, those grades that include the vast majority of whiplash injuries and complaints. Having meticulously sifted through the objective evidence on whiplash, the task force considered that most persons with WAD I–III have a relatively benign disorder that resolves spontaneously in days or weeks and requires very little treatment.

The illustration of whiplash (Fig. 1–1) is taken from an article on common whiplash in the *Journal of Musculoskeletal Medicine.* The WAD IV injury demonstrated is certainly not common whiplash. Such alarming pictures have helped whiplash masquerade as a serious condition.

Although I have examined many cases of whiplash, I have never seen a WAD grade IV, and very few cases of grade III. My whiplash patients belonged to WAD grades I or II, although they had not followed the expected course of recovery. Four or five years after their accidents, they still complained bitterly of symptoms and still received all sorts of treatments for their complaints. This is a common finding. Whiplash claimants with non-demonstrable injuries often take far longer to recover than accident victims with a fractured or dislocated neck.

Although various types of physical injury have been proposed as explanations for whiplash symptoms, no actual injury has been demonstrated to adequately explain the long-term persistence of such symptoms. The failure to find any such injury is not for want of trying. Investigators using an assortment of new techniques repeatedly claim to have discovered yet another whiplash-induced injury but none of these claims has withstood the test of time. No specific whiplash injury has been found because it is highly unlikely that any such injury exists. Then why is so much time and money spent in looking for and treating non-existent injuries? I hope that in the following inquiry into this question you will acquire some revealing insights into the ways in which patients, healthcare practitioners, and lawyers interact.

2

Whiplash and Poor Science in Medical Journals

A great deal of intelligence can be invested in ignorance
when the need for illusion is deep.
– Saul Bellow

As a prelude to its investigation of whiplash, the Quebec Task Force on
Whiplash-Associated Disorders planned to review all the whiplash literature. The members of the task force were soon overwhelmed. They
decided to focus their attention on whiplash material published
between 1980 and 1993, but even with nearly three decades of whiplash
publications discarded, 10,382 publications remained. Of these, they
found only 62 to be "relevant and scientifically meritorious."[1]

In the past two decades the scientific quality of many medical journal articles has improved greatly. Editors of reputable journals have
become much more particular about scientific methodology and the
appropriate statistical analysis of data, and they now send submitted
articles out for peer review. While most whiplash articles published
after 1980 are somewhat improved, those published earlier were
appalling. It was this fallacious early whiplash material, however, that
became the factual basis for court judgments on the prognosis of
whiplash. In the copycat way in which courts tend to work, these judgments now serve as precedents for current court decisions.

American naval doctors were the first to describe the harmful effects
of rapid acceleration upon the neck. In the years after World War I,
the United States navy turned some of its pilots into human slingshots
by catapulting planes from the decks of battleships and cruisers. The
pilots got sore necks and, in some cases, momentary blackouts causing
them to dive into the sea. The navy lengthened the cockpit seatbacks
to prevent the backward extension of pilots' necks and so solved the
problem.[2] Although this acceleration/deceleration injury had not yet
been christened "whiplash," the sore neck and the blackouts were
undoubtedly due to the "whiplash" effect.

Harold Crowe, an American orthopaedic surgeon, claims to have
been the first person to use the dreaded term "whip lash" in relation

to neck injury. He did so in 1928 when presenting eight cases of neck injury to a meeting of orthopaedic surgeons in San Francisco.[3] Thirty-six years later, Crowe ate crow: "This expression was intended to be a description of motion, but has been accepted by physicians, patients and attorneys as the name of a disease; and the misunderstanding has led to its misapplication by many physicians and others over the years."[4]

"Whip lash" first entered the medical literature in 1945 when Arthur E. Davis, an orthopaedic surgeon from Erie, Pennsylvania, provided a description of the whiplash mechanism. "Starting with the fact that the great majority of injuries of the cervical spine are in the nature of a 'whip lash,' and accepting the meaning of the term 'whip lash' as a hyperflexion followed by a spontaneous extensor recoil, the nature of a great variety of injuries of this section of the spinal column becomes understandable."[5] Davis then described 134 cases of neck injury caused by front-end collisions, falls from a height, diving accidents, and severe blows to the head, all of which he ascribed to 'whip lash' – a veritable carnage of neck injuries that he and his partner had seen over the previous twenty-two years. Eleven of these victims died within a few days of the accident; their autopsies revealed "irreparable pulpefaction of the cord."

In retrospect it is clear that such gross injuries were caused not by whiplash but by forces acting directly upon the head or neck. In front-end collisions before the days of seatbelts, the car occupant was thrown forward, hitting his head on the steering wheel, dashboard, or windshield. This impact hyperextended the neck – a potent cause of severe neck injury.[6] (Seatbelts have greatly reduced the occurrence of such catastrophic neck injuries.[7])

Davis's contribution to whiplash was soon forgotten, but he made one observation that is of interest to the present-day reader. He reported that his patients with severe neck injuries recovered well. Even in cases of severe sprain, the necks stopped being painful within a week: "Full recovery has occurred for the most part. Several patients showing complete signs of paralysis on entering hospital have recovered complete or nearly complete function." When compared with recent studies of minor neck injuries, these results are nothing short of amazing. Clearly, the prognosis of neck injuries has taken a marked turn for the worse in the last half-century. However, fifty-five years ago, neck injuries were still perceived as akin to injuries in other parts of the body; they had not yet been accorded the status of a special injury from which recovery is deemed unlikely. Doctors had not yet turned neck injury into a dreaded fashionable injury worthy of much medical sympathy and a generous compensation package.

It was James Gay, an orthopaedic surgeon from White Plains, New York, and Kenneth Abbott, a neurosurgeon from Columbus, Ohio, who in 1953 helped whiplash come into its own. They used the term "whiplash" to describe an injury to the neck sustained by the occupant of a vehicle involved in rear-end collision. Their famous article published in the *Journal of the American Medical Association (JAMA)*[8] began: "Interest in whiplash injury of the neck was aroused by the frequency with which this type of injury was encountered in neurosurgical practice and by the chronic nature of the symptoms that were observed after an accident that appeared to be of little consequence." In contrast to Davis, who had attributed "whip lash" to head-on impacts, most of Gay and Abbott's fifty cases involved a rear-end collision, the majority of which occurred at traffic lights.

Gay and Abbott describe whiplash injury as a strain of the neck from which recovery is often delayed by a "psychoneurotic reaction." It was perhaps their incorporation of this neurotic reaction as an integral part of whiplash that more than anything has accounted for the syndrome's astounding success. Recovery of injured muscles and ligaments is, of course, the norm, but when compensation is pending recovery is frequently delayed. Such delay is often attributed to a *neurotic reaction*, the presence of which is used as an argument for reducing or denying compensation.

Gay and Abbott gave whiplash both a psychological and physical explanation for this neurotic reaction, a double whammy with which to justify all neurotic behaviour. By way of psychological explanation they wrote:

The complication that was most distressing for both patient and physician was a persistent psychoneurotic reaction. More than half of the patients in this series (26 cases or 52 per cent) were seriously handicapped in this way. In our opinion, the circumstances inherent in a whiplash injury make all persons prone to the development of a disturbing emotional reaction.

The accident involved a sudden, violent and unexpected jolt that was a disturbing experience. Since the victim was seldom incapacitated immediately after the accident, there was opportunity for development of considerable hostility toward the offending motorist.

By way of physical explanation, Gay and Abbott introduced the spectre of whiplash brain damage. D. Denny-Brown and W. Ritchie Russell, distinguished British neurophysiologists, had previously demonstrated that acceleration/deceleration forces can produce brain injury even in the absence of any direct head impact.[9] Gay and Abbott quoted this classic study in support of the possibility that "multiple oscillations of the head and neck" could cause injury in various parts of the brain, thus giving rise to an assortment of neuropsychiatric disorders including a "neurotic reaction" consequent upon brain pathology.

Denny-Brown and Russell suggested that careful evaluation could disentangle these two aetiologies, noting that a concussion syndrome improves in the succeeding days following an accident, whereas psychoneurosis "occurs with full intensity late in the convalescent period." It sounds plausible, but sorting out such uncertain symptoms is no easy matter. Whiplash clinicians are kept so busy trying to distinguish the physical and psychological causes of the neurotic symptoms that they fail to question whether the neurotic symptoms are even related to the accident. Many people have neurotic symptoms, accident or no accident. As I will demonstrate later, many whiplash victims have a history of neurotic-type difficulties before their accident, and so it is not surprising that they continue to have similar symptoms after the accident.

To add to their lack of credibility, Gay and Abbott amazingly got the whiplash movement of the head the wrong way round. They described "the mechanics of [whiplash] injury [as] a sudden and forceful flexion of the neck" followed, in some instances, by several other less violent oscillations of the neck in alternating flexion and extension." They accepted unquestioningly the then current belief that in a rear-end collision the head is first pushed forward by the impact of the collision before rebounding backward (see Fig. 2–1). It is, of course, the other way round. Any reader who has doubts can readily prove it himself. Go quietly up behind a sturdy friend, grasp his or her shoulders and give a sharp but gentle push forwards. The head goes backwards.

Gay and Abbott's description of the multiple oscillations of the head in the action of whiplash gives a terrifying impression of the head and neck being shaken to pieces. Again, they were wrong; these multiple oscillations of whiplash only occur in Tom and Jerry cartoons! Two reliable investigations show that after hyperextension the head simply returns to the upright position.[10]

Surgeons are better at mechanical dynamics than psychological ones. Since Gay and Abbott got the mechanical dynamics of whiplash wrong, perhaps they got the psychodynamics wrong as well. I think they did. Having hostile feelings toward a driver who has delivered an unexpected jolt, and having an unexpectedly uncomfortable stiff neck may be both distressing and inconvenient, but neither combined nor separately do they seem a sufficient cause of a prolonged neurotic illness.

The late Ian Macnab, a Toronto orthopaedic surgeon and one of the world's first authorities on whiplash, neatly summed up the whiplash situation: "In terms of the law the striking vehicle was invariably at fault,

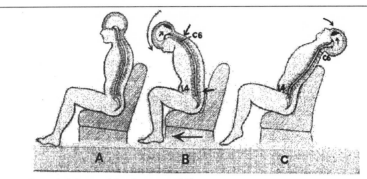

A: Normal sitting position in automobile
B: Collision from behind thrusts body in position of acute flexion, with maximum stresses at lower cervical and lumbar spinal regions;
C: Position of extension usually follows acute flexion posture. There may be more than one oscillation of the neck in alternate flexion and extension. Shading of the brain indicates that a concurrent concussion of the brain occurs from mechanical deformation or the influence of acceleration/deceleration.

Fig. 2–1   The fathers of whiplash get the mechanics of whiplash the wrong way round

and this took away the burden of proof of liability. The injury sustained rarely presented objective stigmata of an organic lesion. The blameless client incapacitated by subjective symptoms, the existence of which could neither be proved or disproved, was manna for the plaintiff's attorney, pestilence for the defence attorneys and represented a paid vacation for the unscrupulous patient ... Whiplash lent an evil connotation to the injury, and many patients became more disabled by the diagnosis than by the injury."[11] Macnab wrote these words in 1971. Insurance statistics show that in 2001 most whiplash victims are still content to settle for the price of a paid vacation, but since some whiplash plaintiffs and their attorneys now think big, the paid vacation may be more along the lines of a well-financed early retirement.

Arguments continue, exemplified by the seatbelt question. The reduction of auto accident deaths following the introduction of seatbelt legislation certainly attests to the effectiveness of seatbelts in reducing such deaths. But even since then whiplash experts have claimed that, by restraining the torso, seatbelts predispose to the development of whiplash. Of the thirteen medical journal articles or letters that deal with this problem, twelve suggest that seatbelts predispose to whiplash. But the methodology (or total absence thereof) used by their authors is so bad and their evidence is so lacking that no reliable conclusions can be drawn.[12]

Members of a group of Swiss whiplash experts were the only
researchers to have used appropriate methodology to study the effects
of seatbelts upon the incidence of whiplash. They reported that seatbelts appear to lessen the incidence of whiplash, but the number of
cases in their study was too small to yield significance.[13]

Whiplash had inauspicious beginnings. Harold Crowe introduced
the term but then regretted it. Davis then wrongly attributed severe
neck injuries to a "whip lash mechanism," while Gay and Abbott got
the whiplash mechanism the wrong way round. Studies with faulty
methodology abounded. With this concatenation of bloopers at its
conception and early life, it is not surprising that the subject of
whiplash remains clouded in confusion.

Since no one ever dies of common whiplash, autopsy material by
which to determine the site or nature of any supposed whiplash neck
injury is seldom available. Evidence for the existence of such injuries
must be obtained by indirect means, including animal and cadaver
experiments, and various clinical investigations.[14]

Whiplash claimants are usually pleased to submit to all manner of
investigations since by doing so they augment their injury status.
Because insurance companies are forced to pay the costs of these
investigations, the care of whiplash claimants is lucrative and their
caretakers can afford the latest in expensive investigative equipment.
New electrical recording devices, imaging techniques, and other wonders of the electronics industry are routinely deployed in the investigation of the hypothetical whiplash injury. They reveal abnormalities
that are then presented as authoritative explanations for whiplash
complaints. But there is a catch. These investigations are faulty. Other
clinicians become suspicious and eventually some perplexed investi-
gator is galvanized into undertaking the time-consuming and expensive task of organizing a well-conducted controlled study.

The results of these controlled studies are monotonously the same
– *whiplash plaintiffs have the same rate of abnormal findings as do the ordinary populace.* The whiplash "experts" had not bothered to use normal
people for comparison. Meanwhile, huge numbers of whiplash victims
have been needlessly treated, lawsuits settled on the strength of biased
information, and whiplash's reputation as a cause of demonstrable
physical injury becomes entrenched a little more deeply in the public
psyche. Undeterred, the whiplash experts simply move on to yet more
modern technology.

While whiplash plaintiffs are prepared to submit to endless investigations, they cannot be used for actual whiplash simulation experiments, so animals were used instead.[15] Macnab, for example, used
anaesthetized rabbits, dogs, and monkeys to simulate whiplash. He

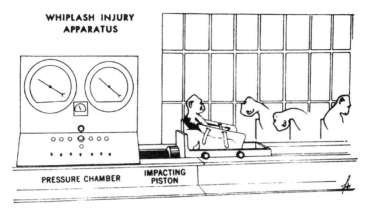

Fig. 2–2 Senseless slaughter
Ommaya's machine for simulating whiplash in monkeys. The piston delivered accelera-
tion forces of much greater magnitude than are normally involved in human whiplash.
The information obtained from these experiments is totally misleading.

strapped each animal supine to a steel tray with its head and neck protruding over the tray's edge. He attached the tray to two guide rails
and dropped the animal from 2 to 40 feet down an elevator shaft. On
hitting an object at the bottom of the shaft the tray and the body of the
animal came to a sudden halt, but the head continued downwards,
mimicking the hyperextension of whiplash. Macnab found that the
lesions produced by this procedure were remarkably constant, their
severity varying with the length of the fall. The lesions consisted of
torn and bruised muscles and ligaments, damaged intervertebral discs,
and spasm of the vertebral arteries.[16]

In another whiplash simulation experiment, Jack K. Wickstrom
and his colleagues from Tulane University, New Orleans, placed
monkeys in a plastic cylinder with the head and neck projecting over
the top. They fastened the cylinder in a vertical position to a movable
carriage by which they rapidly accelerated the monkey forward.
Thirty-two per cent of the monkeys sustained brain damage, 57 per
cent spinal cord damage, 11 per cent ligamentous injury, and 2.3 per
cent disc damage.[17]

Ayub Ommaya and his colleagues, at the National Institute of
Neurological Diseases and Blindness, Bethesda, Maryland, in yet
another animal study, strapped rhesus monkeys onto a fibreglass chair
mounted on a rigid carriage. The carriage moved freely on roller skate
wheels along a 20-foot track. A rear-end collision was mimicked by an
impulse delivered by an air-compression device at one end of the track
(see fig. 2-2). The monkeys sustained "gross haemorrhages and con-

tusions of the brain and upper cervical cord."[18] Other whiplash investigators, using a variety of accelerating devices to induce severe brain damage in their experimental animals, followed suit.[19]

The results of these animal studies profoundly influenced people's beliefs about human whiplash. In "Whiplash Injury of the Neck: Fact or Fancy," Braaf and Rosner, the leading New York whiplash experts in 1966, wrote: "Experimental reproduction of whiplash in monkeys has shown that significant disc and joint damage is always associated with this type of injury. In addition, the muscles and fasciae of the neck, the cervical roots, the sympathetic nerves, as well as the vertebral artery, may be traumatized."[20]

Where information on the underlying whiplash injury was missing, many authors on human whiplash used information from animal experiments to fill in the blanks. In fact, it is unusual to find medical articles on whiplash that do *not* refer at some length to these experimental findings. I have referenced eighteen such articles, but there are hundreds more.[21]

There is, however, a problem with all these experiments: Animal and human whiplash are two very different conditions. Many of the animals were rendered unconscious for several hours, and, on recovery of consciousness, some were left paralysed or had obvious signs of brain damage or other unmistakable evidence of injury. The experimenters produced gross haemorrhages and contusions both in and over the surface of the brain and upper cervical cord. Human whiplash victims, on the other hand, are not rendered unconscious. Characteristically they leave the crashed car without apparent injury, and it is unusual to find any objective signs other than a stiff neck – or even a stiff neck.

Why are the results of animal and human whiplash so different? The answer is that the investigators typically employed forces of around 130 g to simulate whiplash,[22] about ten times greater than the forces involved in a typical rear-end collision.[23] Even using these enormous acceleration forces the experimenters sometimes had difficulty in producing injury. Wickstrom and his colleagues first selected Belgian hares as their experimental animal on the supposition that hares have particularly vulnerable necks. However, despite accelerating the animals at over 150 g – a rate of acceleration that left some of the animals stunned – they produced no observable injury of the neck.[24] Necks are tougher than whiplash experts would have us believe!

The hallmark of chronic whiplash is the persistence of subjective complaints for which no adequate physical cause can be found. Animal whiplash is not human whiplash. John Norris, a neurologist at the University of Toronto, states the position nicely in a letter to the

Lancet: "The experiments in animals are irrelevant to the syndrome, since monkeys cannot complain of the symptoms of whiplash. The extrapolation from experimental injuries, sometimes severe enough to avulse tendons, is invalid, since whiplash does not occur in severe injuries. In fact, this syndrome is commonly seen in patients with no head injury and with a well-supported headrest on their car seat ... Much of the confusion has arisen from observations of orthopaedic surgeons who know too little psychiatry, or psychiatrists who know too much."[25]

Whiplash experts have continued to ignore these words of wisdom. Even into the 1990s they have cited these experiments as justification for their ongoing search for whiplash brain and neck injuries. For example, The Australian whiplash experts Barnsley, Lord, and Bogduk write: "Careful animal experiments have demonstrated haemorrhage in and around the brain from acceleration injuries without direct trauma to the head".[26] La Rocca, editor of *Spine*, comments: "The intervertebral disc injuries found in whiplash experimental animals suggest an injured disc is probably a significant and frequent component of the human acceleration injury as well, and if so, helps explain why the clinical course is often protracted."[27] Bruce Pennie and Lindsey Agambar, orthopaedic surgeons from Merseyside, England, discuss the "important injury" that many whiplash patients sustain:

The pathological basis for the clinical features [of whiplash] is not clear; a sprain of the musculoligamentous structures of the neck is inevitably one component, but cannot explain all the above features. Animal studies have been carried out to elucidate the possible pathologies in the limited situation of acceleration/deceleration injuries.[28] These [animal] studies demonstrated surface haemorrhages and contusions of the brain stem, extradural, subdural and subarachnoid haemorrhages, muscle damage, ligament ruptures, avulsion [separation] of the disc from the vertebral body, retropharyngeal hematoma, intralaryngeal haemorrhage, haemorrhage in the muscle layers of the oesophagus, damage to sympathetic nerves, haemorrhage and inflammation in the thyroid glands and retro-ocular hematoma.[29]

Medical articles can work wonders in court. Charles Frankel, a surgeon from Charlottesville, Virginia, writing in the *Journal of the American Medical Association* (which he refers to as THE JOURNAL), illustrates their use:

Some recently reported cases have shown how effectively articles on whiplash from THE JOURNAL can be used in cross-examination of defence medical witnesses. It may be proper for plaintiff's counsel to test the knowledge and accuracy of defendant's physician on cross-examination by reading pertinent extracts from THE JOURNAL pertaining to whiplash and to ask whether he disagrees with what has been read. Confronted with the authority of THE JOURNAL, most physicians on the witness stand would be inclined to agree with what has been written therein. This, of course, is influential in reducing the weight of adverse testimony even when a physician disagrees with what has been stated in THE JOURNAL. Attorneys may effectively demonstrate to the factfinders (the jury) that the physician is disagreeing with a widely accepted authority.[30]

Ommaya's misleading article was published in the *Journal of the American Medical Association*, and even a quarter of a century after its publication, while in the witness box, I have had his article quoted at me by disgruntled plaintiff lawyers. Recent editions of Science Citation Index show that Ommaya's articles are still cited around the world in medical publications in support of whiplash as a significant cause of brain injury.

The *Journal of the American Medical Association* is undoubtedly "a widely accepted authority" but when it comes to whiplash it has published nonsense. I have already quoted the *JAMA* article with the preposterous statement about a collision of a car travelling 10 mph in which "the head snaps back with the equivalent of several tons of force" (see chap. 1).[31] If the head really snapped back with a force of several tons, it would come right off the body. These scientifically specious articles certainly have allowed the medical profession to capture billions of dollars of insurance money by treating the symptoms of non-existent whiplash injury.

It took nearly three decades for the avid American obsession with whiplash to reach Britain. Michael Livingston, a British-trained family physician working in Vancouver, is interested in the problem of whiplash and social copying. He points out that it usually takes new syndromes about three years to cross the Atlantic, but with whiplash there was a thirty-three-year interval between the publication of the Gay and Abbott article and the publication of the first whiplash study in any major British medical journal – an article by G.T. Deans in the *British Medical Journal (BMJ)*.[32]

Whiplash was not initially a subject of interest in the United Kingdom. Until the 1980s, the British National Health Service provided the lion's share of healthcare in Britain, paying its physicians either by salary or on a per capita basis. The last thing any British physician wanted was more work.

Times change. The National Health Service began to falter in its ability to cater to the sick, and many people turned to private medical insurance to obtain their healthcare. Since private insurance pays physicians for each service rendered to a patient, British doctors developed an interest in the lucrative work generated by whiplash. Britain has two long-established and influential medical journals: the *BMJ* and the *Lancet*. These two prestigious journals, quoting some extremely dubious whiplash studies, quickly brought British doctors up to date on the long-term prognosis for whiplash.[33] Orthopaedic surgeon K.M. Porter, in a 1989 editorial for the *BMJ*, "Neck Sprains after Car Accident: A Common Cause Of Long Term Disability," wrote: "Sprains of the neck occur in 15 per cent to 30 per cent of car occupants examined soon after their accidents, but in the longer term about 60 per cent experience neck sprain." Porter advised that "pain, suffering, and disability after acute neck sprains may be reduced by doctors recognizing that these injuries, especially those that occur after rear-end impacts, may cause long term disability."[34]

Then a 1991 *Lancet* editorial, "Neck Injury and the Mind," commented: "Injuries of the neck are commonly caused by rear-end traffic collisions ... When symptoms of pain and disability persist from these lesions they are often deemed to be emotional in origin; sometimes the patient is thought to be malingering. Radanov and colleagues now provide evidence that favours a different view."

Bogdan Radanov and members of his group of whiplash experts from Switzerland, using sophisticated but flawed statistical techniques, had reported that rear-end collisions caused significant injury to the brain resulting in cognitive impairment. (I will examine the claims of these Swiss experts in detail in chapter 10.) In keeping with whiplash-promoting articles, the *Lancet* editorial presents the alarmist findings of monkey whiplash studies, and it paves the way for brain injury compensation: "Those difficulties could arise because of impaired attention span in the presence of pain or perhaps because of subtle organic cerebral dysfunction related to the cervical sprain injury."[35]

The average award for whiplash in the United Kingdom for the five years prior to 1989 was around £6,000.[36] Following these two editorials in the British journals, some claims shot up into six-digit numbers.[37] A 27-year-old English housewife and packer, for example, who had been a passenger in a rear-ended stationary taxi, developed chronic pain. I provide her history as it appears in the law report.

In consequence of the accident the claimant developed a chronic pain syndrome for which there was no organic basis but which caused her pain across the top of her right shoulder and the right side of her neck down her right arm as far as her wrist. The pain was worse when she undertook any activity.

She had pins and needles in the fingers of her right hand. She had limited movement of her neck. She was unable to carry anything except for a small clutch bag. She was unable to wear a shoulder bag. She could not carry out housework or return to her job as a packer. On medical advice, she underwent various treatments including physiotherapy, acupuncture, local anaesthetic injections and steroids. She took painkillers regularly and was referred to a psychiatrist for assessment and therapy. She also attended for neurological investigation.

All treatments were to no avail. She remained seriously disabled. In cases of long-standing chronic pain disorder the psychiatric prognosis is gloomy. There was a possibility of improvement but it was not likely. Since childhood the claimant had a left hemiparesis [weakness of one side of body] leaving her with a left arm that was virtually without useful function. The judge found the complainant was not a malingerer and there was no real chance of a sufficient recovery to permit her to return to work and lead a normal life.[38]

The judge awarded her £314,772 (US$700,000), including £39,000 for the costs of a future resident nanny. There are many overworked young mothers to whom the prospect of quitting a dull job and having a resident nanny must appear as unimaginable bliss. Peer modelling in whiplash among both patients and practitioners is potent.[39] Predictably, many other unhappy housewives gratefully followed suit, as a 1997 editorial in the *British Journal of Bone and Joint Surgery* pointed out: "Whiplash injuries of the neck appear to have increased dramatically; they are common in both clinical and medico-legal practice."[40]

So now, like the United States, Britain also has a flourishing whiplash litigation industry, and British medical journals are busy publishing articles on whiplash. Current estimates suggest that the annual cost of whiplash in Britain has reached £3.1 billion (US$6.2 billion).[41]

Apart from dropping animals down an elevator shaft, Macnab was a sensible thoughtful surgeon who was perplexed by the problem of persistent whiplash symptoms. Five years after performing his animal whiplash experiments, he wrote: "There is a remarkable paucity of information in the literature in regard to the basic underlying lesions resulting from extension-acceleration injuries of the cervical spine."[42] In the years since he made this observation, bone scans and other modern investigative techniques have been developed that can readily reveal the various kinds of brain, skeletal, and soft tissue injuries produced in animal whiplash. These lesions are NOT present in patients with chronic whiplash symptoms. In this way, Macnab's statement remains as true today as when he wrote it. There is still a remarkable paucity of information on these underlying lesions, though it is becoming clearer that this paucity of information exists because no such lesions exist. The whiplash lesion is a medico-legal illusion.

Nevertheless, an immense amount of medical literature remains devoted to ingenious attempts to find, explain, and prove a physical or disease basis for whiplash symptoms. Both in the healthcare practitioner's office and in the law courts, so much attention is focused on the physical mechanism of whiplash injury that scant attention is paid to whiplash beyond these arenas. However, when it is not complicated by the presence of doctors and lawyers, whiplash is an injury of little consequence.

3

*Bumper Kisses
and Whiplash Severity*

A hidden connection is stronger than an obvious one.
– Heraclitus, *Fragments*

It might reasonably be supposed that the severity of an auto collision neck injury would bear some relationship to the severity of impact, and in severe impacts it does. A person is much more likely to be killed or sustain a severe neck injury if his car is rear-ended by a bus travelling at 50 mph than if a preoccupied driver in a mini-compact rear-ends him while dawdling down the road at 5 mph. However, in common everyday minor rear-end collisions there is no correlation between the size of the impact and subsequent whiplash complaints.[1] In North America about a third of highway collisions, even if they are small, are followed by a claim for whiplash compensation.

Intentional collisions are a different matter. Stock car racers and demolition derby drivers, who are repeatedly involved in major collisions, seem immune to the development of ongoing whiplash symptoms.[2] In the early 1960s, when the whiplash epidemic was being established in Canada, Phillip Melville, a Toronto psychiatrist, pointed out the odd fact that collisions on public highways often cause whiplash but collisions in demolition derbies rarely do. Derby contestants drive reinforced older American cars fitted with seatbelts and standard head restraints. Their goal is to immobilize the other cars and be the operator of the last car able to move under its own power.[3] Since collisions occur at speeds of up to 50 mph, these derbies provide an impressive example of the resilience of the human neck – a telling observation that most healthcare practitioners have managed to ignore.

Henry Berry, a Toronto neurologist, made the first formal study of whiplash – or rather its absence – among demolition derby drivers. He studied 20 drivers aged 19 to 48 years who had participated in the sport for an average of 6.8 years. With an average of 45 hits per derby and almost 6 derbies a year, a derby driver tallies up about 1900 collisions during his career, about 25 per cent of which are described as severe (i.e., nearly 500 severe collisions).

Three-quarters of the drivers in Berry's study reported symptoms of pain and discomfort in the neck and shoulders within the first few hours, or one to two days after a derby. The symptoms lasted a few days. One driver, who had suffered acute back pain when his car was hit on the driver's side door, spent three days in hospital and remained off work for a month. There were no reports of dizziness, headache, numbness, poor memory, or anxiety, symptoms which are now strongly associated with highway collisions. Berry concludes: "The demolition driver and the accident victim are largely similar in respect to age, general health, mode of impact, speed of collision, the blows and strains to which they have been subjected, and damage to the vehicle. They are also similar in that they may or may not have a warning of collision. Apart from gender, the greatest difference is that of context; in the one, the driver is there for the purpose of competition in a sport; in the other, the passenger or driver is an unwilling victim of another's failure or carelessness."[4]

I am not an aficionado of stock car racing, but in my medico-legal practice I see so many plaintiffs claiming permanent disability following a mere *fender bender*, that watching our local stock car races was reassuring. The drivers have horrendous collisions, but the officials at the track laughed at my suggestion that the drivers might be vulnerable to whiplash. These drivers do not get whiplash. Neither do fairground bumper car riders, even though bumper car collisions occur at the same speeds as collisions that cause whiplash in highway accidents. Furthermore, bumper cars have no head restraints to prevent hyperextension of the neck and are especially designed to be elastic in their collision behaviour – a property that is claimed to increase whiplash neck damage.[5]

Over 2000 real or simulated collision experiments have attempted to produce the symptoms of common whiplash. All have failed, even though the forces employed were often greater than those experienced by most whiplash claimants.[6] In such experiments it is relatively easy to induce transient neck discomfort or pain, but this pain disappears within a few days. The bodies of the volunteers for these experiments behave in the way nature intended them to – they recover.

The development of persistent, or chronic, whiplash symptoms following collisions on public highways varies according to time, place, and the circumstances of the accident. In countries where whiplash is regarded as a significant injury, persistent whiplash symptoms are common.[7] In the United States, for instance, where whiplash is a "fussed-over" injury, between 14 per cent and 42 per cent of claimants report chronic pain.[8] In contrast, chronic whiplash symptoms have been reportedly uncommon in Singapore.[9] New Zealand and the province of Victoria in Australia are communities similar in size and affluence. In the mid-1980s, although both had similar rates of rear-end collisions, whiplash claims were found to be eight times higher in Victoria – a difference probably explained by dissimilar levels of compensation. Victoria paid out three times more for whiplash injury than did New Zealand.[10]

Similar discrepancies occur among Canadian provinces. Until a few years ago Saskatchewan had ten times more whiplash claims per capita than Quebec.[11] The government of Quebec has a vigorous "*No crash, no cash*" policy, realistically insisting on objective evidence of vehicle damage and actual injury before paying benefits.

Persistent whiplash only becomes a problem after people have heard of it. It was unknown in Russia in 1970 when Melvin Belli, past president of the American Trial Lawyers Association, was invited to lecture on the management of back pain at the Institute of Traumatology in Moscow. (That an American lawyer should lecture on backache is not as surprising as it may seem since, as many people point out, the management of painful backs in the United States is now more a legal than a medical problem.) After his lecture, Belli asked the Russian doctors (most of whom spoke English) how they diagnosed and treated whiplash. No Russian doctor at the lecture even recognized the term, let alone conceived of it as a medical entity.[12]

Belli and the Russian doctors finally concluded that whiplash was absent from the Soviet Union because, having fewer cars, Soviets had fewer rear-end collisions to cause it. This was an improbable conclusion because other countries with sparse traffic conditions (Iceland, for example) seem to have no shortage of whiplash,[13] and some countries with a great deal of traffic have hardly any. In traffic-congested Greece, for instance, the ubiquitous rear-end collisions are considered as inconsequential as jostling in the crowded markets, and little compensation is awarded to anyone involved.

A group of surgeons at the University of Patras in Greece followed up 140 patients who had sustained a soft tissue neck injury in auto collisions. They examined the patients within two days of the accident and again at one, three and six months. At the one-month follow-up, 91 per cent of the patients were free of symptoms, and within three to six months all patients had become symptom-free. In their 1997 report, the authors comment that these recovery rates when compared to those from other countries are "tremendous."[14] They are, indeed, tremendous, though Greeks are not constitutionally immune to whiplash. In countries where whiplash is perceived as a serious health problem, Greek immigrants make claims with such alacrity that whiplash and backache have sometimes been dubbed "Greek disease."[15] The effects of whiplash seem to depend less on the exposure of people's necks to rear-end collisions, than on the exposure of their minds to the allure of whiplash compensation.

The most striking example of the allure of compensation comes from a Norwegian study by the team of Harald Schrader.[16] When a terrible epidemic of whiplash disability suddenly arrived in Norway, these suspicious investigators wanted to know more about the course of whiplash when it was uncomplicated by the availability of compensation. They picked Lithuania as a suitable place for their study, as that country has no personal injury insurance and therefore no financial incentive to develop whiplash. In fact, even in 1996, most Lithuanians, like the Russians two decades earlier, had not even heard of it.

Schrader and his colleagues obtained from the police the names of 202 Lithuanian drivers involved in rear-end collisions of varying severity within the previous three years. In 11 per cent of cases the impacted car was a wreck and could not be driven; the others had either moderate or mild damage. Forty-four per cent of the crashed vehicles had seatbelts and 59 per cent had head restraints. Some of the drivers had sustained obvious injury in the collision. Each driver was matched for age and gender with a control from his home town who had not been involved in a collision. Without disclosing the purpose of the study, the investigators sent health questionnaires to the accident subjects and the controls.

Thirty-one per cent of the accident subjects recalled having had neck pain within a few days of the accident, but in all cases said it was transitory, lasting at most a week. Thirty-five per cent of the accident victims reported current neck pain, but so did 33 per cent of the controls. Fifty-three per cent of the accident victims had headaches, but so did 50 per cent of the controls. These results revealed no statistical difference between accident victims and controls. The authors concluded that none of the accident victims had acquired disabling or persisting symptoms as a result of the rear-end collisions. When they were told of the purpose of the investigation, the participants couldn't believe that anyone would think that an accident that occurred a year or more previously could be the cause of a health problem. The Lithuanian accident victims were more concerned about their rear-bumpers than about their necks.[17]

Few whiplash studies have used such a scientifically acceptable methodology as that employed by the Schrader team. Instead of being gratified at this improvement, however, the "whiplash community" responded to the Norwegian study with hostility. The editors of the *Lancet*, in which it was published, received a barrage of indignant letters denigrating the study. Ivar Bjørgen, a psychologist and fellow Norwegian, complained, for example, that it was unfair to compare Lithuanian and Norwegian whiplash since, as few drivers in Lithuania have car insurance, the police are called to evaluate every accident, whereas in Norway the police are called only if there is personal injury. Norwegians who are identified as having whiplash are therefore more likely to be seriously injured and have a worse outcome.

Bjørgen also suggested that the higher incidence of whiplash in Norway was to be expected since seatbelts are worn more in Norway than in Lithuania, and they predispose to whiplash. He added that even if 44 per cent of the Lithuanians claimed to be wearing seatbelts, they are so sceptical about giving out information to the authorities that they could not be trusted to tell the truth anyway. "In general," Bjørgen writes, "it is very risky to draw conclusions based on a questionnaire with no control and no objective measurement or medical investigations," and dismisses Schrader's conclusions as "personal, unproven beliefs."[18]

Bas de Mol and Tom Heijer, from the Delft University of Technology Science Safety Group in Holland, add their rebuttal: "Schrader and colleagues justify the selection of Lithuania as a study location by using the popular prejudice that the legal system has in fact created this disability. In our opinion, unsafe traffic is to blame ... One could conclude erroneously from reading this paper that rear-end collisions do not generate an injury hazard."[19] Croft, the California chiropractor who reported a 57 per cent incidence of low backache in whiplash victims (chapter 1), and his colleague, Michael Freeman, complained that Schrader and colleagues had investigated 202 Lithuanian individuals who were involved in car accidents but had not studied Lithuanians with whiplash.[20]

Radanov, the leader of the Swiss group of prolific authors of whiplash articles mentioned in chapter 2, complained that there was "bias potential in the study" since the principal author stressed that the study was prompted by "an explosion of chronic whiplash cases in Norway."[21] Harold Merskey, the psychiatrist member of a group of whiplash enthusiasts from the University of Western Ontario, attacked Schrader and his colleagues for relying on the victims' accounts of the pain two years or so after the accident. Merskey argued that: "The recollection of pain after such a time interval is unreliable." To support his position he cites a study of women's recall of back pain at various time intervals after childbirth, which showed that as time goes by women's recall of pain becomes less accurate. Schrader's whiplash victims must have similarly forgotten their pain. "Thus," stated Merskey, "the measurement method for evaluation of the initial symptoms is profoundly unsatisfactory."[22] He reinforced his attack: "Unfortunately, the Schrader et al study is vitiated by unreliable measurements, inadequate power and mishaps of selection in case material. It provides no justification for the claim by the authors cited above and might just have proved the opposite."

Schrader and his Norwegian colleagues, it seems, had cut too close to the quick. Like frightful Vikings from the past, they had threatened to wreak havoc with the profitable whiplash industry. Despite their critics, however, they remained unbowed. In fact, they confirmed their findings in a second whiplash study designed to take any legitimate criticisms into account.

The second study, again in Lithuania, employed an even more refined methodology. Using current daily police records, they identified 210 consecutive victims of rear-end collisions and mailed them out questionnaires within seven days of their accident. Follow-up questionnaires, evaluating the intensity of headache and neck pain were mailed out at two months and one year post-accident. They again matched their subjects with controls.

Forty-seven per cent of the accident victims reported initial pain: 10 per cent only had neck pain, 19 per cent only had headache, and 18 per cent reported both neck pain and headache. The average duration of the initial neck pain was three days, the longest duration was seventeen days. The average duration of headache was four and half hours, the longest-lasting was twenty days.[23] After a year, there were no significant differences between the accident victims and the control group in the frequency and intensity of symptoms. The investigators also found a dose-response relationship between the force of the impact and the severity of the symptoms. With extensive damage, 52 per cent of the subjects reported initial pain compared with 10 per cent when the damage was minor.

Schrader and his team concluded that, without insurance, involvement of the therapeutic community, litigation, and preconceived notions about whiplash, the symptoms of acute whiplash are self-limiting and brief. Further, chronic whiplash either does not exist or is rare.[24]

Another aspect of whiplash litigation fever is the question of the direction of the collision impact. Collisions come from all directions, but the connection between the direction of impact and the likelihood of developing whiplash has changed over the years. Ninety-two per cent of the original Gay and Abbott patients were in rear-end collisions and for the next three decades such collisions remained the predominant cause of whiplash.[25] For example, in 1971, Macnab, in reviewing over 500 whiplash patients, reported that rear-end collisions were by far the most common cause of whiplash and also reported that these claimants took much longer to recover than those injured in side or head-on collisions.[26]

Although Macnab suspected that lawyers rather than neck injuries were mostly responsible for persistent whiplash symptoms, he was perplexed by his findings: "If neck pain following accident is pure neurosis, why do patients commonly get neurotic if their head is thrown backward and rarely get neurotic if it is jolted forward or sideways? Surely these findings suggest that the persistence of pain after forced extension of the neck is related in some way to the fact that the neck can, and may, move beyond physiologically permitted limits."[27]

In 1978 Janecki and Lipke, orthopaedic surgeons at the University of Rochester, New York, in justifying whiplash "litigation fever," pointed out that hyperextension of the neck is an injury mechanism that leads to "limited function" of the neck "for prolonged periods or indefinitely," and that it is the people in rear-end collisions who sue, whereas people in side or front-end collisions "rarely institute lawsuits." These surgeons emphasized that "the assumption that whiplash syndrome occurs only in neurotic or litigation-minded patients should be discouraged."[28]

Times change and so does whiplash. In 1991, Pennie and Agambar, surgeons from Merseyside, England, reported on 151 whiplash patients. Seventy of these patients were in rear-end collisions but 81 were in collisions described as "other." The authors concluded that: "The associated signs and symptoms did not vary with the accident pattern, nor did the time taken for patients to recover."[29] The English, perhaps seeing whiplash with fresh eyes, discovered that an impact from any direction can engender a whiplash claim.

Normally, the larger the dose the greater the response, but with whiplash it seems that the larger the bump the smaller the whiplash. In a study of 30 consecutive accident victims admitted to Mater Misericordiae Hospital, Dublin, following collisions severe enough to cause fractures,[30] investigators questioned the patients about neck and jaw pains both at the time of admission and six weeks later. Only 2 out of the 30 collision victims had any neck symptoms. One, a front seat passenger, had fractures of the femur and the cheekbone, and the other had a fracture of the femur and a head injury with facial lacerations. Both complained of neck stiffness on admission and at the six-week assessment. Since these were the two patients who had sustained injuries to the face, it is likely that their neck injury was secondary to a direct blow to the head. Pennie and Agambar conclude that the symptoms of neck sprains are less influenced by mechanical factors than by other considerations.[31]

Whiplash is preventable. Lengthening pilots' seat backs eliminated whiplash in pilots catapulted from ships.[32] In human whiplash experiments, head restraints were so effective that, even with impact velocities of 44 mph, study volunteers reported only slight neck discomfort.[33] When it comes to highway collisions, however, head restraints seem to have little effect. An executive from Ford Motors commented: "We have not found one guy whose life was saved or who even avoided a sprained neck [by the use of a head restraint]."[34] No doubt Ford did not want to bear the cost of installing head restraints in their cars so the executive's opinion may have been biased. Nevertheless, the Ford executive was partly right: head restraints have not dramatically reduced whiplash complaints in the way that experts expected. Head restraints soon showed diminishing returns. Why could this have been so?

A study of neck injury claims in the United States by the Insurance Institute for Highway Safety found an 18 per cent reduction in claims involving cars with head restraints.[35] Other studies have been more equivocal. A study from Yorkshire of patients attending a casualty department following a traffic accident showed that head restraints reduce whiplash, but the difference was too slight to be statistically significant.[36] The experts scratched their heads about the disappointing results of head restraints. Perhaps something was wrong with head restraints, but even if head restraints are improperly positioned,[37] it seems reasonable to suppose that they should have made a bigger blip in the whiplash statistics.

At first glance, the statistics do not make sense, but with a second look they do. Head restraints do prevent hyperextension of the neck in high-impact rear-end collisions and so reduce serious neck injury. However, most rear-end collisions are not high-impact. Most whiplash complaints derive from inconsequential collisions in which little or no neck damage – with or without head restraint – is likely to occur. Head restraints cannot prevent an injury that is not going to happen.[38]

The belief nevertheless persists that an actual physical neck injury is the cause of the high rate of whiplash claims. One large Japanese insurance company, for example, hoping to reduce its claims, is spending a billion yen (US$10 million) on a search for an effective head restraint.[39] It will be surprising if a new head restraint is any more effective against our whiplash epidemic than nose posies were against the bubonic plague.

Inconsistencies also abound in rates of recovery from whiplash. Severe injuries heal quickly and minor injuries can take forever. Air force personnel forced to escape with ejector seats from disabled planes are subjected to huge acceleration forces and, not surprisingly, they sustain various spinal injuries. Twenty per cent of Swedish Air Force flyers rescued after ejection by catapult had spinal fractures and disc injuries. But, unless they had multiple limb fractures as well, these air force personnel were soon flying again.[40] A second Swedish Air Force study showed that pilots who had previously sustained spine fractures or disc injuries did not become prematurely disabled or have excessive spine problems.[41] In contrast, minor – or even non-existent – whiplash injuries acquired on our roads frequently lead to permanent disability, and minor whiplash injuries are claimed to predispose to future spinal problems.

In comparison to the tort system of auto insurance, no-fault insurance greatly restricts access to payment for pain and suffering. In 1995, Saskatchewan, a province with a high whiplash claim rate, changed from the tort system to no-fault auto insurance. A study of whiplash claims in the months before and after this change provided an opportunity to access the effects of insurance payments for pain and suffering upon whiplash complaints. David Cassidy and the other authors of this excellent study found a 28 per cent drop in whiplash claims despite a coincidental increase in the number of vehicle-damage claims and kilometres driven. They conclude: "The type of insurance system has a profound effect on the frequency and duration of whiplash claims ... claimants recover faster if compensation for pain and suffering is not available."[42] Investigators whose studies threaten the whiplash industry, are in for a bad time; I describe the fallout for the authors of this study in chapter 18.

In most developed countries rear-end collisions are widely regarded as the most dangerous of collisions, but in terms of causing death (the most objective measurement available) they are the least so. Figure 3–1 below shows the percentage of fatalities for various types of traffic accidents. Rear-end collisions are at the bottom, causing less than one death per 1000 rear-end collisions.[43] You may think it odd that rear-end collisions kill so seldom when they *injure* so often, but, when it comes to compensable injuries, this oddity is, in fact, the norm: the less severe the injury, the more vociferous the complaints.

There is something miraculous about whiplash. Humans are different from all other living creatures (or at least we like to think so) in that we can think in symbols. This singular ability certainly has its uses, but it also complicates our lives for we easily confuse symbol and substance. Bumper touches bumper; magically a flesh and blood wound appears in the neck. Whiplash! Word is made flesh, irrespective of

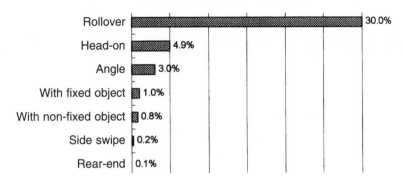

Fig. 3–1   Rear-end collisions seldom kill
Although often portrayed as the most dangerous of collisions, rear-end collisions are the least dangerous of all collisions. The table shows the percentage of fatalities by type of collision. Fatalities from rear-end accidents are way down at the bottom.

whether the infliction of such miraculous injury is compatible with the laws of physics. Two examples illustrate this whiplash miracle:

A 30-year-old Canadian sued for a whiplash injury allegedly sustained at the entrance of an underground parking garage where he had been involved in a lengthy discussion with the garage attendant about where to safely park his smart new Lincoln Continental. A young man in a small Fiat behind the Continental became uncontainably impatient. He edged his Fiat forward until he was bumper to bumper with the Continental – and pushed.

The Lincoln driver was indignant! He complained of a painful neck. His friends, finding him upset and distressed, took him to the emergency department and the whole process of being a whiplash victim began. Consultations, reports, MRIs – the lot! In no way could a small car from a standing position accelerate a Lincoln Continental at anywhere near the rate that the Lincoln would normally accelerate itself from a stoplight. The plaintiff's pride had been hurt, but only by the supernatural suspension of the laws of motion could his neck have been damaged. Highly paid and presumably intelligent physicians and lawyers all behaved as if his hurt feelings were a corporeal injury.

A second example of whiplash transubstantiation comes from the recent Toronto subway crash. The Toronto Transit Commission (TTC) had maintained an exceptional safety record and its subway control systems were considered so foolproof that the subway cars were not designed to withstand collision. Then, on the afternoon of 11 August 1995, the unthinkable happened: a train travelling between 30 and 35 mph crashed into the rear of a stationary train. The front and rear cars collapsed into each other and both ballooned out into the tunnel, putting the thirty or so people in those cars at enormous risk. Only minor or insignificant damage was caused to the five other cars of each train, and within an hour of the accident TTC personnel had escorted the 200–300 uninjured passengers off the trains, along the tunnel to safety. Three people had been killed, and the thirty identified injured were transported to hospital.[44]

Two weeks after the crash, lawyers launched a $55 million class action suit against the TTC on behalf of the train passengers. They warned that the $55 million was "only the tip of the iceberg."[45] One hundred and seventy-one injury claims were submitted. Mrs O, a 37-year-old mother of two children, was chosen as one of two "representative claimants"; she was carefully cross-examined.[46]

One of about a dozen people in the last car of the striking train, Mrs O was quietly dozing facing the front of the train when the collision occurred. She recalled being woken by a loud metallic bang and a sudden jolt. I quote the transcript of her cross-examination:

Question: Okay. What happened to you after, when the train stopped?
Answer: I was thrown forward.
Q: Were you thrown out of your seat?
A: No. The bar on the seat in front of me saved me from being thrown right out of the seat.
Q: Did your buttocks leave the seat?
A: Yes, they did.
Q: And you contacted a metal bar in front of you?
A: Yes, I did.
Q: That was with your hand or …
A: My leg.
Q: Okay. And then you fell back into your seat, I take it?
A: Correct.
Q: And then what happened?
A: That was about it. I just sort of like sat there. Nobody knew what had happened …
Q: All right.
A: So, I just sort of sat there waiting.
Q: Did you expect the train to start again?
A: Yes.
Q: You just thought it was a sudden stop?
A: Yes.

There followed a discussion about the lights flickering. Mrs O agreed that the lights stayed on.

Q: How about the other passengers on the train? Did you notice what they were doing? Were they doing the same thing, just waiting for the train to start up again?

A: Basically.

In the discussion about what happened next, Mrs O indicated that it was only when the personnel walked through the train that she realized something must be wrong. After she had described the orderly evacuation of the passengers through the rear door of the train, the questioner moved to her injuries.

Q: Now, you mention in your affidavit that you received moderate injuries?

A: Yes.

Q: Is that correct?

A: Yes.

Q: In general terms, can you tell me what happened to you? What injuries did you sustain?

A: It was whiplash, the pressing of a disk out of the neck onto nerves and tendons, into my shoulder.

Q: Okay. Are you still suffering from these injuries?

A: Yes.

Q: Has your doctor told you how long he expects you to have these injuries?

A: The ... well, we've sort of talked about it. The actual injuries themselves they figure are healing, but we have recurrences all the time so it's something ... he says there's no way of knowing when the recurrences will stop.

Q: Okay. He's given you no time with respect to that?

Mrs O agreed that she had sustained no psychological injury in the accident. There was further discussion as to whether she had encountered any commercials, either on radio or in the newspapers, with respect to lawyers seeking accident victims – "crash victims" as they were called. Mrs O denied it.

I have quoted extensively from this transcript because it documents a common problem. Data about the crash show that the train travelling at between 30 and 35 mph collapsed into the rear car of the stationary train, coming to a halt in a distance of 51 ft. The train's rate of deceleration was about the same as that of an automobile when braked moderately hard. Such a deceleration might be enough to propel an unbelted passenger forward in his seat, and Mrs O's description of how she slipped forward on the train seat is consistent with that rate of deceleration. This level of deceleration can be the cause of injury from a "secondary collision," especially if the person hits something hard or sharp, but it is extremely unlikely to cause an acceleration/deceleration injury to the neck. Few vehicle passengers get whiplash when a car driver slams on the brakes.

The acceleration of the forward train was equal but opposite to the deceleration of the second train. All the passengers in the train, except for the thirty or so in the two severely damaged cars, experienced the same levels of acceleration/deceleration force as did Mrs O. Altogether approximately 40 per cent of the 171 TTC claimants alleged "whiplash injury." Oddities happen in medicine, and perhaps Mrs O really did injure her neck in the accident, but for 40 per cent of the claimants to have done so would have required the suspension of the laws of physics.

Whiplash physicians expend inordinate energy in searching for neck injuries when the wound is one of symbol and not of substance. Crazy as this may seem, there is method in their madness. While it is certainly nonsensical to accept that necks vary in their vulnerability to injury from year to year and from place to place, there is nothing non-sensical about the search for mythical neck injuries. The search for *symbolic neck injuries* is handsomely rewarded. When it comes to making easy money, both for the claimants and the professionals involved, whiplash is, indeed, a miracle. It is a miracle that works wonders because of our human propensity to convert psychological distress into physical symptoms.

4

Sanitizing the Symptoms
of Distress

Our lives are but toil and trouble; they come to an end like a sigh.
– Psalm 90

Neurosis is always a substitute for legitimate suffering.
– Carl Jung

Many patients complain to their doctors of symptoms for which no physical explanation can be found. Such symptoms are described as *somatoform*, and an understanding of somatization and somatoform illness helps make sense of whiplash and many problems of medical care. Soma is Greek for the body, and somatization implies the conversion of mental distress into symptoms generally associated with a physical disorder. A somatoform or psychosomatic disorder is psychological distress masquerading as a physical illness. Since the symptoms are psychologically engendered, no actual physical disease is present.[1]

Epidemiological studies indicate that the majority of symptoms seen in family practice or even in general medical clinics are somatoform.[2] In one large British family practice, for example, over 50 per cent of the patients with psychiatric problems initially presented with somatic complaints.[3] Excellently designed population studies demonstrate the ubiquity of such psychiatric problems. A survey taken in the skyscraper jungle of midtown Manhattan and one in a quiet rural seaside county in Nova Scotia both gave the same results.[4] One-fifth of each of both populations had mental symptoms severe enough to cause significant impairment of functioning, a further three-fifths had some symptoms of emotional impairment, and only one-fifth were found to be psychiatrically well. In another study, between 10 and 20 per cent of the patient population of forty-six general practices in Greater London were found to be mentally ill or disturbed.[5]

Since it is almost universal for psychological distress to be expressed and experienced as physical symptoms, it is hardly surprising that psychologically distressed people often believe themselves to be physically ill. Many people actually prefer it that way, since any suggestion of a mental disorder makes them uncomfortable. As doctors also prefer to see illness in physical terms, both patients and doctors seek out physical explanations for unwanted symptoms – explanations that regularly turn out to be wrong.

Perhaps a short digression will be useful. It illustrates both the pitfalls of carelessly attributing an illness to a particular cause and the reasons for much of our discomfort with mental disorder. It involves sin, sex, and sickness.

For centuries, mental illness was often attributed to possession by the devil, and sufferers from it were treated accordingly. Then, as science began to loosen the devil's grip on Christendom, "self-abuse" became the "scientific explanation" for mental illness. For four centuries, the Church had disparaged the normal and useful childhood and adolescent activity of masturbation, but our Victorian forefathers became mesmerized by it.[6] They claimed that it caused not only mental illness but moral degeneracy as well.[7] Even the nineteenth-century English psychiatrist Henry Maudsley, although known for his enlightenment and humanity, joined his contemporaries in their abhorrence of masturbation.[8] In a lecture to the august Harveian Society he demonstrates his views: "The miserable sinner whose mind suffers by reason of self-abuse becomes offensively egotistic, a deceitful liar, and in fact, morally insane." While noting that most self-abusers are fortunately impotent, he pitied the "outlook for any child begotten of such degenerate stock." He described the downfall of an 18-year-old youth and concluded: "Once the habit is formed and the mind has positively suffered from it, the victim is less able to control what is more difficult to control, and there would be almost as much hope of the ... leopard changing his spots, as of his abandoning the vice. I have no faith in the employment of physical means to check what has become a serious mental disease; the sooner he sinks to his degraded rest the better for himself, and the better for the world which is well rid of him."[9] In retrospect, the youth suffered from schizophrenia.

Of course, Maudsley was wrong. If he had collected 200 or so young people and divided them randomly into two groups, had successfully managed to prevent the members of one group from masturbating while ensuring that those in the other group did, and, using unbiased observers, had found a significantly higher incidence of mental illness in the masturbating group, he could then, perhaps, have claimed self-abuse to be a cause of mental illness. Even so, there would still have been doubts. In a milieu of conviction that masturbation is both sinful and dangerous, guilt and anxiety amongst the masturbators might of itself have become an aetiological agent for mental illness.

But randomized controlled trials (RCTs), an important tool by which to reveal any causal connection between two events, had not yet been invented. Schrader, in his second Lithuanian study, used such a trial.

(For readers unfamiliar with RCTs I have provided an example of their use in Appendix I. Believing that something causes illness is not a sufficient reason to make it so.)

Prejudices die hard and, since mental illness remains a frowned-upon condition, under the circumstances it is prudent to attribute the symptoms of psychological distress to a physical illness.[10] Once a suitable illness has been chosen, no one wants the ruse discovered, so even the gentlest suggestion that the illness may have a psychological origin is often greatly resented.[11]

Although most doctors now accept, at least in theory, that somatoform symptoms are signals of mental distress couched in acceptable physical form, some doctors, especially plaintiff experts, strongly disagree. They argue that the absence of a demonstrable underlying physical cause to explain the presence of symptoms is not a reason to ascribe these symptoms to a psychological cause. They are, of course, right: it is a breach of logic to attribute symptoms to a psychological source just because a physical source cannot be found for them. Indeed, many symptoms for which no physical cause can be found may well turn out to be physical in origin, our investigative techniques being still too insensitive to demonstrate the relevant abnormality.

Nevertheless, there is overwhelming evidence that many people, when psychologically distressed, develop and complain of physical symptoms.[12] It is not clear, however, how this translation from psychological distress to physical symptoms occurs. Maybe people simply opt, either consciously or unconsciously, to exchange their psychological complaints for more acceptable physical ones. Perhaps depressed and anxious people pay more attention to everyday symptoms which, under happier circumstances, they would ignore. Or again, perhaps psychological distress causes physiological processes to go haywire, resulting in all sorts of physical symptoms. Most likely all these illness mechanisms occur.[13] Anyway, whatever the exact mechanism, many of us, when in psychological distress, develop somatoform symptoms. Those of us who do so a lot are known in medical parlance as "somatizers."

Lees-Haley and Brown are American research psychologists who have studied the prevalence of head injury symptoms. They had difficulty assigning particular symptoms to a head injury without first knowing how frequently those symptoms occur in claimants with no history of head injury. To obtain this information, Lees-Haley and Brown collected a sample of 170 personal injury claimants with no history of head injury, who were making claims for psychological injury such as sexual harassment or wrongful dismissal, and matched them for gender, age, and class with a group of 50 controls from a general

Symptoms	Claimants (%)	Controls (%)
Anxiety and nervousness	93	54
Sleeping problems	92	52
Depression	89	32
Headaches	88	62
Back pain*	80	48
Fatigue	79	58
Concentration problems	78	26
Worried about health	30	74
Irritability	77	38
Neck pain*	74	30
Impatience	65	36
Restlessness	62	18
Feeling disorganized	61	24
Confusion	59	16
Loss of efficiency with everyday tasks	56	16
Shoulder pain*	74	30
Memory problems	53	20
Dizziness	44	26
Sexual problems	41	6
Numbness	39	12
Nausea	38	34
Word-finding problems	34	20
Hearing problems	29	18
Trouble reading	24	12
Bumping into things	21	20
Speech problems	18	16
Impotence	15	4

Fig. 4–1   Everyone has symptoms: litigants have more
The prevalence of head injury-type symptoms in personal injury litigants without head injury (sexual harassment etc.) compared to a control group of patients attending a family practice. The symptoms marked with an asterisk are not "head injury" symptoms; the investigators added them to the questionnaires to act as "distracters."

family practice.[14] The subjects and controls completed a questionnaire about whether they experienced head injury symptoms such as headaches, dizziness, and difficulties in concentration. As is often done in this kind of study, the authors added some "distracters" (symptoms that are not associated with head injury) to their questionnaire. Figure 4–1 shows the results.

You will see that symptoms of all sorts are common. Even patients attending their family physician reported high rates of both head injury symptoms and musculoskeletal pain – neck, shoulder, and back pain. The claimants involved in personal injury litigation reported even higher rates of these symptoms – so high that their rates of *head injury symptoms* were about equal to those found in patients who had actually sustained a severe head injury. Lees-Haley and Brown found that the very fact of going through litigation doubles the normal incidence of neck pain, back pain, and shoulder pain. The lesson to be learned from this study is that the presence of symptoms is an unreliable way to assess for the presence or absence of any actual underlying injury or disease. Added to this difficulty is the problem of suggestibility. We are all suggestible; even the thought that something is wrong soon produces symptoms.

An account in *Science,* "The Dump that Wasn't There," illustrates how readily a belief that something is wrong can generate symptoms. Frayser, a blue-collar residential neighbourhood of Memphis, Texas, is the centre of a large chemical manufacturing industry. In 1976 a woman reported to the County Health Department that toxic chemicals in the environment were giving her family rashes and other illnesses. The next year she reiterated her complaint, and by the summer of 1979 other residents were complaining of rashes, headaches, urinary problems, heart disease, and cancer. Then a former health department employee claimed he knew of an old chemical waste dump in the area. Reports of illness escalated and the citizenry panicked. One local political activist called for evacuation of the neighbourhood.

After an extensive search by the authorities, no dump was found. Most people settled down, and their symptoms abated or at least stopped bothering them. A few residents continued to believe that they had unusual health problems. The author of this account concludes: "The spectre of this ghost dump will continue to haunt epidemiologists confronted with other self-reported increases in illness."[15]

Edward Shorter, a professor of history at the University of Toronto, has traced the changes in somatoform illness over recent centuries. He coined the term "the symptom pool," to designate somatoform symptoms that both doctors and patients regard as indicative of physical disease. The symptom pool changes from year to year and from place to place. Shorter writes: "As the ideas of either party about what constitutes legitimate organic diseases change, the other member of the duo will respond. Thus the history of psychosomatic [somatoform] illness is one of ever-changing steps in a *pas de deux* between doctor and patient."[16]

Not only are the steps of this *pas de deux* continually changing but now the dancing partners are changing as well. The media and the legal profession are rapidly ousting the physician as the patient's dancing partner. Lawyers, journalists, broadcasters, and TV personalities are becoming the arbiters of illness. Physicians have certainly had their ample share of peculiar ideas about what causes illness, but lawyers and members of the media are even more imaginative. Exotic ideas about symptoms and the causes of sickness keep the public in a frenzy of hypochondriacal concern. Shorter's *pas de deux* has become a veritable caper.

In recounting how the symptom pool has metamorphosed, Shorter begins with the nineteenth century. Since doctors believed that seizures and paralysis were organic in nature, somatizing patients of that time who wished (intentionally or otherwise) to present their doctors with medically acceptable symptoms suffered from seizures and paralysis. Then science progressed. Physicians gained a greater understanding of the brain and the nervous system and, with the aid of the newly invented electroencephalogram (EEG), they were able to separate genuine seizures and paralysis from the simulated symptoms of their somatizing patients.

With their cover blown, somatizing patients moved their game elsewhere; chronic fatigue and pain proved more dependable. There were, and still are, no objective tests by which sceptical physicians, employers, family, or friends can challenge either the presence or the severity of these subjective symptoms. The patient remains in control, the final arbiter of his condition. Today's symptom pool is murky with pain and fatigue, though the designated cause of these symptoms varies according to the person's situation, the caregivers' concerns, the lawyer's suggestions, and the media's disease of the month.

While some somatizers develop their symptoms only when under psychological stress, others carry them throughout their lives: illness becomes a way of life. Psychiatrists call this condition "somatization disorder." Timothy Quill, a New York physician, provides a not untypical description of such a patient which was published in *JAMA*.[17] The patient's medical history is long, but then the medical histories of somatizing patients usually are.

A 74-year-old woman was referred by her gastroenterologist for primary care. Her chief complaints were severe headache and weakness that persisted for more than six months. Her recent evaluation by a neurologist had included two CT scans of the head, two EEGs, nerve conduction studies, and a muscle biopsy, none of which was definitive. She spontaneously offered that she was not depressed and that there must be a physical reason for her distress. She warned that other doctors had falsely believed that she had psychological problems, only to be proved wrong when the proper tests had been obtained or the proper surgery undertaken.

In the past year she had been evaluated by a cardiologist for chest pain, and a pulmonologist for shortness of breath. The evaluations included an echocardiogram, two avionics, a stress-thallium test, a cardiac catheterization, an upper gastro-intestinal tract series, a barium enema examination, two endoscopies, two colonoscopies, pulmonary function tests, and two ventilation-perfusion scans. Each physician believed her to be a diagnostic puzzle, but they gave tentative diagnoses of coronary artery spasm, bowel artery spasm, inflammatory bowel disease, and microscopic pulmonary emboli. Her more remote history showed over 30 operations, often for vague indications, beginning at the age of 24 years with a Caesarean section. She carried over 50 separate medical diagnoses but no psychiatric diagnoses. The specific data on which her diagnoses were based were vague and conflicting. She was taking six prescription medications regularly, including a narcotic painkiller.

She described having had a "hard life" and a long marriage to an alcoholic husband who had physically abused her. She had worked hard since childhood, the only respite being periods when she was ill.

Her physical examination showed a thin, downcast woman, who seemed remarkably well despite her medical ailments. With the exception of the numerous surgical scars all over her body, her examination results were within normal limits. She had biologic signs of depression but adamantly denied feeling depressed. All the laboratory investigations were normal.

Quill comments on how frequently "highly skilled physicians repeatedly fail to recognize patients' somatization disorders." "These patients," he writes, "use symptoms as a way to communicate, express emotion, and be taken care of. Instead of recognizing the disorder and exploring psycho-social contributors to illness, non-psychiatric physicians tend repeatedly to pursue organic possibilities through multiple tests, procedures, medications, and operations. The dollar costs of this strategy are only exceeded by its potential for iatrogenic harm."[18]

Patients often put symptoms to good use, using sickness as a wonderfully manipulative tool. Perhaps this ability comes naturally to us, for unlike most other creatures, we remain dependent on parental care for an inordinately long time. As children we have ample opportunity to learn the gentle art of being looked after. Nothing turns on parental concern faster than a few symptoms. When the world is not going our way, some of us remain past masters at upping the ante until we obtain the care response we want.

Of course, the tactical use of symptoms only works when there is a caring other to respond. There is no point in having somatoform symptoms if no one is going to bother. Somatoform disorders were rare in concentration camps,[19] but given a caring environment – the family, social security systems, and the courts – they can work like a charm. Doctors, like patients, tend to interpret symptoms as signposts to physical illness. At medical school they are taught that particular disease processes produce particular symptoms, and they learn which tests to request to confirm a suspected diagnosis. But medicine is not so straightforward and most of the time there is nothing to find. Physicians play safe and investigate anyway.

Doctors have a love/hate relationship with somatoform symptoms and the patients who present with them. Some doctors, especially those who like results, are soon irritated by the waste of time and money involved in looking for something that is not there. Some find these somatizing patients an interesting psychological challenge. But for many, these patients are easy money.

The easy money is, of course, nothing new. In Regency England, to give just one example, hungry young physicians set up their practices at fashionable seaside resorts and soon became wealthy. F.S. Skey, a celebrated Victorian London surgeon, recalled the time when "all the seaside towns were crowded with young ladies … who were confined to the horizontal posture, and wheeled about on the shore in Bath chairs [wheel chairs], on the supposition that they were the subjects of spinal disease. They were placed under much medical and dietetic discipline … Brighton, Worthing, Hastings, and other places on the South Coast were largely tenanted by these unfortunate females." Skey commented on the "absurdity of inferring that pain alone, which locates itself with remarkable precision in hysteria on a given vertebra, can indicate the presence of organic disease of the bone without collateral evidence in its favour."[20]

Somewhat nearer to our own time, in 1927, Francis Peabody, in addressing Harvard medical students about their future practice, reminded them of the advantageous fact that approximately half of all patients "complain of symptoms for which an adequate organic cause can not be discovered. Numerically, then, these patients constitute a large group and their fees go a long way toward spreading butter on the physicians' bread."[21]

Somatoform patients have always helped keep the medical profession well heeled, and in this respect, medical practice has not changed over the years; in some ways it has become worse. Doctors now have sophisticated tools at their disposal and seemingly unlimited government and insurance resources to fuel such searches for treatable pathologies. The fact that lawyers are poised to launch malpractice suits against any physician foolhardy enough to overlook organic pathology adds an incentive for these investigations.[22] All this attention soon confirms the patient's belief that he is ill, and whiplash patients are particularly easily convinced. The whiplash victim holds all the cards. If something is wrong, then the other driver caused it. The insurance company will have to pay up! With so much going for it, it is no wonder that whiplash quickly became a fashionable illness – one of many.

5

Copycats and
Fashionable Illnesses

Physicians see many "diseases" which have no more real existence
than an image in a mirror.
– Karl Marx[1]

Your mind is fine; it is all in your body.
– A very reassuring physician

"Whiplash syndrome" is an example of an illness actually induced
by society, in general, and by physicians in particular.
– Ferrari and Russell[2]

Just as germs spread diseases, so do ideas. Like some microbes, ideas
can be so virulent in their pathogenicity that they soon create epidemics.[3] Copycat pseudo-illnesses thrive in the work place but, as the
so-called "fashionable illnesses," they are common in the community
at large. "Occupational mass psychogenic illness" usually occurs
against a background of anxiety and resentment. The first recorded
outbreak of an epidemic of this type illustrates how dramatic such illnesses can be. It occurred in a Lancashire cotton mill the year after the
introduction of the power loom, an innovation that caused great concern and financial distress to textile workers of Northern England.
The following account is taken from *Gentleman's Magazine* in 1787:

On the 15th of February 1787, [a girl] put a mouse into the bosom of another girl, who had a dread of mice. The girl was immediately thrown into a fit,
and continued in it with the most violent convulsions, for twenty-four hours.
On the following day, three more girls were seized in the same manner; and
on the 17th, six more. By this time the alarm was so great, that the whole work,
in which 200 or 300 were employed, was totally stopped, and an idea prevailed
that a particular disease had been introduced by a bag of cotton opened in the
house.

On Sunday the 18th Dr St Clare was sent for from Preston; before he arrived
three more were seized, and during the night and morning of the 19th, eleven
more, making in all twenty-four. Of these, twenty-one were young women, two

were girls of about ten years of age, and one man, who had been very much fatigued with holding the girls ... The symptoms were anxiety, strangulation, and very strong convulsions; and these were so violent as to last without any intermission from a quarter of an hour to twenty-four hours, and to require four or five persons to prevent the patients from tearing their hair and dashing their heads against the floor and walls. Dr St Clare had taken with him a portable electrical machine, and by electric shocks the patients were universally relieved without exception. As soon as the patients and the country were assured that the complaint was merely nervous, easily cured, and not introduced by cotton, no fresh person was affected.[4]

Doctors had not yet separated psychogenic seizures from genuine epileptic fits. Seizures were in the symptom pool of the time and would have been perceived as symptoms from which it was legitimate to suffer.

Like everyone else, workers resent having changes foisted upon them – a dislike that generates frequent psycho-social epidemics.[5] In an early example of changing office technology, the British Civil Service 150 years ago replaced quill pens with steel nibs. Immediately, large numbers of civil servants developed pain and fatigue in the arms; some became disabled.[6] Eventually, however, the civil servants accepted the nibs and it was business as usual.

In the early twentieth century, the invention of the telegraph keypad was followed in both Britain and the United States by an epidemic of telegraphists' cramp. In Britain, 60 per cent of the work force reported symptoms, and a national committee was established to investigate its causes. After appropriate deliberations, the committee concluded that a nervous instability in the operator combined with the rapidity of the keypad movements overwhelmed the nervous system, causing a "nervous breakdown." Once the hubbub cooled down, telegraphers comfortably tapped out their messages; but the nervous breakdown remained a popular explanation for mental illness.[7]

Repetitive strain injury (RSI) all began soon after the widespread introduction of the computer with a disastrous epidemic that hit Australia in 1983.[8] For many years repeated wrist movements had been a recognized cause of tenosynovitis, a relatively uncommon but authentic painful inflammation of the tendon sheaths. But repetitive movements had not caused long-term health problems.[9] Then, by some oddity of Australian medical bureaucratese, tenosynovitis and arm pain were reclassified as RSI; discomfort attributable to repeated wrist movements became a compensable disease.

Coincidental with this change in medical nomenclature, Australians, like workers in many other parts of the world, had been nurturing a smouldering dislike of computer screens, and, in particular, a focused anger at foreign multinational companies who were rumoured to have dumped outmoded keyboards on the Australian market.[10] Keyboard operators complained of arm pains – so much so that in some sectors of the public service 30 per cent of workers were affected and replacement employees also soon came down with it. In some offices work came to standstill. Health service payments to pharmacists fell so far behind that the government was forced to abandon most of its fee processing systems.[11] RSI, irreverently known as "kangaroo paw," spread to other Australian workers, including teachers, nurses, and process and assembly line workers. Even school children developed it.[12]

It spread like wildfire, particularly in the Australian Public Service, and overwhelmed the responsible authorities into total acceptance of the condition.[13] Doctors emphasized the importance of the early recognition of the disorder, and the government created committees and organizations to investigate it. RSI was found to be a work-related injury and the government took measures to reduce the injury by substantially reducing the workload of any workers considered at risk. As more palliative measures were introduced, the worse the RSI became.[14]

Geoffrey Littlejohn, an Australian rheumatologist, documented the epidemic: "The costs to the community were enormous. Payments for compensation, medical and legal fees, and attention to *ergonomic factors in the work place* ran into hundreds of millions of dollars per year. Patients developed intractable, chronic pain in the neck and arm, and significant disability resulted. Patients left work and did not return for many years. Routine household duties became untenable, and the stress within families resulted in many divorces and gross family disharmony. Australia, a modern, proud, and vigorous country had never seen such a disabling public health problem in its recent history."[15]

I will describe later how this Australian epidemic was brought to an end, but first let us look at fashionable illnesses, the pseudo-illnesses not related to the workplace. In addition to the basic somatoform symptoms that allow psychological distress to be expressed and perceived as physical illness, fashionable illnesses have some characteristic features. Like fashions in general, they usually have panache and class, reflecting current community concerns and the latest scientific discoveries. Often, too, they allow people low on social clout to vent dissatisfaction. They are useful when circumstances dictate the need to control family, friends, employers, or the world in general. They are particularly handy for lawsuits and, like fashions in general, they often make fortunes for their creators.

A handful of these illnesses – past and present – will illustrate their common characteristics. The once popular illness of hypoglycaemia, or low blood sugar, is an excellent example. To appreciate the usefulness of this copycat illness it is first necessary to know about panic attacks. Between 1.5 and 3 per cent of people at some time during their life experience sudden feelings of impending doom and terror.[16] These episodes are now recognized as "panic attacks," a discrete psychiatric disorder, that, although horrible, is not dangerous. The diagnosis of panic attack usefully makes sense of what is otherwise a confusing experience for both patient and doctor.

But there is a problem. While panic attack sufferers want their unpleasant episodes acknowledged, they don't want the psychiatric label that goes with them. A solution was at hand – low blood sugar, inducing the release of adrenaline (nor-epinephrine), which produces symptoms identical to those of a panic attack. Some doctors obligingly claimed that these unfortunate patients did not have a psychiatric condition: they had hypoglycaemia. In the 1950s, 1960s, and 1970s they turned hypoglycaemia into a fashionable illness. Popular books confirmed that the illness was real.[17]

Of course, the fact that hypoglycaemia causes the symptoms of panic attack does not mean conversely that people with panic symptoms have hypoglycaemia; they usually don't. Psychiatrist Charles Ford and his colleagues at the University of California studied 30 volunteers who considered themselves hypoglycaemics. The subjects' attacks were unrelated to low blood glucose levels. "Many patients appeared to be experiencing acute emotional distress. However, they denied this distress or attributed it to the somatic problems; they displaced their psychological discomfort to concerns and pre-occupation with physiological processes. Their personal histories [however] revealed a close relationship between the development of the symptoms and external precipitating stress [such as] marital discord, separation, divorce, job change, and the death of a close relative."[18]

"Environmental hypersensitivity," a more recent example, is an illness in which sufferers become "allergic" to the chemicals of the modern world. *Silent Spring,* Rachel Carson's powerful book on the lethal effects of pesticides on wildlife,[19] made people wonder if humans would be the next to be silenced. Rather than be silent, some people became loudly vocal about the fact the chemicals of the modern world were killing them. "Twentieth-century disease" or "total allergy syndrome," the names by which this fashionable illness was first known, was first identified in the early 1950s and then extensively popularized by the media in the early 1980s. Like many fashionable illnesses, the affliction has many fear-inspiring names – over twenty, in fact, includ-

ing chemical AIDS.[20] Large numbers of people report themselves to be
its victims. Its many symptoms include fatigue and irritability. Since the
alleged indiscriminate potential of modern chemicals to cause disease
has spread to moulds as well, its victims often prefer the all-inclusive
name of "environmental hypersensitivity."

Toronto psychiatrists Donna Stewart and Joel Raskin assessed 42
patients who claimed to have this illness. They found that "the patient
feels incapable of living in the modern world, perceiving that he or she
is having allergic and life-threatening reactions to many substances
including clothing, furniture, construction materials, food, water and
even the air." The more severe cases secluded themselves away in a
"natural environment." They avoided visitors, particularly sceptical
doctors, who might have been wearing nylon underwear or have had
their clothes cleaned with a substance other than natural soap. Stewart
and Raskin found all their subjects had well-recognized psychiatric
conditions, including depression, anxiety disorders, and schizophrenia; some also had long histories of ill health.[21] Other investigators
have since confirmed their findings.[22]

It is certainly not for want of looking, but no consistent physical,
laboratory, or immunological abnormalities confirm the presence of
any actual allergy.[23] I do not wish to imply that some modern chemicals do not pose an enormous hazard to health; I would be among the
first to have the use of some chemicals banned, for there are very
legitimate reasons to suspect that they are harming us.[24] Neither do I
want to imply that people do not become allergic to moulds or various chemicals, but then the person demonstrates ample objective evidence of such an allergy. In contrast, the victims of environmental
hypersensitivity attribute their numerous symptoms to chemicals in
the absence of any objective evidence that these chemicals are causing them harm.[25] Pesticides make for a silent spring, but offices can
also become silent if too many of their occupants claim environmental-
hypersensitivity-related disability.

Like all fashionable illnesses, environmental hypersensitivity is con-
tagious. The Halifax Environmental Health Centre, established in the
early 1990s by the Nova Scotia government, specializes in the treatment of environmental hypersensitivity. Advocates from this centre
and UPDATE, the environmental health magazine published by the Nova
Scotia Allergy and Environmental Health Association, soon began
waging what became dubbed "the Halifax holy war" against perfumes
and they persuaded the Halifax municipality to ban all perfumes from
public buildings. Exposed to such high pressure publicity, nearly 800
citizens of this small provincial capital have, in the last two years,
required treatment for this new illness and this despite the fact that

most of the chemicals that are its alleged cause had already been out-lawed from Halifax.[26] (Oddly, despite their refined health concerns, Haligonians continue to dump their untreated sewage into the harbour. It is much cheaper to ban scent than to build sewers.)

Not only does environmental hypersensitivity provide cover for psychological distress and bestow the benefits of illness; it is profitable as well, particularly when victims initiate lawsuits against international chemical corporations. The story of UFFI illustrates just how profitable these illnesses can be.

UFFI, or Urea Formaldehyde Foam Insulation, was introduced into Europe in the 1950s and into North America in the 1970s. Faced with an energy crisis, the American and Canadian governments subsidized its use in home insulation. Then in the late 1970s it was rumoured that UFFI was giving off toxic formaldehyde fumes, and the foam was soon making people ill by the ambulance load.[27] In 1980 Canada banned the use of UFFI and one year later the United States followed suit. Everyone's fears about it were confirmed.[28]

The plight of the unfortunate inhabitants of the 700,000 houses that had been insulated with UFFI was highly publicized. Television screens showed "houses being bulldozed, families forced to move into trailers, and the UFFI contractors wearing gas masks." About 20 per cent of the inhabitants of UFFI-insulated houses reported symptoms – headache, loss of appetite, allergies, fatigue, and aches and pains, many cases culminated in total disability.[29] Lawyers, in clover, launched lawsuits totalling billions of dollars against both national governments.

Subsequent investigations showed, however, that homes insulated with UFFI had only slightly higher levels of formaldehyde than other homes and that these levels were trivial when compared to those encountered by workers in industrial settings and by generations of doctors in the dissecting room.[30] Extensive examination of people exposed to formaldehyde or the other products of UFFI revealed no significant laboratory or physical changes. On the grounds of insufficient evidence of UFFI being a health hazard, the ban was lifted in the United States.[31]

The history of fashionable illnesses associated with fatigue began in 1869, when George Beard, a gifted, hypochondriacal electrotherapist from New York, introduced the concept of neurasthenia – Greek for weak nerves. This once extraordinarily popular fashionable illness had much the same symptoms as twentieth-century disease, and was also attributed to the modern world, although not to its chemicals but to its social changes. Fashionable illnesses keep pace with science, and at that time Edison's electrical machine was still very new. If a circuit in one of these electrical machines was overloaded by too many light bulbs, then all the light bulbs went dim or the whole machine failed. By analogy, the brain supplied "nerve-force" to the body and naturally, if it was overloaded, it too soon failed.[32]

American brains were becoming overloaded by the pace of industrial life: "steam power, the periodical press, the telegraph, the sciences, and the mental activity of women ... the miseries of the rich, the comfortable and the intelligent [had] been unstudied and unrelieved."[33] The educated and upper classes ("brain workers rather than muscle workers") required more nerve force for their brains and hence were the most vulnerable to neurasthenia. Women were particularly vulnerable, especially female brainworkers, since (in the patriarchal worldview of those times) women had less "nerve force" to begin with, making their brains more vulnerable to its depletion.[34]

Beard took enormous care to present neurasthenia as a physical condition and to separate it from any seemingly similar mental conditions. He pointed out that epidemics of mass hysteria, like those in the middle ages that "spread like a fire on a prairie," were psychological in nature. Neurasthenia was physical, the overtaxed brain having become "dephosphorized" and run down like a used-up battery.[35] The battery had just been invented, and high concentrations of phosphorus had been found in the brain, so both were subjects of contemporary scientific interest. Like a discharged battery, the overtaxed brain required complete rest and time for recharge. It could take "months to make up the deficiency" induced by injudicious exercise or excessive use of the brain.[36]

Neurasthenia influenced the medical profession enormously. Fifteen to 30 per cent of patients seen by physicians in the southern states in the early 1900s were diagnosed as neurasthenics.[37] After the publication in 1881 of Beard's book *The American Nervousness: Its Causes and Consequences*, neurasthenia skipped rapidly across the Atlantic, "where it propagated like an epidemic. Neurasthenia was on everybody's lips. It was a most modish illness."[38] Its symptoms were numerous: pains; fatigue; fears of lightning, responsibility, open or closed spaces, or contamination; inability to make decisions; sensitivity to hot or cold, or to changes in the weather; idiosyncratic responses to food, medicines, or external irritants; vertigo and dizziness, and even dental caries.[39]

Neurasthenia soon became so all-embracing that it overstepped itself, and the sceptical began to see its symptoms for what they were. Neurasthenia no longer indicated to the world at large that something was physically wrong with the brain; it indicated that something was wrong with the mind.[40]

The somatizers, who had dropped neurasthenia like a hot brick, transferred their allegiance to more explicitly physical conditions. Psychiatrists are used to picking up the pieces of their shattered patients, but in the case of neurasthenia they picked up a whole disease. They adopted this abandoned illness and used its name to designate a common psychiatric disorder. Neurasthenia remained in the psychiatric lexicon until 1980.[41]

Fatigued somatizers needed a new diagnosis. They attributed the cause of fatigue to viruses. They developed "chronic fatigue syndrome" (CFS) in North America and "myalgic encephalomyelitis" (ME) in the United Kingdom. Both conditions had much the same symptoms as neurasthenia had had – "Old wine in new bottles."[42]

In the United States, the epidemic of chronic fatigue began in 1934. There was a large polio epidemic at the time and when 198 employees of the Los Angeles County General Hospital became ill it was assumed that their illness was an atypical form of polio. Although some hospital staff, who had been exposed to polio patients, complained of headaches, fatigue, and muscle pains (all symptoms of polio) there was something wrong. The staff did not have the characteristic cerebrospinal fluid changes found in polio, they had no real paralysis, and none died. The medical authorities were perplexed as to the cause of this mysterious illness, and the media gave detailed publicity to the hospital outbreak. Then Americans who had not been anywhere near Los Angeles also complained of these symptoms; they have continued to do so ever since.

Chronic fatigue syndrome has gone from strength to strength. Hillary Johnson, a leading American reporter, writes, "It is now [1996] estimated that between 1½ and 2 million Americans are suffering from this extraordinarily debilitating disease, with disastrous consequences to their professional and personal lives." Noting that less than a fifth of CSF sufferers ever fully recover from the illness, Johnson criticizes "the extraordinary failure" of the National Institute of Health and the Centers for Disease Control to protect the public health from this disabling condition.[43]

In Britain, the epidemic of chronic fatigue started fifteen years later than its American counterpart. In the mid-1950s, an apparent viral illness featuring muscle pains and severe fatigue hit 292 members of the staff of the Royal Free Hospital in London. Again the illness was well publicized by the media, and, in a familiar pattern, people all over the country soon came down with it; many are still doing so.

The Royal Free epidemic was first christened "encephalomyelitis" (inflammation of the brain and spinal cord), and then, because, unlike most cases of brain and spinal cord infection, no one died and no pathological changes were found, the illness was renamed "benign myalgic encephalomyelitis" (myalgic = painful muscles). Its victims soon dropped the "benign," claiming that there was nothing benign about it, so the condition is now known simply as "myalgic encephalomyelitis" or ME. Shorter comments, "The disease label alone was a triumph of the longing for organicity over science."[44]

Toward the end of the 1980s, the Centers for Disease Control, having consistently failed to find the mythical virus that was this disease's purported cause, rescinded its cherished viral aetiology. The victims of fashionable diseases have a love-hate relationship with science. Their diseases cloak themselves in the language and concepts of science, but then reject the need for scientific validation. CFS victims were enraged at the humiliating loss of status of their disease, but fortune was on their side. At the end of the 1980s, conventional medicine focused on the acquired immunodeficiency syndrome or AIDS. AIDS left its victims in a chronic state of exhaustion and vulnerability to any infection. In the typical way that fashionable illnesses have of acquiring serious-sounding pathology, CFS quickly incorporated this concept. The chronically fatigued promptly renamed their illness "chronic fatigue immune dysfunction syndrome" (CFIDS), a condition satisfactorily endowed with all the pathological glamour of AIDS, but nicely desexualized and respectable.[45]

Fibromyalgia (a new name for fibrositis) shares many of the features of CFIDS. Its victims have severe muscle aches and pains, unrefreshing sleep, and constant exhaustion. So similar are the symptoms of fibromyalgia and CFIDS (CFS) that their sufferers decided in the late 1980s that they are the victims of the same disease. Then in 1990, at a national conference in Ohio, it was agreed that CFIDS and ME are also one and the same illness.[46] Now CFIDS, ME and fibromyalgia have coalesced into one conglomerate of pain and exhaustion. Following this merger, whiplash victims who suffer from similar symptoms often in one fell swoop lay claim to all these debilitating conditions.

Actually whiplash had already acquired a whole range of symptoms in its own right, so this takeover was more a consolidation of assets than a new acquisition.[47] In 1958, five years after whiplash was born, Braaf and Rosner, the surgeons at the Lebanon Hospital in the Bronx and inveterate itemizers of whiplash symptoms, reviewed their findings from over 1000 whiplash cases. Here is a small sampling of the symptoms they attributed to whiplash in their much quoted article: "Constant fatigue, general irritability, poor concentration and memory, mood changes, feelings of tension, depression, confusion, general anxiety, profuse perspiration, pallor, flushes, labile hypertension or hypotension, faintness, momentary blackouts, tremor, insomnia, frequency of micturition, and development of periodic or permanent intolerance to certain foods and drugs."[48] The food and drugs included chocolate, cake, meat, raw fruits, orange juice, alcohol, and aspirin. This is almost an identical list of substance intolerances to which Beard had previously attributed "the fast pace of modern life."

From the medico-legal point of view, lists of this sort are a goldmine. They provide lawyers with symptoms over which they can litigate and healthcare practitioners with the ability to charge insurance companies for treating practically any symptom of which a patient might choose to complain. Further, Braaf and Rosner warn against "the common tendency to dismiss [these symptoms] as being psychoneurotic or irrelevant to the injury."

In conventional epidemics of flu or other infectious diseases, it is the old, the young, the frail, and the poor who are the most vulnerable. Serious morbidity and death from such infectious diseases occur equally in men and women. Epidemics of neurasthenia, CFS, ME, RSI, hypoglycaemia, environmental hypersensitivity, and whiplash are different. Like a rapist on the prowl, these fashionable illnesses most commonly take women between the ages of 20 and 40, and, unlike the majority of victims of infectious disease epidemics, the victims of psycho-social epidemics are not primarily the poor and underprivileged; in fact, their victims often come from the middle classes.

In Ford's study of alleged hypoglycaemia, for example, 64 per cent of the subjects were middle-class women with an average age of 37.6 years.[49] In Stewart and Raskin's study of environmental hypersensitivity patients, 83 per cent were women, their average age was 38 years, and all were well educated from the middle and upper classes.[50] In the Australian RSI epidemic so many of the victims were women that the illness became a *cause célèbre* for feminist organizations, including WRIST (Women's Repetitive Injury Support Team).[51]

Emil Kraepelin, the pioneer German psychiatrist, observed that neurasthenia was "confined largely to the professional and clerical callings and to women of the middle classes."[52] Less fortunate women were working a fourteen-hour day, some no doubt catering to the upper-class neurasthenics who were taking the prolonged rest cure of doing nothing, while others worked in the detestably polluted conditions of mines and factories, the very thought of which would implode the immune systems of the present-day environmentally hypersensitive. These underprivileged workers seem not to have developed neurasthenia, or if they did, they certainly had no time to be ill with it.[53]

Victims of CFS and ME, like the neurasthenics before them, are mostly young to middle-aged women from the middle and professional classes.[54] The gender differences for whiplash are even greater, a fact that is strikingly odd. Men drive more recklessly, spend much more time on the road, and are killed and seriously injured in collisions in far greater numbers than are women, yet, paradoxically, it is women who develop whiplash – the ratio of whiplash victims being two-thirds women to one-third men.[55] On an actual risk basis, women are about ten times more likely to suffer from whiplash than are men.[56] Not much has been written about the age and class distribution of whiplash, but what little there is suggests that middle-class women between the ages of 20 and 40 are the most frequent victims.[57]

Epidemics of ME, CFS, environmental hypersensitivity, disabling fibromyalgia, and persistent whiplash do not occur in the industrially undeveloped countries. Fashions and affluence go together and fashionable illnesses are no exception. Before the days of the welfare state, only the well-off could afford a fashionable illness. Fashionable illnesses have, in part, remained the prerogative of the well-to-do, although, as sickness benefits and compensation payments have made the luxury of pseudo-illness more accessible, these illnesses have trickled down the social pyramid. Trickle-down economics may be a dubious way to distribute wealth, but it certainly works well with illness.

I have, perhaps unkindly, used the word "victim" to designate the sufferers of fashionable illnesses. I have done so deliberately, because these sufferers are quick to adopt the victim role and they frequently apply this term to themselves. They often see themselves in double jeopardy: being harmed not only by someone or something but also by the world and, in particular, by members of the medical profession, who inflexibly refuse to recognize the validity of their suffering. Sufferers of fashionable illnesses consider themselves victims with neither redress nor acknowledgment.

However, as well-educated members of the middle and professional classes, these victims are often vocal advocates for their own anguish. Despite their fatigue, from Beard onwards, literate victims of fashionable illnesses have displayed inexhaustible energy when it comes to writing, arranging meetings, and proselytizing on behalf of their particular fashionable illness. In what they see as an unresponsive world, they vigorously articulate resentment.

Despite the many physicians who clearly accepted the validity of neurasthenia (and the no small number who even claimed to have it themselves), Beard complained that the medical profession were indifferent to neurasthenia. "Physicians," he wrote, "imitating the unscientific example of the laity, have denied the existence of such symptoms."[58] Many present-day physicians still do accept a physical basis for neurasthenia's various updated versions.[59] But some doctors do not –

and a blot on the landscape and a disgrace to their profession the sufferers of these syndromes consider them to be. Following Beard's precedent, victims aim much of their copious literature – ostensibly scientific and otherwise – at the unbelieving doctors and their callous disregard for such illnesses.

In many developed countries, the fashionable illnesses have their own periodicals. Canada has three for the fatigue illnesses: the *Nightingale*, the *MEssenger* and the *CFIDS Chronicle*. Many of their articles are directed at sceptical physicians and the reluctance of insurance companies and compensation programs to validate the syndromes they represent as legitimate illnesses.

Sometimes patients with CFS and other fashionable illnesses do indeed get short shrift from doctors who dismiss their symptoms as "just a neurotic fuss." Psychiatrists are often more prepared than other medical professionals to accept the reality of psychogenically induced fatigue states, but to a patient with a fashionable illness sympathy from a psychiatrist is worse even than downright rejection by a physician.

Claire Francis, president of the ME Action Campaign and Britain's most famous ME sufferer of our time, puts this contempt for psychiatrists in a nutshell. "Psychiatry," she writes, "is the dustbin of the medical profession."[60] Being sent to a psychiatrist is tantamount to "being blackballed." Few CFS patients want to go anywhere near one.[61] To them, the "good psychiatrist" is the psychiatrist who finds nothing wrong and declares the sufferer psychologically normal.[62]

The relationship between a doctor and a patient with a fashionable illness has all the ingredients of a disaster. In order to provide compensation or support, insurance companies and government social services require medical validation of the illness. As an American commentator pointed out, using the diagnostic criteria of the Centers for Disease Control, 19,000 American adults are currently estimated to have chronic fatigue syndrome. In contrast, 5 million Americans think they have it.[63] The 4,810,000 remaining Americans who *think* they have it but lack the features required to validate the diagnosis are dependent upon the medical profession to rubber-stamp their self-proclaimed diagnosis.

Doctors, like most other people, well know on which side their bread is buttered; they prefer to remain on the good side of their patients and are usually quick to authenticate any required diagnosis. A recent example of just how willing doctors are to do so comes from Winnipeg. As a form of protest, 107 police officers called in sick on the same day. Faced with the threat of losing a day's pay, 91 officers produced a doctor's note certifying that they were sick.[64] The newspaper report mentions nothing about the other 16 officers, perhaps they did not have the gall to ask their physician for a note, or perhaps their physicians turned them down.[65] Sick notes may keep administrators happy, but such notes are usually meaningless.

Some physicians have a thriving practice in applying the rubber stamp, and rubber-stampers can be found among the most venerated of physicians. On my way to work every morning, I pass the Ontario College of Physicians and Surgeons. Even on the coldest days of the fall of 1996, outside the building there was a sizable crowd of placard-waving demonstrators. A physician was up before the discipline committee for serious breaches of professional conduct. He appropriately lost his licence but his grateful patients were rallying to his support.

Some doctors, perhaps out of a sense of scientific integrity, out of bloody-mindedness, or even, as the claimants for fashionable illnesses sometimes maintain, because of payments from insurance companies, refuse to validate these pseudo-illnesses. Doctors are gatekeepers to the very tangible financial, political, social, and emotional advantages that accrue from sickness. As St Peter must well know, a gatekeeper's job does not make for easy relationships. Effective medical gatekeepers receive few accolades from their patients.

Fashionable illnesses become a way of life, often mixed with strong religious overtones. In "The Gifts of CFIDS," an article in the *MEssenger*, an ME victim writes:

I have faith in the Lord and faith that he has a plan for me and maybe CFIDS is part of that plan, so that I may help others and make a difference in someone's life. I have courage. I have courage to face those who don't believe in CFIDS. Courage to face the doctors who doubt us. Courage to make a difference and be heard ... I'm determined to educate and spread awareness on CFIDS. I'm determined to help others in their struggle and ease someone else's load ... I have knowledge. Years of searching gives you knowledge ... Most of us with CFIDS should have honorary medical degrees ... My husband loves me. He fell in love with me, even though I am sick ... He has heard from those who "don't believe in CFIDS" and has defended me against them ... I have happiness. I have a great life ... Yes, I have many special things in my life because of CFIDS ... I have appreciation for all the good in my life. Appreciation for every moment I'm not in pain. Appreciation for the love and support of my family and friends. Appreciation for all the good doctors who care and stick by us, and the researchers who search every day for a cause, treatment and cure ... I like the person CFIDS has made me. How about you? How many blessings has CFIDS given you? Take some time and count them. You just might be surprised.[66]

Entrapment by an invalid lifestyle is common. The longer and more profound a person's disability, the greater the need for unequivocal authentication of the physical nature of the illness. Responsible members of the medical profession have difficulty providing authentication when no evidence of any disability exists.

Patients with fashionable illnesses and the practitioners who treat them have interdependent goals: one for the patient and one for the practitioner. For the patient, treatment must substantiate a physical basis for the supposed illness. In our society, nothing defines the diagnosis more than treatment: "No treatment, no illness!" The treatment of fashionable illnesses is meant to impress but not to cure. The more expensive, the more experimental, the more imperative, and even, perhaps, the more uncomfortable a treatment is, the more satisfactorily it fulfils its task. "Oh, she must have a terrible neck if she has to have this electrical treatment every day!" If at first you don't succeed, try, try, try again, but don't try too hard! For the practitioner, successful treatment must provide an ongoing opportunity to treat. The very last thing that either side wants is for the treatment to work; such an outcome for both parties would defeat its whole purpose.

Axel Munthe, in his engaging book *The Story of San Michele,* gives an example of the usefulness of an illness that won't recover. In the 1880s, as a young neurologist with a fashionable practice in Paris, Munthe reassured his wealthy clients that "their symptoms were due to organicity and not just nerves." Munthe reported: "What they all liked was appendicitis ... Appendicitis was just then much in demand among the better-class people on the lookout for a complaint. All the nervous ladies had it on the brain if not in the abdomen, thrived on it beautifully and so did their medical advisors."[67] Then James Simpson discovered chloroform and Joseph Lister the aseptic surgical technique; the recalcitrant appendix could be safely removed. People soon lose sympathy for anyone suffering from a condition which, if desired, could be cured. A new disease was required for the fashionable world. Munthe provided it – COLITIS.[68]

Despite the fortunes spent on fashionable illnesses, they seldom remit.[69] Perhaps the best indication that treatments for them do not work comes from the victims themselves, whose constant and recurrent complaint remains: "No treatment works!" This therapeutic failure does not discourage victims from demanding more treatment or governments and insurance companies from providing funds for its continuance.[70]

Fashionable illnesses can be effective problem-solvers.[71] Some of my whiplash litigants made effective use of these illnesses. Mrs B's case serves as an example.

Mrs B was aged forty when I examined her in 1994 on account of a claim for permanent disability following an alleged whiplash injury sustained four years

previously. She is a married woman with two sons. She and her family reported that before the accident she had led an idyllic life on a small holding in
rural Ontario. Seldom did she have occasion to leave her ideal homestead but,
on a rare outing when her husband was driving her to the hairdresser, the
family car was involved in a rear-end collision. No damage was done to either
vehicle. Neither the police nor an ambulance was called to the scene of the
accident.

Following this accident, Mrs B and her family claimed that the accident had
destroyed her life. She had developed constant headaches and her memory
was gone; she had such fearful neck pains that sleep was impossible. Her
fatigue was so great that she was forced to spend much of the day in bed, and
her husband, who had been employed with a real estate company, was forced
to quit his job to take care of her.

With difficulty, the defence lawyer obtained Mrs B's medical records. These
records were extensive, and with their help it was possible to reconstruct Mrs
B's past personal and medical history. She was an only child. Her father had
been an alcoholic and her parents separated when she was three years old.
Her father paid no child support and her anxious mother struggled to earn
sufficient money for their needs. Miriam performed well at school, but there
was no money for her to go to university. On leaving school at 18, she took a
job as a clerk with the provincial government. At 20, she married [Mr B], a
junior executive ten years her senior. Their first son was born six months after
the wedding, and the couple bought a small house in Toronto. Mr B had a
drinking problem that made the marriage turbulent from its beginning.

It was reported in the records that Mrs B disliked her job. She always worried about her health and for many years she had felt the need to control her
carbohydrate intake to prevent hypoglycaemic attacks. She often had hypoglycaemic symptoms on her way to work and, on having an attack, she would
return home. She was absent from work several days each month. She left her
job when her first son was born.

In 1982, on hearing about the effects of UFFI, she suddenly realized that the
insulation in their house was making her ill. The family became more solicitous of her and her husband initiated legal proceedings against the federal
government. The family was forced to move to an apartment. While in the
apartment, the family doctor's notes showed, there were constant family problems on account of Mr B's binge drinking and her eldest son's drug use. The
younger son was in trouble for petty vandalism at school.

In 1988 the part of the apartment building in which the B family lived was
renovated, which created dust and paint fumes. These pollutants extended
Mrs B's allergy from UFFI to other chemicals as well. She developed environmental hypersensitivity. Again, the family became increasingly solicitous of
her. She received neutralizing solutions and other treatments from a clinical
ecologist but all without benefit. The family decided to leave the unhealthy

city. With the help of a financial settlement from the apartment owners for having been the cause of Mrs B's difficulties, the family moved to their present house in the country. In the country all had gone well with the family apart from Mr B's excessive drinking bouts with his colleagues at work.

After the rear-end collision, Mrs B's symptoms showed no signs of improvement and her husband was forced to remain permanently at home to provide the care that his wife needed.

Mrs B's case has a number of features common to the lives of patients with fashionable illnesses. Several aspects of her life were unhappy: she came from a broken home, she had had marital and family problems, had never liked her job, had panic attacks, and was agoraphobic. She moved from one fashionable illness to another – hypoglycaemia, allergy to UFFI, environmental hypersensitivity, and chronic whiplash – in order to explain or perhaps justify her psychological distress. Her symptoms kept her family in line and helped out financially.

Fashionable illnesses run remarkably true to form. Epidemiologists use Australian RSI as the benchmark of psycho-social epidemics. How does the Western world's whiplash epidemic compare to that model? The two epidemics have much in common, except that the Australian RSI epidemic was relatively brief, while the worldwide whiplash epidemic has dragged on for nearly half a century.

After the Australian epidemic, several authors identified the factors that had fostered it and the measures that brought it to an end.[72] RSI was compensable. Physicians were seeking a physical cause for it, and their patients' complaints were accepted uncritically at face value. Patients gravitated to lawyers and physicians who were sympathetic to the notion that RSI was a physically induced condition. Physicians, reluctant to see any dishonesty in the complaints, provided their patients with numerous physical treatments and encouraged them to define themselves as ill.

David Bell, a psychiatrist from New South Wales, Australia, describes the contribution of the medical profession to RSI: "Perhaps the most devastating iatrogenic contribution of all was the many and varied attempts to treat RSI as a physical illness, which aided the community to accept the condition as an "injury." Splints and slings [substitute collars for whiplash] became the hallmark of RSI. Surgery was undertaken until the poor results persuaded even the proponents of RSI that it was inadvisable. The newfound experts developed therapeutic empires with a vigorous entrepreneurial spirit that was undeterred by the ineffectiveness of their treatment methods."[73]

In another account, Paul Reilly, a British rheumatologist, provides a succinct description of the early days of the epidemic: "The media, unions, medical, paramedical, legal, governmental and self-help groups went into overdrive. The incidence increased in proportion, as if interest in the condition was actually contributing to its prevalence."[74]

In the mid-1980s, when the penny dropped that social factors rather than physical injury were the cause of RSI, the epidemic was quickly terminated. The media, which had at first promoted the epidemic, found news value in demonstrating its spuriousness. Popular current affairs programs featured factory workers discussing the ways in which they had exploited RSI, and TV programs showed American video-screen operators at work at their terminals with no distress or concern about wrists. The Australian government reduced compensation for the condition, and courts found the association between RSI and the complaints of pain to be unproven.[75]

Despite the previous intense litigation, compensation, and publicity, most RSI sufferers are now back at work, many at their previous job doing the same activity and using the same equipment as before. Ex-sufferers now seldom talk of RSI or consult their doctors about it unless they still have unfinished medico-legal business. Not all their symptoms have disappeared, but complaints about them have diminished significantly and most persons have returned to a normal or near normal lifestyle.[76]

In responding to my gentle inquiries about RSI, Australian colleagues look sheepish. They are much relieved that their secretaries no longer require one hour of rest interspersed with each hour of typing. Even their secretaries seem pleased to have dispensed with the prophylactic regime. People can get on with their work, reports now go out on time, and all that remains of RSI in Australia is an embarrassing *frisson* in the memory.

Doctors and other healthcare practitioners, although unable to cure fashionable illnesses, can be extremely effective in creating them. Australia's catastrophic epidemic is over, but elsewhere in the industrial world healthcare practitioners, along with personal injury litigation lawyers, the media and office furniture manufacturers are still quietly aiding the spread of RSI.

In Canada a lengthy article on RSI headlined "Keyboard Injury 'Can Ruin Lives' Specialist Warns" appeared in a national newspaper, the *Globe and Mail*. The reporter discussed the physical nature of RSI and the need for frequent breaks to prevent its occurrence. He reported that in 1993 cases were increasing and that lost time, compensation claims, and medical treatment might cost billions of dollars. The reporter then goes on to write about his own situation: "After I began work on this story, I realized that I too – a *Globe and Mail* reporter for

14 years – was developing symptoms. My arms and hands eventually went numb, forcing me to seek medical help. In fact, I was not able to type these words. An editor acted as my hands, making it possible over the period of several days to organize the material and write the story. It is not clear how many other Canadians are in the same boat. More than three million use computers regularly, but no one collects statistics on RSI."[77] We are all suggestible. This *Globe and Mail* reporter seems to have had the medical student syndrome: he caught the symptoms of the disease he was studying. I wonder how many of his readers caught it also?

An RSI epidemic simmered in Britain for several years with an ongoing battle between the believers and the sceptics. The *Times*, under the headline "Screens of Protest over Rules," reported in 1992 that Britain would introduce rules to fulfil her obligations to the European Community's directive to protect employees from RSI.[78] The next year, the *Guardian*, under the headline "RSI ruling may only delay claims avalanche," reported that in a test case it was ruled that "RSI is meaningless and has no place in the medical books."[79] Nevertheless, on a visit to England in 1994, I found two architect friends at work designing ergonomically correct desks and chairs to decrease the risk of RSI.

A British rheumatologist confirms the dramatic increase in the incidence of RSI in Britain: "The overall pattern is proving very similar to that of Australia in the 1970s and 1980s. A failure to understand the complex and multifactorial basis of chronic pain syndromes on the part of medical and paramedical practitioners is helping to promote and perpetuate the epidemic. So are the adversarial legal system, sensationalism in the media, and faulty beliefs in those experiencing upper limb discomfort. We have not learned [yet] from the Australian experience, and the epidemic is still on the increase."[80]

Public-sector organizations such as the Inland Revenue Service, the BBC, and the Post Office are the hardest hit. The majority of the stricken employees are women, but males in newspaper and other media offices now claim to have it as well. As in Australia, the self-employed, although they may be glued to a computer, rarely suffer from it.[81] The United States caught it as well. *Time* magazine in "Crippled by Computers" reports on the case of Grant McCool, a veteran journalist. A few months after being transferred to New York City as an editor, he came down with it.

That's when the trouble started. After typing on his computer keyboard for hours a day over several months, McCool developed excruciating pain in his hands; some mornings he would awake with his arms throbbing and burning.

"The doctor told me to stop typing immediately," recalls McCool, 32. He hasn't written or edited a story on deadline since. Nor has he been able to clean house, carry heavy objects, or play squash. He cannot even drive a car, as controlling the steering wheel with his injured hands is impossible.

McCool suffers from a severe case of cumulative trauma disorder, a condition that results from the overuse of the muscles and tendons of the fingers, hands, arms, and shoulders. More commonly known as repetitive stress injury (RSI), this condition brings pain, numbness, weakness, and sometimes long-term disability, and it now strikes an estimated 185,000 U.S. office and factory workers a year. The cases account for more than half of America's occupational illnesses, compared with about 20 per cent a decade ago.

McCool joins hundreds of telephone reservationists, cashiers, word processors, and journalists who are suing computer manufacturers for having caused their disability. Some journalists have claims of $1 million or more. *Time* estimates that the annual cost of RSI in the United States is already about $7 billion. *Time* accompanied its article with illustrations of the best typing posture to prevent RSI and wrist splints to help treat it.[82]

In 1996 a federal jury in New York ruled against Digital in a product liability suit and awarded three middle-aged women $5.8 million compensatory damages for musculoskeletal injuries arising from the use of Digital's keyboards. Digital reports that it knows of thousands of similar suits against IBM, Apple, AT&T, and other computer manufacturers.[83] Repeated movements, especially when combined with long hours, tedium, and poor ergonomic design, can undoubtedly cause discomfort. These ordinary everyday pains, when authenticated by possible physical diagnoses, glamorized by media hype, and fostered by litigation and financial incentives, soon become disabling. It is easy to make people sick in droves. It seems likely that anyone who has sufficient knowledge of RSI to promote it is also likely to know how the Australian epidemic came to an end, but no squeak of such constructive information seems to have reached the popular press outside Australia.

The whiplash epidemic crept so slowly upon us that it convinced the world of whiplash's authenticity. Even epidemiologists interested in fashionable illnesses were slow to acknowledge it as one of their own. Given the right circumstances, however, whiplash can take hold in a country as fast as any other fashionable illness. It did so in Norway.

Until the early 1980s few Norwegians had heard of whiplash, and few older neurologists could recall having seen a case before 1980. Then, in the second half of the 1980s, complaints of whiplash injury came thick and fast. In 1993 about 13,000 Norwegians gave notice of real or alleged chronic disability from whiplash, and about 8,500 received financial compensation. By 1994 the cost of whiplash insurance claims per inhabitant was three times higher than in Sweden, Norway's immediate neighbour.[84] Norway, with a population of 4.5 million, now has an organization of 70,000 whiplash patients who claim to be disabled by it.[85] By 1996 Norway led the world with its rate of whiplash disability.[86]

Special circumstances helped to accomplish this record. Schrader (the Viking rocking the whiplash boat) identifies these circumstances. Norway has a stable and prosperous economy that can sustain generous disability payments. Even without whiplash, Norway's disability rate is extraordinarily high. About 10 per cent of its working-age population receive a disability pension, mostly on the basis of such subjective complaints as pain, depression, or anxiety. Norwegian physicians have a long tradition of taking their patients' complaints at face value, and their patients, believing it is the doctor's duty to be supportive of their interests, have a custom of being particularly unpleasant to doctors who fail to do so. Lodging whiplash disability claims is in keeping with customary Norwegian illness behaviour.[87]

Norway has lots of trees, and newspaper is cheap. It easily holds the world record in newspaper readers, with about seven times more independent newspapers per million inhabitants than most industrial countries. News is needed, but in a peaceful country with few inhabitants, a robust economy, and little crime there is little to write about. Critical reports of the health system in general, and of arrogant, ignorant, and careless physicians in particular, are a staple of the Norwegian press. The Norwegian media already had an especially soft spot for fibromyalgia and CFIDS.[88] Fifteen per cent of employed Norwegians work in the health sector, about three times more than most developed countries.[89] With such heavy investment in ill-health perhaps it is not surprising that whiplash, once arrived in Norway, quickly found a snug home in which to flourish.[90]

Whiplash literally did find a snug home. Whiplash gets into funny places: one American doctor found it in the ankle joints.[91] Then a prominent Norwegian whiplash physician, a hero of the whiplash patient organization, discovered it even in the female genitalia. After all, the uterus also has a neck; it too gets whiplash. In a newspaper interview, this doctor expresses pride in his gynaecological investigations and, on the strength of his new groundbreaking findings, he compares himself to Galileo Galilei.[92] *Per ardua ad astra!*

Patient victim organizations do not like "heartless, unsympathetic, and obdurate" physicians who question the legitimacy of their particular disorder. They are always after the heads or, more catastrophically, the professional licenses of the medical sceptics. The Norwegian whiplash patient organization tried to sue Schrader for his Lithuanian study, but since no grounds could be found on which to do so, the suit was dropped.[93]

Soldiers are the latest group of people to become regular victims of copycat illnesses. "We have kicked the Vietnam syndrome," exulted President Bush in 1991, but while he uttered these jubilant words, the symptoms of the even more pesky Gulf war syndrome (GWS) was quietly incubating.[94] Nearly 80,000 out of the 700,000 American and 45,000 British soldiers who served in the Gulf claimed compensation for the symptoms of debilitating chronic fatigue, along with memory loss, muscle aches, and other symptoms attributed to chemicals or disease to which they were exposed in the Gulf war.[95] The development of such a syndrome was probably inevitable. From the American Civil War onwards soldiers, after their involvement in wars or peace missions, have complained of unexplained symptoms, but the rates at which soldiers fall victim to post-war syndromes has increased.[96] Armies are always rife with stories of catastrophes and the Internet now spreads rumours even faster. The anxious swap symptoms.

The Gulf war veterans were exposed to months of uncertainty and inaction cooped up in desert heat awaiting an attack with chemical and bacteriological weapons – the sort of experience that would undermine the morale of the most seasoned troops. The troops were anxious, but soldiers cannot get scared; they develop symptoms instead. When symptoms are compensable they persist.

Any cancers or birth defects in the veterans or their families were attributed to chemical exposure, but the incidence of these occurrences is no greater than in the control groups of troops who were not involved in the war.[97] Two veterans thought they were shrinking.[98] Some veterans' wives now complain that their husbands are so contaminated with chemicals that their semen burns when it comes in contact with their skin or vagina. Some wives and other family members have even contracted GWS from their husbands.[99] One English nurse, who developed fatigue six months after her husband returned from the Gulf, argues that the condition cannot be psychological since too many people are suffering from the same symptoms.[100] In fact, true physical illness demonstrates the normal biological variation, whereas the symptoms of a fashionable illness tend to run much truer to form.

As with other fashionable illnesses, some doctors were – and still are – determined to find an organic cause for the soldiers' complaints. Jonathon Bernstein, a Cincinnati allergist, contacted nearly 100 veterans with burning semen syndrome (BSS). He states that although it is a formidable task to link BSS to specific Gulf war exposure, he is optimistic that it can be done.[101] Preordained by such John the Baptists, many Messiahs are claimed as the true cause of GWS.[102] Despite a plethora of studies and investigations, little convincing evidence has been found to validate any of the claims.[103]

For governments held responsible for compensating post-war syndromes it is a no-win situation. If they early on deny that a claimant has suffered harm, they do so in the absence of evidence, but by ordering of tests and careful investigations they admit the possibility of harm and allow the power of suggestion to work its alchemy. Inevitably, all the negative results will be attributed to a cover-up by the powerful at the expense of the victim. The veterans unite in righteous anger against the heartless authorities who deny financial responsibility. One English veteran refers to the Ministry of Defence as "pig-ignorant and uncaring";[104] the American veterans are equally contemptuous and angry towards the army and government authorities.[105]

As the years slip by and no physical cause is found to legitimate the symptoms of GWS, the suffering veterans are locked into a debilitating battle more precarious to their health than the Gulf war itself – wounds of resentment from which they may well not recover. America now has invaded Afghanistan. It is interesting to speculate what form the Afghanistan war syndrome will take.

Sometimes other people's oddities give a clue to one's own. In chapter 3, I noted that the symptoms of chronic whiplash are virtually unknown in Singapore.[106] These symptoms are not absent because the people of Singapore do not develop somatoform illness; they just have a different set of symptoms in their symptom pool.[107] Our own pool is made murky by pain and fatigue, but the Chinese have a dragon of a symptom in their pool.

Koro is a conviction that the penis is disappearing into the abdominal cavity, an unfortunate occurrence generally considered fatal. Not surprisingly, *koro* is accompanied by much panic. Working as a junior doctor in a London hospital, I remember that the arrival by ambulance of a Chinese man with his penis tightly wired in place by two chopsticks caused quite a stir.

An epidemic of *koro* occurred amongst the Chinese in Singapore in October 1967.[108] It followed a newspaper report alleging that eating pork from pigs inoculated with anti-swine fever vaccine caused *koro*. Pork sales plunged and the number of *koro* cases seen at the Singapore General Hospital swooped up. Some doctors stressed publicly that *koro* should be treated with injections, acupuncture, and other measures. The Ministry of Primary Production, alarmed by the acute drop in pork consumption, issued a statement that their vaccine was harmless to men, a response that only succeeded in confirming their worst fears. The *koro* cases mounted, and within a week, 97 such cases were seen in one day alone at the Singapore General Hospital.

An expert medical panel explained in a public announcement that *koro* was the result of fear and not a physical disease, and that none of the victims seen until then had come to any harm. The number of cases dropped off. After a month there were none. The authors, in concluding their report, commented: "How easily public fears can be caused by injudicious propaganda and statements, and how easily too they can be assuaged ... Newspapers, television, and radio are powerful tools in these circumstances."

Why did this Singapore epidemic fizzle out after a month when our whiplash epidemic has lasted so long? The fact that *koro* is of necessity a male disorder, and that fewer men are victims of fashionable illnesses, is easily counterbalanced by the greater propensity of men to worry about their penises than women about their necks. The *koro* epidemic ended quickly because there was nothing in it for the professions. Given more time, Singapore lawyers might have initiated litigation against the pig farmers and the vaccine manufacturers, which would have helped to keep the epidemic going, but for healthcare practitioners a disease like *koro* is just an inconvenience; in fact, it is a downright nuisance. It presents as an emergency – as likely as not in the middle of the night or at meal times – and its treatment cannot be scheduled into regularly ongoing and lucrative appointments. The authorities and the medical profession quickly united and competently ended the epidemic. Singaporean penises stayed where they should!

RSI and whiplash, unlike *koro*, are ideal fashionable illnesses for both patients and professional healthcare practitioners. In Australia, however, patients and healthcare practitioners so enthusiastically fostered RSI that its epidemic grew large enough to play havoc with the Australian economy. As soon as its cause was understood, the Australian government stepped in to terminate it. In contrast, whiplash has been with us for so long that we have learned to live with it. Many doctors and lawyers make their living by it, and the public appears to enjoy this high stakes lottery. Even insurance companies make money out of it. There is no pressing reason for governments to be greatly concerned, and lots of their citizens have a keen interest in perpetuating it. The costly and quixotic search for a physical explanation of whiplash symptoms seems destined to continue unabated.

PART TWO

The Quest for the Mythical Whiplash Injury

6

The Enigmas of the Human Spine

The whiplash industry seems to be doing more, but helping less.
– Michael Livingston[1]

Back pain is an illness in search of a disease.
– Williams and Hadler[2]

Low back pain is to Worker's Compensation
as neck pain is to the auto insurance industry.
– W.O. Spitzer[3]

Injury to the spine is held responsible for a great deal of trouble. Whiplash is blamed for disabling pain at the top end of the spine and industrial injury for disabling pain at its lower end. The two conditions have so much in common that I will examine them together.

First, I cannot emphasize strongly enough that both low back pain and neck pain are extraordinarily common. Up to 60 per cent of adults experience at least one episode of back pain each year.[4] In Ontario, my own neck of the woods, at any given time, one out of ten people report serious back pain.[5] Healthcare practitioners are very involved in the management of low back pain. It is the most common reason for visiting an orthopaedic surgeon, a neurosurgeon, an osteopath, or a chiropractor, and the second most common reason for seeking care from a family physician.[6] Neck pain occurs so frequently that, statistically at least, a person in the community at large is no less likely to have neck pain than someone involved in a collision four weeks previously.[7] When someone has been in a collision or has "injured" his back at work, pain is attributed to a spinal injury. Whether such "injuries" are in the neck or the low back, they have similar recovery rates.[8] In every industrial setting studied so far, between 5 and 10 per cent of low back pain cases progress to become more or less permanent. The figures for whiplash neck pain are the same.[9]

Although failure to recover from whiplash or an occupational low back injury is usually attributed to some structural damage of the spine, the evidence that such injuries actually exist is slight or often non-existent. In keeping with medical concepts of the structural causes of back pain, pre-employment x-rays began to be used in the 1920s to identify anatomical abnormalities that might make the back of a new employee susceptible to injury. But pre-existing abnormalities were found to correlate poorly with subsequent complaints of back pain.[10]

Complaints of pain in the aging spine are exceptional. Most musculoskeletal problems worsen with age, and advancing years certainly weaken the back's capacity to withstand strenuous activity. Yet younger employees report back problems at the workplace more often than do their older co-workers.[11] Manual labour is usually considered to predispose to back problems, but workers in light occupations experience back pain at almost the same rate as workers in heavy occupations.[12] Of course, once someone has developed low back pain, heavy work becomes a different matter. It may be possible to sit and collect parking lot payments all day with low back pain, but quite impossible to dig for burst water mains.

Keeping physically fit is often considered a panacea against backache, but even this is uncertain. Studies have shown that firefighters and Swedish nurses who kept physically fit had fewer complaints of back injury, but other studies have found little or no association between fitness and backache.[13]

While it is unlikely that the extent of back pain or its underlying pathology has changed much in the last forty years, our response to it has changed enormously. Where back pain was previously accepted as a fact of life, it is now perceived as a work-related injury.[14] In the United Kingdom, days lost through low back disability increased more than tenfold in the period from 1955 to 1999 (see fig. 6–1).[15]

Much the same pattern can be seen in the rest of the developed world. Sweden, despite having the world's most comprehensive and available health service, led the world in its escalating back disability rates. In 1970 one per cent of the working Swedish population was off work with back pain for an average of 20 days; by 1987, 8 per cent were off work for an average of 34 days. During this period there was a 6000 per cent increase in the number of Swedes receiving permanent disability pensions for low back pain. Back pain was costing more than 5 per cent of the Swedish gross national product and for a while it seemed that back pain was going to bankrupt Sweden's social and medical services. Then the Swedish government reduced compensation payments for back pain and Swedish backs improved.[16]

Although previous statistics for disability due to whiplash neck pain are unavailable, it is clear that disability attributable to neck pain, like

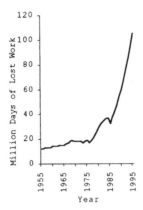

Fig. 6–1   Backache takes off!
Starting in the late 1950s, an epidemic of disabling back pain hit the developed world.
The graph shows workdays (in millions) lost in the United Kingdom each year because
of back pain.

low back pain, has increased dramatically. Disability from both now
stands at epidemic proportions.[17]

The same practitioners, physicians or otherwise, treat both whiplash
neck pain and occupational low back pain. They usually attribute the
pain to an underlying injury, the common diagnosis being a non-specific strain or sprain. Despite years of intensive search, however, no
convincing physical cause has been found to explain the ongoing pain
of whiplash or occupational low back pain in about 97 per cent of
cases.[18] Costly investigations and treatments continue, but so does the
pain. Low back pain plagues the work force of the industrialized
world, and neck pain plagues the auto insurance industry.[19]

Chiropractors are orthodox medicine's main competitors for the care
of the spine. In 1996 there were 23,000 licensed chiropractic practitioners in the United States compared to 17,250 board-certified orthopaedic surgeons.[20] Chiropractors, medical practitioners, and osteopaths
vie with each other in seeking out hypothetical spinal injuries to treat.
By their intensive search for alleged structural abnormalities of the
spine, these various practitioners have managed to convince themselves
and practically everyone else that neck and back pain is due to a physical injury. Of course, a litigant with whiplash pain or a worker with low
back pain does not need much convincing that he has a physical injury
in undisputed need of both treatment and compensation.

Exactly what injuries are all these healthcare practitioners looking
for, and how do they go about finding them? I will start off with the

claims of the "way out" alternative caregivers and work through to those of orthodox physicians. I am critical of these alternative practitioners, but do not jump to the conclusion that I am medically biased against them: I am equally critical of the medical practitioners who hunt endlessly for spinal injuries.

Alternative healthcare practitioners tend to see health problems in terms of wide general principles and universal forces, and their perception of whiplash is no exception. Theresa Cisler, a chiropractor from Tucson, Arizona, advises: "The physician must first assume that whiplash is not an injury isolated to one region of the body. Therefore isolating certain tissues or regions of the body may be too confining an approach."[21] In a similar vein, J.H. Harakal, an osteopath from Dallas, Texas, writes: "There is a palpable unidirectional force present in or about the person who has sustained inertial injuries."[22] Monique Harriton, the author of *The Whiplash Handbook,* herself a victim of four rear-end collisions, comments: "Hands-on health providers do not share the distrust of whiplash patients which is present among some medical doctors. Cranial osteopaths, for example, can detect the perturbation caused by the car accident through palpation of the skull."[23] While such "perturbation" of the skull and "palpable unidirectional forces" provide dubious evidence for structural damage in whiplash injury, they cause utter confusion in the minds of judge and jury alike.

Chiropractors usually explain spinal injury in terms of subluxation, but like unidirectional forces and perturbations, these subluxations seem more metaphysical than structural. When used by orthodox physicians, "subluxation" is a term indicating an incomplete dislocation of a joint. The joint capsule, when damaged by either disease or injury, permits the displacement of the joint surfaces. Chiropractors use the term differently. Subluxation is central to chiropractic. Daniel Palmer, the late-nineteenth-century founder of chiropractic, taught that subluxation of the vertebral joints interferes with the body's expression of the "nerve force," and that such interference is the cause of disease. Diseases were prevalent in the nineteenth century, and so, therefore, were subluxed joints. Palmer advocated their realignment.[24]

Each disease required attention to different combinations of vertebral subluxations. Malaria, for instance, required adjustment to the fourth dorsal vertebra, while diphtheria required realignment of the third, fifth, and seventh cervical vertebrae. Although Palmer's approach to disease was relatively simple, chiropractors managed to outdo even conventional medicine's scientific-sounding terminology. To help in the diagnosis of subluxations, B.J. Palmer, Daniel's son, invented the electroencephaloneuromentimpograph, a machine that occupied the whole of a large room.[25] (The machine has now fallen into desuetude.)

From a scientific point of view Palmer's ideas are incomprehensible; but from the perspective of the good health of the patient, they were useful. Medical treatments, though usually presented as scientific, are often far from sensible. In Victorian times, not only were many medical treatments useless, they were often toxic or highly addictive as well. Chiropractors' manipulations, although not free from harm, were a blessed alternative to conventional care. Over the years since Palmer first elaborated his theories of disease, chiropractors have become proficient manipulators of joints, often giving relief from stiff necks and uncomfortable backs. However, present-day chiropractors have inherited their founder's preoccupation with subluxation – and a controversial legacy it has proven to be. "Subluxation" must be a confusing term even to chiropractors, for they provide totally conflicting definitions for it.[26] Some see it as a hallowed word that defines their profession, while to others it is an impediment to sensible care.[27]

Some chiropractors claim to detect subluxation with their fingers, though the evidence is that they probably can't.[28] Chiropractors seem just as prepared as their conventional colleagues are to expose their patients to unnecessary radiation. They reinforce the intuition of their fingers with numerous x-rays of the spine, but as David Drum, a distinguished Canadian chiropractor, reports, "Most subluxations visible on x-ray are not 'chiropractic' (this is reducible with adjustment)."[29] Perhaps it is churlish for a physician to comment on the financial dealings of a rival profession, but as the Medicare allowance for the manipulative treatment of any particular intervertebral joint becomes exhausted, subluxations unaccountably move up and down the spine.[30]

Chiropractic fails to provide confirming evidence of actual structural damage, but the concept of subluxation certainly helps convince patients that the collision pushed their neck vertebrae out of alignment and that their necks, like the front wheels of a car after collision, stand in urgent need of realignment.

When it comes to the investigation and management of neck and low back pain, conventional medicine is seldom any more reliable than chiropractic. In fact, because the results of invasive treatments are potentially very harmful, the final outcome of care may sometimes be worse.[31] Despite the wonders of scientific medicine, neck and low back pain leave modern medicine singularly defeated. The three popular medical explanations for back and neck pain attributable to trauma are sprain, ruptured intervertebral disc, and injury to the facet (zygapophyseal) joints. These three pathologies are variously championed as the hidden culprits of chronic whiplash and low back pain. None of them are convincing.

Why should neck and back sprains fail to recover when sprains in other parts of the body usually heal without trouble? For instance, there is nothing special about neck ligaments and muscles that can account for their failure to so. During surgery on the cervical spinal cord, neurosurgeons inflict severe trauma on neck muscles, fascia, ligaments, periosteum, bone, and joints, and yet within a few weeks the tissues have healed and the patient's neck is mobile and pain free.[32]

What about the notorious discs that seem so given to slipping and rupturing? An intervertebral disc is a fibrous cushion separating two vertebral bodies. Each vertebral body has a top and bottom end plate to which the adjacent disc is attached. The periphery of the disc forms a tough fibrous ring (the annulus), while the inside of the disc is filled with a gelatinous material. Discs do not actually slip but they may become separated from the vertebral body endplate or, like old tires, may bulge or rupture.

Sprains, ruptured discs, and injured facet joints (which I will discuss later) loom large in physicians' minds but, unless there are objective indications that something actually is amiss, the chances of finding a patho-anatomical explanation for the pain that stands up to scientific scrutiny is small. For the back, the usual quoted figure is 3 per cent.[33] One leading Swedish back expert puts this figure as low as 0.1 per cent; that is, there is a one in a thousand chance of finding a scientifically acceptable explanation for occupational low back pain.[34] Since little serious scientific work has been done on whiplash pain, it is not possible to provide similar estimates for the neck, but in the case of common whiplash, there is no reason to suppose the success rate would be any higher.

These are humbling success rates. As a way of managing such discomforting uncertainty, Galen, the great second-century Greek physician, suggested to his colleagues that they intersperse their prescriptions of various herbs and obscure animal parts with Egyptian hieroglyphics. With any luck, the suitably impressed patient failed to notice that his physician did not actually know what was wrong with him. Our legacy from this psychological ploy is the "R/" in front of prescriptions; the body of the R represents the eye of Horus, the Egyptian God of Healing, and the little slash beneath it symbolizes the tear he shed for Osiris, his cruelly murdered father.

Modern day practitioners, faced with a similar predicament of knowing little more about the causes of back pain than do their suffering patients, adopted a similarly obfuscating technique. They have given non-specific low back pain a host of imposing names: lumbar sprain, lumbar strain, lumbago, sciatica, discal hernia, discopathy, facet syndrome, lumbar myositis, ligamentitis, minor intervertebral displacement, dysfunction of the intervertebral joint, fibromyositis, fibrositis, fasciitis, myofasciitis, articular hypomobility and hypermobility, discarthrosis, metameric cellulotenoperiostomyalgic syndrome, posterior branch syndrome, rhizopathy.[35] The length of the list reflects the brevity of what is known about the causes of low back pain.

When examining your back, a physician looks for limitation of movement, muscle spasm, tenderness, or other such accepted signs of injury, but their elicitation often has little actual significance. Signs such as immobility, stiffness, and tenderness vary greatly from one "normal" person to another; also the elicitation of these signs is unreliable. In a telling study, experienced orthopaedic surgeons examining the same group of patients failed to agree on the presence and absence of the eight physical signs commonly used to make back diagnoses. Even when the physical examination was spiced up with gadgets that measure strength and motion, their findings still remained unreliable.[36]

Besides having difficulty with physical signs, orthopaedic surgeons make poor lie detectors. If physicians befuddle their patients with meaningless diagnoses, patients equally befuddle their doctors. In the absence of any clear-cut physical findings, a doctor must rely on what a patient reports.[37] Patients, being human and sometimes having good reasons to lie, may well do so, and physicians find it difficult to detect the simulators.[38] When a patient wishes to exploit neck or back pain, a doctor can usually do little more than rubber-stamp a patient's complaints. For would be simulators, back doctors are putty in their hands![39]

The clinical diagnosis of whiplash is just as unsatisfactory as the diagnosis of ordinary low back pain. Again, sprain is the hidden pathology most frequently diagnosed, but this diagnosis is seldom made on the basis of any clear-cut physical signs. In fact, the purpose of the diagnosis is usually to keep emergency room doctors out of trouble. It is a convenient diagnosis they use to pigeonhole neck pain complaints in collision victims, who show few or no signs of any actual injury. Wily emergency room physicians – and they have to be this way to survive in their jobs – cannot risk sticking out their necks with a diagnosis of "No injury."

A patient who has taken the trouble to go to a crowded emergency room would be irritated by such a diagnosis. If an injury (real, imaginary, or coincidental) is subsequently found, the errant ER doctor will be in for a bad time. A diagnosis of sprain lets the doctor off the hook. If the patient is eventually found to have some other pathology, a diagnosis of sprain is a forgivable mistake. Once again, the ER doctor will have escaped a malpractice suit.

The problem with this ER ploy is that any determined whiplash litigant can finesse this injury diagnosis into long-term disability. The ER doctor diagnosed a *bona fide* whiplash sprain. Everyone knows that whiplash sprains may fail to recover; the courts confirm such unfavourable outcomes every day, so why should this patient's sprain be any different?

Doctors have many investigational techniques to aid in the diagnosis of back and neck pain, but while these techniques are excellent for serious spinal diseases (cancers, infections, and severe trauma for example), they are mostly useless, and indeed often misleading, for the diagnosis of whiplash neck pain and occupational low back pain. Some are more useless than others, and I will start with the most useless.

Brightly coloured thermographs of the neck and back feature in many whiplash medico-legal briefs. Accompanying these artistic creations is a report stating something to the effect that "the results are consistent with a cervical/lumbar myofascial irritation." Such reports impress the court but they do not confirm the presence of any underlying injury. Thermographs, maps of skin temperatures, were introduced into medicine in the mid-1950s to help diagnose breast cancer, but they did not work. On the optimistic assumption that asymmetrical thermographs provide evidence of tissue irritation, the thermographers moved on to back and neck diagnosis instead.[40] A Darwinian process of natural selection soon occurred. Thermographers who could be relied upon to provide positive findings are the ones who stayed in business.[41]

Well-designed studies have now demonstrated that the results of thermographs are virtually meaningless, and many medical academic institutions have condemned their use.[42] But thermograms are still presented in court as solid evidence that a whiplash victim has been physically injured.[43]

Vertebrae show up very nicely on a straight x-ray, but vertebrae are seldom injured in whiplash – and by definition not in common whiplash.[44] The cervical spine is usually curved (the cervical lordosis) and, as medical students, we were originally taught that loss of this curve – a loss that is very visible on x-ray – is due to the spasm of injured muscles. Even though three studies have now shown that this loss of curvature is as common in asymptomatic controls as in victims of whiplash, this belief persists, especially among plaintiff whiplash experts.[45] Straightening of the cervical spine is no longer a certain sign that anything is wrong.[46]

Degenerative bony changes also show up well on x-ray, but there is a poor correlation between the presence of symptoms and such changes. The presence of symptoms in whiplash patients does not predict the finding of an abnormal x-ray, and neither does an abnormal x-ray predict the presence of whiplash symptoms.[47] Of course, the fact that these x-rays are useless for diagnosis does not stop every ER doctor from ordering one whenever a whiplash patient walks through the door. The exigencies of health justify unlimited waste. Such unnecessary x-rays also help make radiologists wealthy.

Imaging techniques such as CT scans, and particularly the MRI, allow the visualization of soft tissues. Bulging, prolapsed, or ruptured intervertebral discs show up nicely.[48] In the minds of many, slipped discs and low back pain go together like bacon and eggs. At the best of times, surgeons have difficulty keeping their fingers out of painful places. In the mid-1970s American neurosurgeons were performing about 200,000 back operations a year, most of which were for prolapsed discs,[49] and on average they made half their income repairing discs.[50] With the introduction of the MRI in the late 1970s, prolapsed discs were discovered all up and down the spine – they were everywhere.[51] Surgeons had a bonanza; they were in up to their elbows. Between 1979 and 1989 discectomy increased by 75 per cent and spinal fusion (another surgical treatment of these nasty looking discs) by 200 per cent.[52]

In properly selected cases the surgical repair of prolapsed discs can be a miracle, but only in about one per cent of cases of low back pain is a prolapsed disc the actual cause of the pain.[53] The operative results of poorly selected surgical cases are disappointing and sometimes disastrous.[54] Such unnecessary surgery spawned a whole new medical literature on the "failed back surgery syndrome."[55] The many bulging discs shown up by MRI and CT scans in the necks of whiplash victims soon convinced the courts that whiplash leaves a trail of damaged discs in its wake – discs all in need of prolonged treatment, and frequently of surgery as well.[56] Remember the basic rule of whiplash investigations: when a new technique is employed to search for a suspected whiplash injury, any positive finding is immediately accepted as confirmation of whiplash damage. It subsequently transpired that matched controls have just as many bulging discs in their necks as do whiplash victims.

Excellent epidemiological studies using MRI and CT scans have now demonstrated that the presence of these bulging and ruptured discs is almost meaningless. Discs break down as part of the normal process of aging; bulging and ruptured discs are often present in people who have never had back or neck problems or any history of spinal column injury.[57] Dutch radiologists used the MRI to study whiplash in a methodical way. They examined 100 consecutive whiplash patients referred to the radiology department and found only one patient with an abnormality on the MRI that they considered whiplash-related. This one patient had some prevertebral oedema (swelling), a condition that soon settles on its own.[58] Clearly, the MRI is of little use in whiplash diagnosis, yet I do not remember seeing a whiplash plaintiff who has not had at least one MRI.

At the same time, doctors are appealing for more of these fabulously expensive scanners, claiming that patients are dying of cancer and other serious illnesses because the necessary MRI machines are unavailable. Medico-legal work is more financially rewarding than routine hospital work, so the whiplash claimants get their necks scanned but the cancer patients have to take their place on the long waiting lists.

While American surgeons and radiologists were busy finding and treating ruptured discs in whiplash claimants, Australian anatomists Taylor and Twomey claimed they had proof positive that rear-end collisions severed the discs from the vertebral endplate.[59] They examined the cervical spine of fifteen victims killed in major rear-end collisions and compared them to discs taken from non-trauma controls. But the Australians are standing on their heads. Impacts sufficient to cause death are not the same as fender benders and bumper kisses that are the cause of most chronic whiplash symptoms. Comparing apples to oranges is not good science, and it is certainly not good sense.

While many whiplash experts continued to espouse injured discs as the culprit of whiplash pain, Bogduk, Lord, and Barnsley championed injury to the facet (zygapophyseal) joints as its hidden cause.[60] These Australian whiplash experts argue that small fractures involving these joints are common but they are missed because plain x-rays are insufficiently sensitive to demonstrate their presence. In support of their claim they cite a study of motor vehicle accident victims in which there were 73 fractures near or around the facet joints at autopsy, only four of which were evident on plain x-ray films.[61]

More standing on heads. This team totally ignored the difference between low-impact collisions that cause common whiplash and collisions sufficiently forceful to cause death. Anyway, to test their hypothesis, Barnsley and his colleagues injected local anaesthetics into the facet joints of whiplash litigants.[62] In pain relief studies there is always the problem of a placebo response: when a person believes that the pain will stop, it usually does. About a third of ordinary patients will respond to therapeutic or medicinal intervention with improvement or cure, but with patients in pain the placebo response jumps to nearly two-thirds. Six out of ten people will respond with pain relief to any drug or procedure that they believe will lessen their pain.[63]

Therefore, simply injecting an anaesthetic into an injured joint to see if the pain goes away is unacceptable evidence that the pain originates in the joint. To circumvent this placebo effect, the Australian team used a long-and a short-acting local anaesthetic alternately. If the patient responded with a short period of pain relief to the short-acting anaesthetic and with a long period of pain relief to the long-acting anaesthetic, the patient was accepted as having had a true-positive response. The study was double-blind, so neither the doctor giving the injection nor the patient receiving it knew whether the anaesthetic was short- or long-acting.

Thirty-four out of 47 patients showed true positive responses. When examined statistically, these results were scientifically more than acceptable. But there is a snag. Anyone who has had a local anaesthetic for dental work knows, even when there is no pain from which to obtain relief, that the anaesthetic has been given. The jaw feels different, a feeling that continues until the anaesthetic wears off. This detectability of the anaesthetic makes the results of the Australian study suspect. Sceptics also point out the injections anaesthetize other tissues in the neck besides the facet joints.[64]

An injury requires a treatment. Dismissing all other conservative treatments of Western medicine and non-insured alternatives (Hindu, Chinese, and Aboriginal), as unproven, the Australian researchers recommend the three-hour operative procedure of radio-frequency neurotomy (cutting of the nerve) to destroy the nerves to these allegedly injured and painful facet joints.[65] Opposing authors Drinka and Jaschob are just as strongly sceptical of this procedure, warning that pain sensation protects joints from damage and that joints devoid of such protection soon wear out and degenerate. They wonder about the long-term future of these "treated" joints.[66]

The uncertainty about injured facet joints, if there ever really was one, is now resolved. In a new imaging technique, an injected radioactive substance that accumulates at injury sites shows up as "hot spots" on a scintigram.[67] Small cracks in bones (much too small to be seen on x-ray), and even recent intramuscular injection sites, are all visible. Injuries around the facet joints, of the kind that Bogduk, Lord, and Barnsley claim are the hidden cause of ongoing whiplash pain, light up like little beacons.

Two studies using scintigrams examined whiplash claimants (55 typical whiplash patients) and found a remarkable absence of any injury. There were no hot spots around the facet joints, the intervertebral discs, or, for that matter, anywhere else in the neck.[68] While these scintigrams should be the death knell of "hidden" whiplash lesions, they are in no immediate danger of extinction, for plaintiff experts simply do not request scintigrams of the neck that could imperil the existence of these mythical pathologies. I have never found one scintigram of the neck in all the medico-legal briefs that I have examined.

It is not that plaintiff experts are reluctant to order scintigrams because of concern about the injection of a radioactive substance into a patient: just the reverse. Whiplash medico-legal briefs contain scintigrams of wrists and other parts of the body ordered on the off chance that the results will turn up evidence of unsuspected injury. No personal injury litigation lawyer wants a scan on the chart revealing the embarrassing absence of any neck injury. If a plaintiff expert unwisely ordered such a scan, its results undoubtedly would be carefully "buried" to protect them from unfriendly eyes. Only treating practitioners and plaintiff experts order investigations; defence experts do not.

Since a physical cause for backache is seldom identifiable, it is not surprising that the numerous physical treatments provided for it seldom work. Nortin Hadler, a distinguished rheumatologist from North Carolina, catalogued 150 randomized trials of medical, surgical, and physical interventions commonly used by the medical community for acute and chronic low back pain. He found all of them to be "without convincing or reproducible benefit."[69]

Manipulation is paired with backache as turkey is with Thanksgiving, but even the effectiveness of manipulation is now in doubt.[70] Physicians and chiropractors from Los Angeles, using a meta-analysis evaluating all the relevant studies in the literature, demonstrated that manipulative treatment is useful only within the first two weeks of an episode of low back pain.[71] Following suit, Dutch epidemiologists in a 1996 review of the randomized clinical trials of manipulation for acute and chronic low back pain (another meta-analysis) concluded that its efficacy has not been demonstrated.[72] It is difficult to know if manipulation for low back pain (and whiplash) is useful or not, but, like the Thanksgiving turkey, it's probably best not to wait too long before having it. It is certainly best not to have it with a chiropractor's dynamic thrust, which I will come to later.

Rest has always been a popular treatment for backache; when doctors do not know what to do, they put the patient to bed. However, even this medical panacea is now in question. In twenty-four randomized controlled studies, bedrest was found to do no good and often to be harmful.[73] Rest, it seems, is also not good for the spine.[74] Discs get their nutrition through movement, and activity has a beneficial influence on muscles, bones, ligaments, and cartilage as well.[75] Richard Deyo, an orthopaedic surgeon from Seattle, and a leading world authority on low back pain, found that in the treatment of acute low back pain two days in bed were better than seven days in bed: the less bedrest the better.[76] Other experimental studies have corroborated that healing (or at least the recovery of low back pain) is enhanced by controlled activity.[77]

In a Swedish study, 100 blue-collar workers at a Volvo plant who had been off work for eight weeks with non-specific low back pain were randomly assigned to either an active or a control group. Workers in the active group were given a half- to full-day program of "back-school," graded exercises under the supervision of a physiotherapist, while those in the control group were not. When compared to workers in the control group, workers in the active group had a 33 per cent reduction in lost time in the current episode of low back pain, and a 40 per cent reduction in subsequent episodes occurring the following year.[78]

In line with these studies, Hamilton Hall, *the* "Back Doctor" who runs the Canadian Back Institute, teaches back exercises to people with low back pain both by way of strengthening the back and providing reassurance that movement will not cause it to break in two. Hadler, on the other hand, argues that such activity only serves to perpetuate the "injury label." He proposes a clean new start by totally abandoning any concept of a structural abnormality of the back that needs to be put right. He considers that "back schools institutionalize the medicalization of low back pain ... No one sees the need for 'common cold schools' or 'flu schools.'"[79] Both viewpoints are supported by well-designed studies.

Since most of us perform exercise programs more by intention than by deed, perhaps the best and most reliable activity is to continue with the normal routine of our daily lives. Members of the Finnish Institute of Occupational Health at Helsinki demonstrated the effectiveness of doing so. Within one or two days of going off work with a diagnosis of low back strain, 186 Helsinki municipal employees were examined, reassured about the benign nature of their condition, and provided with standard analgesic prescriptions. Each patient was then randomly assigned to one of three management groups:

- Two days of complete bedrest;
- One hour of instruction on extension exercises done intensively at home until pain subsided;
- No treatment, but patients instructed to carry on with their usual duties as much as possible.

When followed up at three and twelve weeks, there was better recovery (in terms of pain and functional status), and substantially less time lost from work, in the workers who just got on with their lives.[80]

Without doubt, the surest way of not recovering from backache is to sit around at home doing nothing except worrying about which part of the back is out of joint. The same almost certainly goes for whiplash pain, but sitting around at home doing nothing is exactly what most of the whiplash plaintiffs I have seen in my career have been doing for the previous four or five years of their lives. Of course, every now and again, their insurance companies sent them off to expensive exercise programs, but for one reason or another the plaintiffs usually found a way to escape from the program.

Backs do not respond to physical treatments and neither do necks. Again, there is no lesion to treat, but this does not means there was and still is a shortage of treatments for the neck. The "pull treatment" or traction was for many years one of the most popular. It too had its opponents. Back in 1979 Lawrence Weinberger, a physiatrist from California, wrote of his concern about its detrimental effects:

Neurophysiology does not provide a satisfactory theory that explains the phenomenon of muscular "spasm" which is said to be present in the neck following soft-tissue injury. Lacking knowledge as to whether long-continued intermittent traction – ranging from 10 lb to total body weight pull – is therapeutic or traumatic, such treatments nevertheless are prescribed in physiotherapy departments and at home for months. They are non-physiological and irrational and, in the author's opinion, represent the persistence of several medical myths associated with the rear-end collision. The question is moot whether the intractable complaints following such injuries are not caused, in large part, by the repeated traumas to muscles, disks, and joints produced by strong intermittent distraction.[81]

Attempting to turn humans into giraffes may be harmful, but is probably less so than the "dynamic thrust," the sudden vigorous push, by which the chiropractor attempts to realign allegedly misaligned vertebrae.[82] When vertebrae really are realigned, the spinal cord and its blood supply stand in grave danger of harm. A wide variety of neurological lesions, varying in severity from the "locked-in syndrome" downwards, have been reported following such repositioning of the neck. [83]

Not as dramatically dangerous as the chiropractor's thrust, but perhaps more insidiously harmful is conventional medicine's neck collar. I will let Macnab have the first word about collars: "One often sees the ridiculous situation of a person leaving the emergency with a walking cast applied to his sprained ankle and a rag around his neck as the sole treatment of his sprained cervical spine. Either the lesion is serious enough to be worth treating, or it should be left alone. The only way to treat a severe sprain of the neck is to get the patient to lie down and take the weight of his head off his neck."[84]

The women of Padang in Sumatra wear multiple permanent gold collars. Their necks become so frail that if the rings are removed, the neck collapses, the spinal cord is severed and the woman dies. Fortunately, whiplash collars are far too inefficient to cause any such catastrophe, but the neck, like other parts of the body, is kept healthy by use, and a collar reduces both its strength and suppleness.[85] Even Gay and Abbott in their original description of whiplash, noted that the "constant wearing of a neck support results in atrophy of the cervical muscles and adds the complicating problem of weakened cervical muscles to the patient's problem," a warning that was assiduously ignored. With the arrival of whiplash, "the ubiquitous cervical collar [soon] became socially acceptable, and colours other than white made their appearance on some pretty necks."[86]

Numerous whiplash experts have reiterated Gay and Abbott's warning against the use of a collar for more than a week or so.[87] Even doctors on both sides of the Irish border agree about their detrimental effects. Two Irish randomized controlled studies on the use of collars in acute whiplash, one from St James' Hospital, Dublin, and the other from Victoria Hospital, Belfast, found the same thing. The outcome is better following neck mobilization than after wearing a collar.[88] Despite such longstanding and international execration of collars, however, numerous whiplash studies show that patients continue to wear them.[89] They are an emblem of victimhood and, as such, they are not readily surrendered.

There are, of course, many doctors who roundly condemn all these unnecessary treatments for the neck.[90] To stand the Australians the right way up again, I provide a quote from an Australian physician writing in the early 1970s:

Though the original accident seemed relatively trifling, the patients often have been treated for months or years by the time I see them. Treatment has been conducted variously by general practitioners, general surgeons, orthopaedists, neurosurgeons, neurologists, psychiatrists, physiotherapists and chiropractors. The only common factor is a conspicuous lack of success in the relief of symptoms whichever regime is adopted. Patients are given assorted irradiation from infrared to ultrasound (truly the whole spectrum); traction devised in different ways is employed for long periods or short; manipulation with or without general anaesthesia is employed; almost invariably neck collars are supplied and worn, often for many months, made to measure, or off the shelf; while finally these patients consume inordinate quantities of painkillers, sedatives, hypnotics and tranquilizers of a wide range, frequently for months on end.[90]

Treatment is often paradoxical. "The patient pursues treatment with the same doggedness with which he complains that it does him no good."[92] Since treatments for the relief of whiplash seem guaranteed to make its symptoms worse, it is reasonable to conclude that, whatever else, the purpose of treatment for whiplash is not to bring about a cure.

There can be few gaps wider than that between the treatment whiplash claimants receive and the treatment recommended by the Quebec Task Force on Whiplash-Associated Disorders: Mobilize the neck within 72 hours of the accident, exercise, limit inactivity, and avoid dependence on collars and analgesics. A few million dollars would cover the cost of such treatment for the whole of North America. The difference between this amount and the many billions of dollars actually spent on treating whiplash is the financial enticement for healthcare practitioners to perceive whiplash as a structural injury in need of treatment.

7

The Medico-legal and Psycho-social Spine

Says the one, "How long will the epidemic last?"
Says the other, "As long as we can keep it going."
– William Burroughs, *The Naked Lunch*

The case was only one of these phoney whiplash suits against
the Insurance Company filed by a lady passenger in a taxi collision.
– Saul Bellow, *Humbolt's Gift*

As a small boy I sometimes stayed in the country with my very Victorian grandmother. When it was time to return home she would put me on a train to London. I wanted to be in the first carriage, as close as possible to the smoke, noise, and soot of the steam engine, but she insisted that the carriages in the middle of the train were much safer, an opinion that seemed far in excess of acceptable grandmotherly concern. Having read about nineteenth-century train crashes and the Victorian preoccupation with "railway spine," I now understand better her protective zeal.

Whiplash is not lawyers' first love affair with the human spine. They already had a torrid affair a century ago when railway spine was accepted as a major health hazard. History teaches useful lessons and since whiplash is a replica of railway spine its lessons here are particularly germane.

The world's first railway, the Liverpool Manchester Railway Company, opened in 1830 and on its first day its famous engine *Stephenson's Rocket* ran over and killed the member of Parliament for Liverpool – a portent of the carnage to come. Over the next few decades railways crisscrossed Britain and the world, mangling bodies as they went. Railway accidents of the nineteenth century were what traffic accidents are for us today. Charles Dickens was in two of them and graphically described the wails of the injured and dying.[1]

Railways frightened the Victorians. Queen Victoria would not allow her train to go any faster than 20 mph, while a visiting shah of Persia insisted on an even slower speed, as his doctors feared he might otherwise suffocate. Thomas Carlyle was no braver: "I was dreadfully frightened before the train started; in the nervous state that I was in, it seemed to me certain that I should faint, from the impossibility of getting the horrid thing stopped." Edna St Vincent Millay, an American feminist and poet, was more courageous: "There isn't a train I wouldn't take, no matter where it is going." But few Victorians were as stalwart about trains as was Millay. Railway travel, they considered, caused nothing but harm.

In addition to the many people who indeed were killed and seriously injured in railway accidents, a far greater number were disabled by inexplicable persistent symptoms that often followed seemingly harmless collisions. Even the smallest jolt or collision produced symptoms. Although seldom were there any demonstrated signs of injury, railway collisions and jolts left their victims weak and paralysed. The injured sued the railway companies for compensation, and doctors, as is their wont, produced the necessary explanations for the symptoms. "Physicians," said Immanuel Kant, "think they do a lot for a patient when they give a disease a name." They certainly did a lot when they named "railway spine." The spinal cord, they maintained, had suffered concussion. The "spinal shock" led to wasting of the spinal cord and chronic inflammation of its coverings (meningitis).

Railway spine kept doctors busy. In Britain, John Erichsen, surgeon to Queen Victoria, commented on the legal trend of the times: "There is indeed no class of cases in which medical men are now so frequently called upon to give evidence in the courts of law, as those which involve the many intricate questions that arise in actions for damages against railway companies for injuries of the nervous system alleged to have been sustained by passengers in collisions; and there is no class of cases in which more discrepancy of surgical opinion may be elicited."[2]

S.V. Clevenger, a physician and member of numerous American scientific and medical societies, popularized the condition on the other side of the Atlantic. In his book *Spinal Concussion: Erichsen's Disease; One Form of Traumatic Neurosis,* Clevenger espoused the position that collisions were likely to cause permanent harm to the spinal cord.[3] The word *neurosis* at that time referred to damage to actual *neurones* or nerve cells, since the term had not yet acquired its psychological connotation.

Besides the fact that people like suing for damages, three other factors helped these doctors' views take hold. The first was that railway spine was caused by minor collisions and jolts and, as with whiplash, people rarely died of it. There was little autopsy material available that could be used to refute its supposed pathologies. In the absence of such proof, the authority of the Queen's surgeon carried the day.

The other two factors were the Victorians' obsession with the evils of masturbation and the ubiquity of syphilis. Just as Henry Maudsley attributed schizophrenia to the vice of self-abuse, Victorian neurologists attributed wasting of the spinal cord to this unfortunate "vice." Dr J. Russell from Birmingham in England described the autopsy of "a dead masturbator" in whom he found "small haemorrhages in the cord" complicated by wasting of its substance; in the United States two patients admitted to the Charity Hospital in New Orleans were certified as having died of masturbation.[4]

While masturbation certainly did not cause any pathology of the spinal cord, syphilis most certainly did, and our Victorian forebears, despite their sexual prudishness (or more probably because of it), suffered as much from syphilis as we do from AIDS; in fact, a good deal more so. Syphilis is reported to have "constituted about a third of all human pathology.[5] About 80 per cent of cases of myelitis (inflammation of the spinal cord) were a complication of syphilis but, as the Victorians had no laboratory tests for syphilis, they had no way of linking the spinal pathology to syphilis other than by autopsy.[6]

Given these three commonly accepted causes of spinal cord disease, it goes without saying that if the Victorians had anything wrong with their spinal cords (real or imagined), railway spine was the most popular of the three diagnostic choices. The fact that no one had actually demonstrated the presence of any cord lesions in railway spine was overlooked.

Michael Trimble, a British neurologist at the National Hospital for Neurological Diseases in London, in his book *Post-traumatic Neurosis: From Railway Spine to Whiplash*, gives an excellent account of railway spine. He notes that while the worth of a limb or an eye lost in a railway accident had been clearly established, the concussion of the spinal cord opened up undreamed of clinical and pathological possibilities all of which stood in need of compensation. "The concept that the injured were victims of at best 'shock' and at worst spinal anaemia or meningitis became prevalent."[7]

Some Victorian physicians objected to the unproven concept of railway spine. Herbert Page, a surgeon at St Mary's Hospital, London, clearly understood the psychological nature of the condition. He described the case of a 30-year-old man who, having been awarded generous compensation for an abnormal gait alleged to be the permanent result of a railway collision, was three and a half years later found to be in good health:

That there never was any lesion of the spinal cord the issue of the case has abundantly proved, and we cannot help thinking that such a diagnosis would never have been raised were the influences of the mind upon the body more fully recognized, and were it not regarded as almost a matter of course that injuries received in, and the symptoms seen after, railway collision must be due to 'concussion of the spine' and be followed by chronic meningitis and myelitis, and the irritation of the membranes of which we hear so much but which no man has even seen.[8]

Sir James Paget, a surgeon at St Bartholomew's Hospital, after whom a bone disease and a cancer of the breast are both named, coined the term "neuromimesis" (mimicry of a disease of the nervous system) to describe the symptoms of railway spine and other similar conditions, symptoms which mimic diseases with a genuine pathology. Physicians had difficulty distinguishing between psychogenic symptoms and those of genuine disease, a difficulty that seems endemic among expert physicians even today, in regards to whiplash and other fashionable illnesses.

For years the scepticism of the railway spine critics remained unheeded; the potent combination of the financial interests of the medical profession and the determination of patients to have their symptoms validated easily prevailed. Lawyers outdid themselves in proving black is white – that small collisions cause irreparable damage to the spinal cord. The disastrous epidemic of railway spine persisted for well over half a century. Eventually, railway spine came to the end of the line; the courts "tumbled to the nature of railway spine and it promptly disappeared," though by then the railway spine epidemic had served its purpose. Railways had become safer and travellers were soon abandoning trains for the family car. In the United States whiplash had arrived; an excellent substitute for railway spine.[9] Lawyers and healthcare practitioners had new fish to fry.

Ongoing court battles over whiplash took over from where the ongoing court battles over railway spine had left off. The plaintiff side continued to support an injury explanation. The defence supported a psycho-social explanation, often arguing that all that was needed to bring about cure was a greenback poultice (a thick wad of green dollar bills provided by way of compensation), a curt observation that sent the plaintiff bar into orbit.[10]

To be fair to lawyers, it is not always lawyers that help mess up our spines when there is nothing physically wrong with them. Given the right circumstances, we are perfectly capable of doing it ourselves. Despite the prodigious endeavours made by healthcare practitioners to find the physical causes of ongoing neck and back problem symptoms, relatively little effort has been made to examine the factors other than physical that predispose to their development. There is a

growing recognition that physicians and other healthcare practitioners, with their trauma-based concepts of pain, have managed to create
disease where no disease exists. Empirical evidence is accumulating
that persistent low back and neck pain are linked less with trauma and
physical abnormalities than with various psycho-social risk factors.[11]
What are these risk factors?

A previous history of low back pain puts a person at greater risk for
having it again in the future. However, such a history does not necessarily indicate something is physically amiss with the low back, since a
previous history of chronic pain other than low back pain also increases the risk of future backache.[12]

Coffin nails increase the risk. Smokers are 1.4 times more likely to
report an industrial back injury than are non-smokers.[13] However, it is
unknown whether this greater incidence is a direct effect of smoking,
or whether people who smoke and people who have a tendency to
report industrial low back pain have certain demographic and psycho-
social characteristics in common.[14]

Nasty work makes nasty backs. In the early 1970s it was shown that
negative experiences at work increase complaints of low back pain.[15]
Indeed, "psycho-social factors have a clear influence upon low back
pain, which sometimes may even transcend that of physical factors
related to the occupation itself."[16] Subsequent studies have confirmed
this.[17] S.J. Bigos, from the University of Washington Department of
Orthopedics, is another American pundit on back pain. He and his
colleagues have an ongoing study of backache among the employees
at the Boeing factory in Seattle. They found that, second only to a history of previous low back pain, attitudes towards work (such as work
being of low enjoyment) are the strongest predictors of low back pain
complaints, these factors being more relevant than the actual physical
demands of the job.[18]

A person's state of mind, personality, and psychological problems
predispose to low back pain.[19] Bigos and his team found that strong
tendencies toward somatic complaints and denial of emotional distress
were associated with an increase in low back pain complaints. They
used the Minnesota Multiphasic Personality Inventory (MMPI), a well-
standardized screening instrument for personality derangement.[20]
Investigators at Manchester University, United Kingdom, compared
people with low back pain to matched controls. They found an
increased occurrence of adverse life events – burglaries, illness in close
relatives, court appearances, marital separations, and so forth – in the
few months prior to the onset of chronic low back pain.[21]

Several other studies have provided evidence of emotional causes of
backache. An Australian study showed that anxiety, depression, and

family conflict were greater in people with chronic low back pain than in healthy controls.[22] Similarly, an American study found family conflict to be predictive of chronic low back pain.[23] A study from Duke University Medical Center found that alcoholism and depression are higher in families of patients with chronic low back pain than in those of a control group, while a study from the Department of Neurology, Fort Worth, Texas, reported high rates of abandonment and emotional abuse in the childhood histories of sufferers with chronic back pain.[24] Harried heartstrings, rather than any hypothesized pathology, are a predisposing factor for backache.

Money matters at all levels. Financial disincentives for recovery, and financial incentives for the healthcare practitioner to provide treatment both delay return to health.[25] Complaints of low back pain vary with the ups and downs of the business cycle. In times of high employment, when the danger of losing a job is reduced, time off for low back pain doubles.[26]

Vexation proverbially causes a "pain in the neck," but it can cause backache as well. Lees-Haley and Brown, in their study of baseline rates for head injury symptoms (see chapter 4), found that 80 per cent of litigants reported having back pain even though their litigation was for non-physical injury. Of course, this percentage is likely to be even higher for litigants suing for an alleged back injury.

The beliefs and interests of healthcare practitioners are central to the problem of back pain. John Sarno, a New York physiatrist, puts it well: "The various health disciplines interested in the back have succeeded in creating an army of the partially disabled in this country with their medieval concepts of structural damage and injury as the basis of back pain ... Virtually every patient has come to fear and avoid physical activity under the impression that it is a structural disorder which requires rest and protection."[27]

Constant dripping wears away a stone. The various psycho-social factors predisposing to disability from low back pain add up – a summation that certainly makes sense.[28] A worker is bored with his monotonous job ... he does not like his patronizing boss ... feels depressed, tired and anxious ... his wife and family are making inordinate demands on his time and energy ... he has recurrent episodes of back pain ... without quibble his doctor will validate his need for sick leave. Once on compensation he will suffer only a negligible loss of income. If, because of a recession, his co-workers are laid off, his disability status will protect him from any loss of employment. His doctor will probably prescribe Tylenol #3s and Valium, both of which make him feel better. His masseuse will be kind to him. All things added up, it is sensible behaviour to take sick leave.

That the treatment of low back pain often benefits the healthcare practitioner more than the patient has not gone unobserved. Gordon Waddell, an orthopaedic surgeon from Glasgow, has spearheaded a movement for reform. "Back pain is a twentieth-century medical disaster," is the opening sentence of his 1998 book *The Back Pain Revolution*.[29] Waddell discusses the ingredients of this disaster and what can be done to put things right. He is not alone in his campaign for reform.

The Agency for Health Care Policy and Research (AHCPR) in the United States, the Quebec Task Force on Spinal Disorders in Canada, and the Clinical Standards Advisory Group (CSAG) in the United Kingdom have published practice guidelines for healthcare practitioners based upon the hard evidence of well-designed studies.[30] These guidelines all advocate similar changes in the management of low back pain: a thorough clinical examination and the avoidance of investigations (including straight x-rays unless there is reason to suspect something other than occupational low back pain). They encourage mild exercise (swimming and walking) and discourage the use of muscle relaxants and opioid analgesics. The guidelines also recommend seeking a second opinion before undertaking any major treatment. In a pilot project in which such a second opinion was mandatory, the number of surgeries performed fell by 88 per cent.[31]

If healthcare practitioners actually followed these practice guidelines, backs would cause far fewer problems. However, it is one thing to provide guidelines based on a thoughtful synthesis of scientific information and quite another to persuade physicians and other healthcare practitioners to follow them.[32] With healthcare practitioners, as with patients, social considerations rather than science play a crucial role in shaping decisions.[33]

In the United States, the AHCPR's guidelines were so unpopular with the medical establishment that doctors nearly persuaded Congress to cancel the agency's funding.[34] Asking healthcare practitioners to forgo their incomes and to give Mother Nature – their chief and usually successful competitor, a head start, will be perceived as unreasonable treatment. Lip service will be paid to these guidelines but it will then be business as usual.

For whiplash also, the evidence is that psycho-social factors are crucial to its development. Quite apart from peer-copying and the availability of financial compensation, other personal factors influence its development. Aaron Farbman, a surgeon from Detroit, in 1973 examined the factors he suspected of lengthening the duration of whiplash symptoms. He assessed 136 patients with uncomplicated whiplash in whom the symptoms had lasted from three days to over five years. On physical examination (usually within three weeks of the accident), only 6 per cent of patients showed any objective finding (reduced range of neck movements, muscle spasm, swelling, or tenderness) and 8 per cent had doubtful findings, whereas 86 per cent showed no findings at all. Farbman found no association between the extent of vehicle damage and the duration of symptoms. He found, however, that the severity of symptoms, at least in terms of their duration, close-ly correlated with the presence of four psycho-social variables: emo-tional factors, length of the previous medical history, treatment, and litigation.

From the patients' histories, Farbman identified the "emotional fac-tors": persistent nervousness, use of tranquilizers, pressure at work, serious illnesses, accidents or operations on self or family, care of men-tally retarded child or invalid relative, recent death of loved relative, and history of previous psychiatric care. He then scored the patients in terms of these factors and found that a high score for emotional fac-tors was associated with the prolongation of whiplash symptoms: the higher the score, the longer the duration of symptoms.[35] The results of Farbman's study were ignored by the whiplash industry.

Michael Livingston, the family physician from Vancouver with a spe-cial interest in whiplash, reported on the outcome of 100 consecutive whiplash cases. Using the factors identified by Farbman as impair-ments to recovery, Livingston provided each patient with an early prognosis based on the estimated force of collision and the patient's past history, life situation, clinical findings, and psychological status. He discouraged his patients from consulting a lawyer. Livingston found that the 15 patients whose recovery took longer than six months had a history of many accidents, pre-existing spine complaints, long-standing spine complaints in other family members, significant stress or unhappiness, significant treatments such as spinal operations prior to the accident, or excessive physiotherapy.[36]

Despite the inclusion of these problem patients, most of his patients required only a few office visits, and all recovered within two years. This successful outcome contrasts startlingly with the poor outcomes reported in most other whiplash studies in which attention is directed towards the treatment of a supposed underlying injury. Livingston paid as much attention to his patients as to their necks. It worked.

Marete Karlsborg and her colleagues from the Hvidovre Hospital, Copenhagen, using a sophisticated methodology, largely confirmed Farbman and Livingston's work. Her team intensively investigated, both physically and psychologically, 39 whiplash patients who were consecutively admitted to the casualty department. Physical examina-tion, including MRI scans of the neck and brain and other physical investigations, revealed very few abnormalities. But the investigators found that high stress scores, as measured by questionnaires, and stressful life events (the birth of a baby, the loss of a relative, or a robbery) allowed them to predict the number of complaints at the final neurological examination six months post-accident. The presence of initial neurological signs did not.[37]

There is reason to suspect that from the viewpoint of recovery the management of whiplash is even more unsatisfactory than that of occupational low back pain. In the management of occupational low back pain, compensation boards ameliorate some of the worst abuses of overtreatment and the exploitation of symptoms both by healthcare practitioners and their patients. With whiplash it is a free-for-all. Plaintiff injury litigation lawyers orchestrate the claimant's interminable care. They select healthcare practitioners on the basis of their known success in nurturing symptoms – with multiple investigations, treatments, and rest, rest, and more rest. The longer the plaintiff remains off work the larger the settlement will be and so, therefore, the lawyer's fee.

We are all human; when it is possible to hold someone else responsible for symptoms, it is tempting to adopt an illness that implicates them. In doing so, the process of being a lifelong patient begins.[38] Once we start trying to prove we are injured, recovery becomes unlikely; any diminishment of our pain undermines our claim. Backache does not abolish a healthy self-interest.

8

Putting the Bite into Whiplash

"In my youth," said the father, "I took to the law,
And argued each case with my wife:
And the muscular strength, which it gave to my jaw,
Has lasted the rest of my life."
– Lewis Carroll

Temporomandibular joint disorder, more recognizable as TMJ, is a fashionable illness and, like other fashionable illnesses, it paired up with another one – whiplash. A quarter of the whiplash plaintiffs I assessed had an additional diagnosis of accident-induced TMJ disorder. The marriage of TMJ disorder and whiplash was bad for the jaw. The more lawyers exercised their jaws on the vulnerability of the TM joints, the more debilitated their clients' jaws became. Ms T's TM joints make the point. I reproduce her history word for word from a summary in her medico-legal chart.

Ms T is a 28-year-old married receptionist who had been involved in a rear-end collision six years previously. Little damage was done to her car and she had no immediate effects from the accident. Next day she had a stiff neck and headache. Over the next year, the stiff neck gradually subsided, but the headache remained. Eighteen months after the accident, she returned to work.

Information from her medical file revealed a history of multiple minor somatoform complaints from the age of twelve onwards. As an adolescent, she had been diagnosed as having chronic fatigue syndrome. One year before the accident, she received treatment for TMJ disorder, involving steroid injections to the TM joints, a bite plate, and physiotherapy. According to the patient, the condition had improved. She dismissed this previous treatment as insignificant – "I just needed a mouth guard."

Two weeks after returning to work, on a routine follow-up visit for her TMJ problems, Ms T informed her dentist of the accident. He insisted on a legal consultation. The problems with her jaw increased – she had much more pain; her jaws locked several times each day, where previously this "only happened on rare occasions." Sometimes her jaws would lock while a utensil was in her mouth and she then had to pry open her jaw with another utensil to remove it. She was investigated with arthroscopy and, two years after the accident, she had her first jaw surgery. Three other surgical interventions soon followed. [Between] surgical interventions, Ms T married a supportive husband. Because of increasing difficulty in opening her mouth to talk, she quit her receptionist's job. She was only able to eat bland foods processed in the blender. Her energy levels are down, necessitating that she spends much of her time at home. Mostly, she only leaves home in connection with the ongoing whiplash litigation, or to visit either her family doctor or the emergency department for narcotic injections for pain. Ms T reports her only treatment option left is "a total bilateral jaw replacement."

This is the story of how TMJ disorder became a fashionable illness, how, why, and when it linked up with whiplash, and why Ms T, six years after a minor collision, believes she now requires artificial jaw joints. Some background about the TM joints will help to unravel this mystery.

The temporomandibular joints (TMJs) are the hinge joints that connect the lower jaw to the skull. These joints are small but they can give big trouble. The TM joints, like other joints in the body, can be damaged by injury or disease and then, like other joints, cause pain and other problems. But seldom is any such disease process found in TMJ disorder.[1] The cardinal symptom of TMJ disorder is pain around the TM joints; its salient physical signs are clicking sounds on opening and closing the mouth, sometimes accompanied by difficulty in opening the mouth wide. TMJ disorder was first described in 1934 by an American laryngologist who attributed it to malocclusion from the loss of the back teeth, a common event in the hungry thirties.[2] Other authors attributed TMJ symptoms to nocturnal grinding of the teeth. These explanations do not hold water. Control studies show that many people with TMJ disorder have neither malocclusion nor grind their teeth at night, while many teeth grinders and many people with malocclusion do not have the disorder.[3]

Uncertainty surrounding the cause of any painful ill-defined condition breeds fashionable illnesses. People with TMJ disorder are known as "TMJers," and they often familiarly refer to their condition as "my TMJ." Since experts on this condition (and there are many) seem to like to name TMJ disorder themselves, the condition has many other names but I will stick with just two: "TMJ disorder" and "TMD" which stands for temporomandibular disorder.[4]

As with other fashionable illnesses, clinicians soon took sides, some seeing TMJ disorder as a somatic response to psychological stress and some interpreting it as a psychologically distressing physical disorder in need of investigation and treatment.[5] Well-conducted studies demonstrate that, as with other fashionable illnesses, the distress usually precedes the disorder.[6]

How then did TM joint problems get hooked up with whiplash? As with many other things in medicine, it was mostly a matter of economics. In the 1960s and 1970s municipalities began adding fluoride to drinking water. The fluoride successfully reduced dental caries but it cut back on dentists' incomes as well.[7] If dentists were to remain in business, they needed to become less "tooth-oriented;" they desperately needed a different kind of work.[8] Then, in the strange way that life has of coming to people's rescue, whiplash plaintiffs – backed by seemingly unlimited insurance money – were reported to be suffering from TMJ disorder. Whiplash became the dentists' restoration. The marriage of TMJ disorders and whiplash received a fanfare of publicity that I will come to later. But first, what is the acceptable scientific evidence that whiplash causes TMJ disorder? There is none.

Although there is now a massive literature on whiplash and TMJ disorder, the more reliable material on these disorders is found in peer reviewed medical and dental journals. Information about such journal articles is stored in databases. For the years prior to 1966 this information is only available in printed form in the Cumulated Index Medicus, huge volumes that are tedious to use. Since 1966 the information has been computerized on MedLine, which is a medical researcher's joy. Fortunately for me, whiplash and TMJ disorder did not become associated in the medical literature until 1965 so, except for one article, I could obtain all the relevant journal articles from MedLine. Twenty-two articles are listed that deal with both TMJ disorder and whiplash, some of which are in support of whiplash being a cause of TMJ disorder and others are opposed. I have used the more germane of these articles to illustrate the growing intimacy between TMJ disorder and whiplash. I have tracked their relationship to 1993, the year in which whiplash became forty, though certainly not past its prime.

The first thing to notice is that their relationship, although certainly not lacking opportunity, got off to an unpromisingly slow start. Gay and Abbott's original 1953 article set off an intense search for whiplash symptoms. Clinicians indiscriminately attributed myriad problems to whiplash, yet oddly enough, TMJ disorder was not one of them. Whiplash had already had twelve tumultuous years of medicolegal acclaim before there was any hint that the two kept company. Then in 1965 Victor Frankel, an American orthopaedic surgeon, linked their names together.[9] He studied 40 patients, all with whiplash from rear-end collisions, and found symptoms and signs pointing to a derangement of the temporomandibular joint.[10]

Frankel had an underprivileged clientele and most of his patients had some back teeth missing.[11] He reported that many of his whiplash patients "complained of painful mastication, pain when opening the mouth, clicking in the temporomandibular joints, facial and aural pain, limited mouth opening and deviation of the jaw to one side when opening the mouth." Here is his first case:

BR – 39-year-old-male. His car, halted for a red light, was struck from behind. Typical symptoms of a neck sprain were found and conservative treatment was instituted. At the time of initial admission he complained of some loss of hearing and a sensation of loudness and roaring in the left ear. When examined two months later, he complained of pain at the left side of the jaw. The patient [had no teeth] in the posterior molar region. On opening the mouth, the mandible deviated suddenly to the left as it attained the fully opened position.

Frankel referred his patient to a dental consultant for jaw exercises and the patient gradually improved. Frankel describes the mechanism of injury: "When an automobile is struck from behind, the relaxed passenger is projected forward and his head is snapped back abruptly. The mouth flies open. The stretch reflex (the jaw jerk) of the masseters [a powerful jaw muscle] is evoked; the jaw snaps shut." The TM joint, like the knee, has a cartilage or "disc" between its articular surfaces. Frankel went on to describe in technical but graphic terms how the rapid opening and shutting of the mouth stretches and tears the joint capsule and disc.

Frankel's observations on whiplash-as-a-cause-of-TMJ-disorder went unnoticed, and eight years passed before the next combined entry for whiplash and TMJ disorder. Richard Roydhouse, a dentist from the University of British Columbia, wrote in the *Lancet*: "There is a similarity between some symptoms of whiplash and TMJ dysfunction. Head pains, stuffy noses, plugged ears, blurred vision, sore throats, stiff jaws, and so on, are insufficiently precise to warrant a diagnosis of high probability. The confirmatory signs, such as a clicking TMJ, deviation on opening of the jaw, and a disordered dental occlusion, again may be imprecise because they exist in many persons without symptoms or discomfort." Despite the uncertainties of its diagnoses, however, Roydhouse treated fourteen patients with whiplash symptoms (varying in duration from two days to one year) for a TMJ disorder.[12]

Again, nothing for six years. Then in 1979, Edwin Ernest, a dentist from Alabama, described the case of an 18-year-old woman who, on a regular dental check-up, reported that she had sustained a whiplash one year previously. Ernest found a mild abnormality of her bite. Her post-accident history provides a typical example of how whiplash helps to keep the medical profession in business. "This patient had been under the care of six physicians for vague pain of the neck and shoulders, chronic headaches, ear stuffiness and earaches, and vague pressure behind the left orbit. She received medications, a cervical neck brace, brain scans, and other diagnostic tests from her physicians in order to determine the source of her problem. As a direct result of her automobile accident, the patient was classified as a victim of whiplash by her orthopedic surgeon and physician."[13]

Then Ernest gives the first report in the literature of a bite plate being used to treat whiplash-induced TMJ. The plate met with a not uncommon demise: the patient lost it. Ernest writes of his treatment: "One cannot separate a tooth and its function from the surrounding ligaments, tendons, muscles, and bones. With this knowledge, we are able to communicate with our patients and other health professionals to achieve the goal and intent of dentistry and medicine – better patient care."[14]

Perhaps it was Ernest's somewhat expansionistic article in *General Dentistry* that did it. Anyway, somewhere around this time, twenty-five years after the publication of Gay and Abbott's article, whiplash and TMJ disorders became irrevocably hitched (at least in the eyes of the law). Enthusiastic dentists jumped on the whiplash bandwagon, constructing bite plates by the thousands, and lawyers appointed themselves their bandleaders.

Six year later, there appeared an article by dentists Allen Moses and George Skoog, appropriately first written for the law journal *Trial*. The authors point out similarities in the symptomatology of TMJ disorder and whiplash. "They explain how dentists successfully diagnose, document, and treat cervical whiplash and TMJ disorder, using the latest biomedical instruments."[15]

The entries in MedLine now speed up. Simon Weinberg and Henry La Pointe, oral and maxillofacial surgeons at the University of Toronto, assessed a sample of 28 whiplash patients, 22 of whom were wearing cervical collars. Arthrography (the injection of a radio-opaque into the TM joint) showed that 22 out of 25 patients had internal derangements of the TM joints. In 10 patients these observations were confirmed by surgery. The surgeons wrote: "There appears to be a relationship between acceleration-deceleration type automobile accidents and internal derangements of the TMJ ... The primary structural alteration within the joint occurs at the time of the accident ... The mandible due to its own inertia will move posteriorly less quickly than the cranium. This results in downward and forward displacement of the disc-condyle complex relative to the cranial base ... Arthrographic examination of the TMJ(s) is recommended when the patient's symptoms fail to respond to a reasonable course of conservative therapy." Dramatic drawings illustrate the injury process.[16]

In an entry from the following year, Arthur Kupperman, a dentist from New York, decisively takes Weinberg and La Pointe to task: "I disagree with their proposed mechanism for whiplash-related internal disc derangement. The masseter is one of the strongest muscles in the body and can easily brace the jaw against any extreme force. It is more likely that the eyes would fly out of their sockets than the mandible be displaced in such a proposed manner."[17]

In 1989 Jeffrey Mannheimer and colleagues from the University of Medicine and Dentistry of New Jersey again seek to tie whiplash and TMJ disorders firmly up together. Theirs is one of those "a pound of prevention is worth an ounce of cure" articles, a prescription that had by then become trendy in medicine: everyone required extensive early intervention to prevent future possible problems. Their intent was to foster "an appreciation of the interrelationship of the cervical and craniomandibular architectures as well as the significance of proper evaluation and treatment of the cervical strain and mandibular whiplash injuries. With the coordinated cooperation of properly trained dentists and physical therapists [and] the early implementation of a sequence of integrated treatment plans between the two practitioners, the index of recovery from cervical strain and TMJ dysfunction could improve ... This is the only way to eliminate excessive, costly, and unnecessary treatment."[18]

The next three entries (at least from my point) are all on the side of sanity. Herbert Goldberg, a dentist from Philadelphia, writes:

The information that has been accumulated over the last five years regarding the diagnosis and treatment of myofascial pain dysfunction and TMD is overwhelming in scope. These data are often replete with interpretations based on personal conjecture and the use of questionable diagnostic instruments. Statements have been taken as truth without adequate research or clinical trials. Twenty-eight treatment modalities have been reported. No other body joint has been given such regard.

[The rear-ended patient's feelings and symptoms are validated by] the support of the attorney, physiotherapist, physician and treating dentist ... The patient who is involved in such an accident is typically prepared for TMJ treatment. Long term appliance therapy and physiotherapy for 14 to 18 months without significant improvement is accepted as indicating the severe nature of the injury ... Anterior disc displacement is easy to explain to third parties, since the lay concept is a cap (disc) on the condyle that is waiting to be dislodged. It is therefore the most frequently diagnosed injury and generally accepted without question.[19]

Richard Howard and a group of physician-engineers from San Antonio, Texas, specifically rebut the Weinberg and La Pointe contention that whiplash entails injury to the joint discs. Noting that extension-flexion of the cervical spine is often presented as a causal factor in TMJ injury, they report that they had by computer simulation analysed the forces involved in mild to moderate extension-flexion motion of the neck and found them weaker than the forces routinely encountered in the everyday chewing of food.[20]

Researchers from the Medical College of Virginia Hospitals, in a methodical study followed whiplash patients seen in the emergency department, one month and one year after their accidents. They found the incidence of TMJ pain and clicking following whiplash to be extremely low. They concluded that there is "no clinical evidence of a significant relationship between cervical musculoskeletal injury and the development of TMJ dysfunction." [21]

Then in 1992 Barry Pressman and his radiology colleagues from Cedars-Sinai Medical Center, Los Angeles, presented some seemingly convincing evidence that whiplash damages the TM joints, with "accurate scientific data." These authors used the then newly available MRI scanner to examine 33 consecutive patients (66 joints) symptomatic after a rear-end collision. Like Weinberg and La Pointe, they too found that the majority of the discs in TM joints were in abnormal positions.[22]

Next year, Ronald Levandoski, president of the TMJ Institute of America, again reinforces the cases for TMJ damage: "There appears to be incontrovertible clinical experience reported in refereed journals for the past several decades of a relationship between acceleration and deceleration trauma to craniocervical structures and internal derangement of the TMJ." Levandoski finds that "many whiplash injury victims needlessly suffer with chronic intractable pain and eventually manifest permanent degenerative changes in their TMJs ... from which many patients never recover."[23]

In 1994 researchers from the Royal Melbourne Hospital entered the scene. Noting the uncertain relationship between TMJ disorder and trauma to the head and neck, they analysed the 20,673 traffic injury claims submitted in the province of Victoria for the year 1987 (before the Australians had become aware of the relationship between whiplash and TMJ disorder). Out of a total of 2,198 whiplash claimants, only 12 (0.5%) had submitted an additional claim for TMJ disorder. The authors concluded that, with only one whiplash claimant out of 183 seeking treatment for TMJ disorder, TMJ disorder is an unlikely accompaniment of whiplash.[24]

The last of the MedLine entries is for another study by Howard and the group of physician-engineers from San Antonio. In 1995, having four years previously presented theoretical calculations of the acceleration/deceleration forces acting on the TM joints, they presented hard measurements. Using four human subjects, accelerometers, and high-speed cinematographic techniques to study the effects of an 8 km/h (5 mph) rear-end collision on the jaw, they found the maximum force at the TM joints ranged from 1.6 to 2.2 pounds. They comment that such forces "constitute a minor fraction of the forces experienced at the joint during normal physiological function."[25]

MedLine only extracts articles from reputable medical journals. Even *la crème de la crème* of the medical scientific literature is full of questionable science. Let us look more closely at the science in these articles and the kind of "medical science" it subsequently spawned.

Frankel, having found that 15 out of 40 whiplash patients had TMJ disorder, claimed whiplash was its cause. There is, however, a problem. Frankel treated his patients with neck traction which consists of placing a halter under the chin and around the back of the patient's neck, threading the rope from the halter over a pulley, and putting a heavy weight on the end. Frankel reported that most of his patients were missing their back teeth. The likely explanation for his patients' jaw pain is that after fifteen minutes or so of being pulled by a 7-pound weight, the jaw feels uncomfortable, especially when there are no back teeth to stop the traction strap from squeezing the surfaces of the TM joints too tightly together. Several authors, including Frankel himself one year previously, had reported that neck traction either worsens or causes TMJ disorder, to the extent that cervical traction is now discredited as an acceptable treatment for cervical whiplash.[26]

It seems likely that the neck traction prescribed for the alleged neck injury rather than the whiplash *per se* was responsible for the high incidence of TMJ disorder in Frankel's patients. When treatment causes symptoms, the disease often takes the blame. With his description of the mouth flying open and snapping shut and so damaging the joint disc, Frankel provided an injury explanation for his patients' complaints. Subsequent high-speed cinematography and studies on the forces involved show that the mouth does not even open, let alone fly open with a force sufficient to damage the TM joints.[27] Like Gay and Abbott, with their description of the head oscillating back and forth, Frankel had made up this injury scenario.

Once dentists realized the implications of Frankel's invented concept of whiplash injury of the TMJ joints, the concept caught on with a bang. Much medical whiplash literature is like medieval scholasticism. It matters more that a recognized authority has affirmed something to be true than that it actually is. Once an idea has been printed in the medical literature it can, with good academic conscience, be quoted chapter and verse, and often improved along the way. That is exactly what authors did.[28]

Once something enters the medical literature it can be offered as evidence in court, where it soon "acquires a larger-than-life stature."[29] Medico-legal suppliers, for a price, furnish large colour pictures of torn and tattered TM joints that can be handed in court to judge and jury. The only problem with these pictures is that this TMJ injury does not actually occur!

As you know, whiplash investigators are not partial to the use of controls. If either Weinberg and La Pointe or Pressman and his fellow radiologists had done so they would have found that, at least as far as the position of the TMJ discs is concerned, whiplash claimants are no different from anyone else. Subsequent arthrography, MRI, and autopsy studies of symptomless subjects with no history of rear-end collisions show that it is normal for the TMJ discs to be displaced either anteriorly or into other positions within the joint capsule.[30]

Although most of the articles portray the TM joints as easily damaged, these joints are in fact well protected by strong muscles and ligaments, and, as joints go, they are remarkably injury-proof.[31] To accept that the TMJs are damaged by whiplash requires a suspension of common sense. If, when tripping on the stair carpet, you tear a knee cartilage, you do not need a doctor to tell you something is wrong. It is excruciatingly painful. The TM joints have a richer nerve supply than does the knee, so tearing a TMJ cartilage is even more painful. Any injury to the joint discs will not go unnoticed for several months after the accident.[32] Levandoski sidesteps this problem with the suggestion that, because of the severe life-threatening trauma of the accident, the patient and the emergency physician overlook the initial injury to the TM joints. Injuries are sometimes overlooked in a crisis situation, but not, surely, in whiplash. Characteristically, whiplash claimants have minimal initial pain or distress. Levandoski also suggests that whiplash victims take active steps to forget their injuries – an odd observation since most whiplash claimants seem unusually intent on remembering every detail of their accident.

Besides all the bad science there is a lot of self-serving promotion in these articles. All the proponents of whiplash as a cause of TMJ disorder recommend the further involvement of their own professional discipline. Weinberg and La Pointe recommend arthrographic examination of the TMJs "when the patient's symptoms fail to respond to a reasonable course of conservative therapy." Pressman and his radiology colleagues recommend that "MRI be obtained routinely in patients who have a history of whiplash injury and TMJ dysfunction and/or symptoms." Mannheimer, a physical therapist, commenting that "the overwhelming majority of patients who sustain cervical strains are never referred early enough," suggests "referral within the first one to three weeks to a skilled physical therapist." Levandoski, president of the TMJ Institute of America, warns that failure to refer whiplash patients to a TMJ specialist means that many of them will "needlessly suffer with chronic intractable pain."

Superimposed on this small travesty of science a mountain of illness promotion and bogus treatments was constructed, all stressing TMJ disorder's attachment to whiplash. Whiplash experts distributed flyers to lawyers' offices offering their services for the management of this distressing coupling:

Headaches or neck aches • Dizziness • Earaches • Ringing noises in the ears • Neck pain that will not go away • Clicking noises when opening or closing mouth • Teeth that do not meet right • Hearing loss • Pain when eating • Pain when opening and closing mouth • Difficulty when swallowing – must be treated as soon as possible.[33]

A decade later in 1985, two American professors of dentistry reported on the effectiveness of these types of promotional activities:

During the past ten years there has been an explosion of interest in TM disorders. The TM joint is a popular topic of lay publications, radio and TV reports. TMJ courses now rank among the most popular of dentists' continuing education offerings, and articles dealing with TMJ in professional journals have increased at an exponential rate during the last ten years ... There are now three major societies whose primary interests focus on clinical aspects of TMJ, and last year a new journal devoted exclusively to management of TM disorders was started. Dental practitioners are inundated with TMJ continuing education program advertisements that claim to revitalize faltering dental practices ... The management of TMJ disorders is viewed by some as one solution to the problem of practice "business" ... It appears that the recent interest [in TMJ disorder] is a result of redefining old conditions, increased education of professionals, increased public awareness, and a belief by clinicians that these signs and symptoms should be treated.[34]

As a job creation opportunity, the promotion of TMJ disorder worked wonders. A 1988 edition of *Time* magazine called TMJ disorder the "in-malady" and noted that "some 10 million Americans suffer from it."[35] As with most other fashionable illnesses, women became its most frequent victims, the condition being up to nine times more common in women than men.[36] The hype continued.

As we have already seen, victims of fashionable illnesses champion their own illness. Sharren Carr, a TMJ victim, established MyoData and

---

South Florida Institute for Post-Graduate Health Education

Presents

WHIPLASH
AND
T.M.J. INJURIES

(4-Hour Seminar for Trial Lawyers)
Approved by Florida Bar for C.L.E. Credits*

Instructed By

Dr. Reda A. Abdel-Fattah of Boca Raton, Florida

Graduate Of

Oral-Facial Pain and T.M.J. Disorders Program at the
University of Medicine and Dentistry of New Jersey

Fees: $95 if paid 2 weeks in advance (add $25 for late registration)

Fig. 8–1   Learning to make the best of whiplash
Flyers for continuing legal education (CLE) credits. These courses were held in various locations throughout Florida in August of 1988.

the TMJ & Stress Center to "offer help and hope to fellow sufferers." Carr herself appears on radio and TV stations across the country and writes articles to educate the public. The Stress Center handles suicide calls from TMJ victims and provides information through a newsletter subscription. MyoData also offers support to dentists who want to treat TMJ disorder, and its catalogue advertises brochures, books, slides, charts, and videos on TMJ and whiplash.[37] Its brochure "Dentistry's role in whiplash injury" is touted as an excellent marketing piece to send to attorneys for referrals, one that discusses how damage occurs, symptoms, compensation, and dentistry's role. A yellow flyer from the Center reads:

STARTING OR PROMOTING A TMD PRACTICE?

At last – A two-day seminar that addresses the how-to's of building your TMD practice and ways to make the transition to a diagnostic practice or establish a new one. This seminar is a necessity for TMD doctors and their front office staff.

Integrity Seminars, Inc

presents

The Permanency of Whiplash

Catalog of Resource Materials

Various publications are catalogued including: *Evaluating TMJ Injuries* [240 pages], *Litigating TMJ cases* [412 pages], *Anatomy and Physiology for Lawyers* [376 pages], all published by Wiley Law Publications.

Seminars are held regularly in various states.

Fig. 8–2   Making sure whiplash stays permanent

The treatments employed to remedy TMJ disorder are innumerable and not infrequently disastrous.[38] Harold T. Perry, a director of a TMD and Facial Pain Center and editorial chairman of the *Journal of the American Dental Association (JADA)* reports that over half the patients he sees in clinic have an "[iatrogenic TMJ] disturbance because of surgery, unnecessary [crowns], unwarranted restorations, orthodontics, and most frequently, incorrect splint therapy. These difficult situations seem to arise from the practitioners who have had sporadic, single-concept 'Hilton University' weekend TMD education."[39]

Owen Rogal, executive director of the American Academy of Head, Facial, and TMJ Orthopedics, is an enthusiastic promoter of whiplash as a cause of TMJ disorder. He reported that 80 per cent of victims of motor vehicle accidents with whiplash also have trauma-related TMJ dysfunction from which they may never recover.[40] But even Rogal seems shocked at the results of some of its treatments:

In the name of dentistry, we have seen a whole host of assorted treatments being heralded as "the answer" to the treatment of temporomandibular joint problems. One by one, we've seen them pass in and out of vogue, casting much despair and disillusionment upon the entire field of temporomandibular joint orthopedics.

Among those "cure-alls" have been: cortisone injections into the temporomandibular joint, bite-raising appliances, occlusal equilibration, wiring of the upper and lower teeth together, hard and soft splints, soft diets, nutrition, tranquilizers, spray and stretch exercises, vapocoolant sprays, [various electrical stimulations], ultrasound, arthroplasty, condylectomy, menisectomy, biofeedback, pull forward splints, pivot splints, Gelb splints, maxillary splints, mandibular splints, kinesiology, chiropractic, osteopathic, physical therapy manipulation, cranial-sacral manipulation, Alexander technique, arthroscopy, psychiatric treatment, exercises, rest, orthodontics, crowns and bridges, overlay partials, iontophoresis.[41]

The frenetic professional activity surrounding TM joints motivated epidemiologists to look more closely at these controversial joints. They found that the clicks and discomfort that dentists were using as diagnostic of TMJ disorder are extremely common in non-patient populations. In ten such studies of non-patient populations performed in Western industrialized countries, the prevalence of the signs and symptoms of TMJ disorder ranged from 28 per cent to 86 per cent.[42] Clearly, many people live with the clicks and discomfort and do not bother to report them either to their dentist or their doctor.

You might suppose that these epidemiological findings would have cooled the therapeutic ardour of the TMJ specialists. Not at all: they put these findings to profitable use. The epidemiologists had revealed vast realms of untapped pathology crying out for professional attention. Flyers went out to lawyers advising them of the large numbers of people with TMJ disorder in need of treatment.

A doctor and a dentist in New York went one better. They did not rely only upon epidemiologists to point out the large numbers of people who have TMJ symptoms. They demonstrated that even people with no symptoms and no abnormal clinical findings also have TMJ problems. Using questionnaires, they selected subjects who had absolutely no jaw symptoms. They examined these subjects and selected 26 who showed no signs of any jaw problems. Then, using "advanced bioelectronic technology" (a myo-monitor), they studied the functioning of the jaw muscles and demonstrated *muscle dysfunction* in 81 per cent of the subjects. With virtually universal TMJ pathology waiting in the wings, the public health authorities could dump as many barrels of fluoride into the water supply as they wished; there would still be inexhaustible work for dentists![43] In contrast to the advocates of intervention, other clinicians spoke out against the excessive treatment of TMJ disorder.[44] Consensus among the responsible experts on both sides of the Atlantic seems to be that little is actually understood about the functioning of these joints and that usually the least treatment given to them the better they are.

The least treatment the better! Nevertheless a host of new investigative devices have been developed in the last ten years "to provide objective evidence of temporomandibular joint disease." They include computerized jaw-tracking, sonographic recordings of the noises of the joint, thermography, Doppler recordings of the blood flow within the joint, and electromyographic recordings from the surrounding jaw muscles.[45] Besides an almost total lack of reliability, the one thing all these expensive devices have in common is that they show many false positive results. Like the myo-monitor by which its inventors were able to demonstrate "muscle dysfunction" in 81 per cent of subjects specially selected for the apparent normality of their jaws, these new devices support a diagnosis of disorder when no disorder exists.

Diagnostically hopeless these devices may be, but the International College of Cranio-mandibular Orthopedics seems determined to see them used. In 1987 the College passed a resolution virtually mandating their use. Entitled *Third Party Reimbursement*, the resolution states: "The only truly objective means of such diagnosis, treatment and validation for TMD is electronic diagnosis of the musculature and craniomandibular relationship. The use of the instrumentation and technology presently available consisting of electromyography, [nerve stimulation for relaxation of muscles], and mandibular tracking provide a purely objective compilation of data not heretofore attainable and should not only be encouraged, but insisted upon."[46]

The use of these devices has not escaped responsible concern. In 1994 the American Food and Drug Administration (FDA) convened a panel of sixteen scientists to evaluate these diagnostic devices. They concluded that the devices were not effective for the diagnosis of TMJ disorders and that their use could lead to over-diagnosis and unnecessary treatment. The American Dental Association (ADA) tried to set guidelines for their use in the assessment of insurance reimbursements for whiplash-induced TMJ disorders, but Rogal and other members of the American Academy of TMJ Orthopedics obtained a restraining order in the Federal Court to prevent the ADA from doing so.[47]

Although the wealthy whiplash experts successfully muzzled the ADA, eleven leading Canadian academic dentists, safely above the 49th parallel, spoke out about the *Third Party Reimbursement* resolution: "Statements such as this give the impression that the techniques advocated have been shown, in controlled clinical trials, to be unequivocally superior to the physical examination, analysis of symptoms and conventional treatment. To our knowledge, this is not so. Furthermore, they imply, erroneously, that clinicians who do not avail themselves of this technology do not treat their patients in an acceptable manner. In fact, this argument has been used in a malpractice suit in the United States."

The eleven Canadian dentists conclude their letter: "Thus in our opinion, these instruments [new diagnostic devices] do not yet have a proven value in the diagnosis and treatment of TMD, and their use for purposes other than research could lead to misdiagnosis and over-treatment of patients."[48]

James Berry, editor of *ADA News*, in cooperation with the ADA Division of Scientific Affairs, described TMJ disorder as "dentistry's *hottest* area of unorthodoxy and out-and-out quackery."[49] However, the ADA, per-haps hampered by threatening litigation, has done little to combat the treatment excesses by dentists that result from the use of these devices. Cranio-mandibular centres process the jaws of whiplashed clients in large numbers.[50] Rogal claims to have processed 6000 of them.[51] Insurance companies underwrite the large costs of these investiga-tions. Litigants are pleased to collude, for the greater the attention paid to their jaws the more serious will the courts consider their injuries to be. By the time a patient's jaw has been showered with atten-tion, fitted with splints, or worse, had surgery, he probably very gen-uinely does have TMJ disorder. However, the collision did not cause it!

An editorial in the *Journal of Craniomandibular Practice* – "TMJ impair-ment: the $64,000 question" – states in its opening paragraph: "Doctor, would you give us your professional opinion as to how much physical impairment your patient has experienced? This question, like the ones posed in the old game show, may literally be worth $64,000 to the patient, his attorney, and/or the insurance company involved."[52]

Whiplash's involvement with TMJ disorder is no accident. Much pro-fessional effort has been invested in insuring the stability of their union. Whiplash's marriage to TMJ disorder sharpened whiplash's legal bite, and sharpened it enough that the 28-year-old receptionist who, although almost certainly originally had little wrong with her TM joints, now stands in danger of requiring artificial ones.

9

Whiplash Rescues
Some ENT Surgeons

For every age is a dream that is dying, or one that is coming to birth.
– Arthur William Edgar O'Shaughnessy

This wonderful epigraph was written about the rise and fall of empires; it is perhaps flippant to apply it to the fluctuating dreams of medical practice, yet even in this realm such dreams arise and fall away. Ear, nose, and throat surgeons were once the financial princes of the profession. Tonsils and adenoids made them rich; anxious parents brought their coughing and runny-nosed children to ENT surgeons (laryngologists) to have them out. In the 1930s and early 1940s between one-half and three-quarters of both North American and British children had had tonsillectomies, or, as they have been dubbed, "remunerectomies."[1] Then, in the years following World War II, medicine became, at least in patches, a little more scientific.[2] Epidemiologists collected statistics – uncomfortable data showing that tonsillectomies did not decrease the number of coughs and colds, but they did decrease the child's resistance to some serious diseases.[3]

The tonsils and adenoids are nature's first lines of defence against microbial invasion of the body. It can hardly have been surprising news that it is not sensible to remove them, but good sense is seldom a priority in treatment decisions. In the 1960s, as information about the unfortunate effects of tonsillectomy trickled down to the public through *Readers Digest* and *Ladies' Home Journal*, parents stopped taking their children for tonsillectomies. For ENT surgeons the dream of the good life was evaporating.

Greener pastures were needed. Some ENT surgeons became adept at placing small tubes through children's eardrums for the treatment of chronic middle ear infections; some took up cosmetic surgery; some became interested in allergy and twentieth-century disease. Others opted for whiplash.

Among the symptoms that whiplash patients frequently complain of are dizziness, deafness, and tinnitus (buzzing in the ears), three complaints that are also the cardinal symptoms of inner ear disease or injury. ENT surgeons got a foot in the door. In the United States there are about a million new whiplash cases a year, a number that approximately equals the number of children who had previously undergone tonsillectomy.[4] ENT surgeons tapped into this alternative source of patients, using their new testing device, the electronystagmograph (ENG).

The ENG measures nystagmus, small jerky movements of the eyeball that can indicate damage to the vestibule of the inner ear or its neural connections in the brain. (The vestibule is the half of the inner ear that is concerned with balance. The other half is the cochlea, which governs hearing). Nystagmus can be hard to perceive but after the ENG came on the market in the mid-1960s it became easy to detect and record.[5]

With the help of the yet untested electronystagmograph, ENT surgeons demonstrated that about half of all whiplash claimants have nystagmus. Surgeons then set out on a quest to find the injury that caused it. Whiplash victims suddenly needed extensive investigations and treatment. Some years and many millions of dollars later, it transpired that the ENG results on which the ENT surgeons had based their diagnoses of vestibular injury were meaningless. Half the population at large have the same ENG results as do whiplash claimants. Once again, in their enthusiasm to discover evidence of physical damage, researchers had neglected to use controls.

How did ENT surgeons manage to keep themselves well remunerated while looking for an injury that was not there? Gay and Abbott had reported that subjective vertigo (a grand name for dizziness) is one of the many nervous symptoms that can complicate whiplash. In fact, dizziness is such a ubiquitous complaint, that no one had paid much attention to it. ENT surgeons had shown no interest in whiplash at all. In 1958 Braaf and Rosner, the meticulous delineators of whiplash symptoms, threw in vertigo along with a hodgepodge of other non-specific ENT symptoms: "Rhinorrhea [running of the nose], clogging of one or both nostrils, disturbances of smell and/or taste, [nose bleed], tinnitus, vertigo (especially on movement of the head), temporary deafness, neuralgia of the nose, neuralgia of the ear, irritation or pain in the throat, hoarseness, yawning, and [difficulty in swallowing]."[6]

As the demand for ENT surgery ran short, whiplash dizziness looked more appealing; the surgeons staked out their territory by means of articles on whiplash for medical journals. Since citation is an excellent indicator of an article's impact, I have chosen the most frequently cited for discussion. Again, I have arranged them chronologically to make it easier to follow the way that ENT surgeons seem to have convinced themselves and almost everyone else that whiplash was a cause of vestibular malfunction.

The story begins in 1968 with W.E. Compere, an ENT surgeon from California, who wrote in *Laryngoscope*: "Dizziness is one of the common distressing symptoms resulting from so-called 'whiplash' injuries. In about 50 per cent of these patients complaining of dizziness, abnormalities of the vestibular system can be substantiated by an examination utilizing nystagmography."[7]

Compere discussed some possible causes of whiplash dizziness, noting that injury to the neck, "with or without fracture dislocation," can produce vertigo. He observed that deaths had been reported from chiropractic manipulation of the neck, and that such manipulation can cause brain damage by interference with its blood supply. He raised the possibility that whiplash dizziness was also caused by interference with the blood supply to the brain stem – the part of the brain that has nerve connections to the vestibule – and that this interference was not caused by direct trauma (as in chiropractic manipulations) but by scar tissue and spasm in the injured neck muscles. The shortened muscles compressed the subclavian artery and so reduced blood supply to the brain.

For nystagmus that persisted despite conservative treatment Compere recommended a surgical intervention called "decompression."[8] This surgery involved cutting a neck muscle and making a "meticulous dissection" of the tissues around the subclavian artery and brachial plexus. Ward Wilson Woods, a neurosurgeon from San Diego, California, who had already perfected this operation on 227 whiplash patients, performed the surgery on Compere's patients.[9]

With the new ENG results, Woods and Compere treated ten cases of whiplash dizziness by decompression.[10] In all cases dizziness was relieved as well as "blurred vision, pain and numbness of the neck, shoulder and arm, and difficulty with memory and concentration." The authors concluded: "The ENG provides a new and important method of demonstrating objectively a vertebral-basilar arterial insufficiency of the brain stem following cervical trauma."[11]

Then Joseph Toglia from Philadelphia's Temple University Health Sciences Center, noting that Ommaya in his animal simulation experiments had not examined the inner ear for whiplash damage, looked for such damage in humans instead.[12] Toglia's team used the ENG to search for vestibular damage, and measurements of hearing loss to search for cochlear damage. They examined 116 whiplash patients and 119 head-injury patients. Thirty-seven per cent of the whiplash patients and 36 per cent of the head injury patients had nystagmus (an indication of vestibular damage), and about half of the patients had "frank audiological complaints ... describing various degrees of hearing loss or tinnitus."

L.Q. Pang, an otolaryngologist from Honolulu, also used the ENG to look for inner ear damage in twenty whiplash patients who had been referred for evaluation in the previous two years. Eighty-eight per cent had high-frequency hearing loss and 35 per cent had nystagmus. Pang praised the ENG's capabilities: "Prior to the use of ENG, it was difficult to evaluate the symptoms because there were little or no objective signs to account for their complaints. However, with the ENG, it is now possible to find objective evidence and signs to account for the symptoms of dizziness in a great percentage of cases."[13]

Wallace Rubin an otolaryngologist from Tulane University, New Orleans, commenting on the "tremendous increase in the incidence of orthopedically confirmed whiplash injuries of the neck," used the ENG to confirm vestibular injury in 50 per cent of whiplash patients, sometimes as long as three years after the automobile accident. His whiplash cases must have kept him busy, since he reports that he examined the majority of these patients more than five times during the two years following their injury.[14]

Then in 1973 M. Hinoki and his team from Tokushima University came up with yet another explanation for the "abnormal" ENG findings. In the very early 1970s Japan had a large output of whiplash articles. These researchers noted that there were already three well-supported theories on the cause of whiplash dizziness (the theory of sympathetic nerve irritation, the neck reflex, and the theory of circulatory disorders of the vertebral artery). They added a fourth: "over-excitement of cervical proprioceptors due to whiplash injury."[15] (Proprioceptors are sense organs in muscles and ligaments that measure tension.)

The Hinoki team studied 43 whiplash patients, of whom 21 had vertigo and lumbar pain, and 22 had vertigo without lumbar pain. They used corsets to immobilize the waists of all their subjects. This immobilization improved the vertigo in 17 of the 21 patients with lumbar pain but only in 5 of the 22 patients without pain. On the strength of their findings (though I don't know why) the Hinoki team suggested that treatment of whiplash dizziness be directed towards the lumbar muscles. In particular they recommended procaine injections into tender spots of the soft tissues of the back.

In a 1977 study, Paul van de Calseyde and his team of Dutch colleagues compared the ENG data they obtained from 916 whiplash patients referred to them for medico-legal purposes with the data they obtained from 137 applicants for a pilot's license. The tests were considered positive in 102 out of the 916 whiplash patients (11.1%) and 15 out of the 137 applicants for a pilot's license (10.9%).[16]

Did these Dutch surgeons use the ENG on the pilot applicants to add scientific respectability to their assessments and more guilders to the bill? It would be difficult to find a more *normal* group of controls than applicants for a pilot's licence. The ENG had been in clinical use for ten years and this appears to have been the first time that normal people were tested. The 0.2 per cent difference between the whiplash claimants and the pilot applicants in statistical terms is no difference at all. The surgeons demonstrated convincingly, and evidently to their own surprise, that the ENG results, which everyone had assumed to indicate vestibular damage, indicated no such thing. Normal people showed just as many "abnormal" responses as people who had supposedly been injured.

If science gets in the way of treatment, it has to go. Despite this dramatic demonstration that "abnormal" ENG results are no indication of vestibular damage ENT surgeons merrily continued to report whiplash as a common cause of vestibular damage. Cecil Hart, a maxillofacial surgeon from Northwestern University, Illinois, is one example. Introduced by the editors of *Medical Trial Techniques Quarterly* as having "impeccable medical qualifications," Hart continued to declare the invalidated studies of Woods and Compere, and of Rubin to be confirmation that whiplash causes physical injury. He added: "Traumatic vestibular impairment [from whiplash] continues to be a matter of great concern, to patients, to physicians, and to attorneys. This problem is often accompanied by damage to the central nervous system, which in turn is frequently associated with psychological disturbance. In addition, both these factors can react upon the vestibular system, making the exact evaluation of the impairment more difficult."[17]

Despite the continuing endorsement of ENG's ability to demonstrate the destructive power of whiplash by doctors with "impeccable medical qualifications," the cat had slipped from the bag and ENG results now looked somewhat threadbare in court. It was time for a new diagnostic test for vestibular injury: the ENT surgeons soon produced it. Robert Grimm at the Neurological Sciences Center, and ENT colleagues in Portland, Oregon, used the new technique of moving platform posturography (MPP), by which they were able to diagnose fistulas (holes) in the vestibule. They claimed that these fistulas allowed the escape of fluid in the vestibule (perilymph) and so caused perilymph fistula syndrome (PLFS). This syndrome is, among other things, an alleged cause of dizziness.[18] Grimm and his team needed patients for their research.

Whiplash and minor head-injury claimants have many complaints but no demonstrable pathology. They are the standard human guinea pigs on whom to apply these sorts of new tests. The Portland doctors examined a series of mild head-injury patients, and (lo and behold!) out of 389 patients they diagnosed 167 as having PLFS.[19] Thirty-two of the 102 PLFS patients selected for further review gave a history of whiplash injury without loss of consciousness, while the remaining 70 patients had a direct head injury with or without loss of consciousness. The four most common symptoms attributed to PLFS were "disequilibrium, headache, memory loss and tinnitus," symptoms that are popularly attributed to whiplash.

The surgeons treated all 102 PLFS patients, regardless of their illness duration, with a six-week program of strict bed rest to control fluctuations of pressure across the fistula and so allow for healing. Patients who were not cured by bed rest were offered surgery. Forty-four patients (66 fresh ears) were operated upon and the presence of the fistula was confirmed in 90 per cent of them. The surgeons reported, "Even when diagnosed late, a good-to-excellent outcome was achieved in 70 per cent of the treated patients." I will return later to the subject of these demonstrated fistulas.

As a Canadian chiropractor, Don Fitz-Ritson is the odd man out in this series of ENT practitioners. He comments on the difficulties that chiropractors face in assessing vertigo, including the prohibitive cost of equipment such as the ENG. He describes a poor man's method of assessment. The patient, sitting on a swivel chair, is asked to shake his head vigorously from side to side with his eyes closed. Some patients vomit during this procedure, and Fitz-Ritson sensibly suggests that the doctor stand behind the patient. Induced vertigo indicates injury either to the vestibule or to the muscles and joints of the cervical spine. To differentiate between the two, the patient is asked to close his eyes and rotate the chair with his feet from side to side while the doctor holds his head still. If the patient now suffers from vertigo it will originate from the tissues of the cervical spine.

Fitz-Ritson reports on 235 "cervically traumatized patients" [whiplash] of whom 112 proved positive to his "poor man's assessment." Fifty-seven patients were examined within three months of the accident, and the rest were examined later. Most of the patients had "prominent upper cervical joint fixations as revealed via motion palpation." The patients were given standard chiropractic treatments; after 18 treatments, more than 90 per cent were symptom free.[20]

Still on the search for whiplash pathology, W.R. Oosterveld and his colleague from the University of Amsterdam examined 262 patients with "traffic light disease," 87 per cent of whom complained of some type of vertigo.[21] On assessing the patients six months to five years post-accident with extensive testing including the ENG, they found that over half had nystagmus. When 41 patients were retested one to two years later, the tests remained positive. The authors inferred that there had been "no significant change in the severity of the pathology." They concluded: "The results of our survey emphasize the importance of nystagmographic examinations in patients suffering from central nervous system complaints originating in cervical whiplash injuries." This despite the fact that fifteen years previously their fellow countrymen had shown these results to be meaningless.

Enthusiastic healthcare practitioners catch diagnoses from each other. Soon John Chester, an ENT surgeon also from Oregon, was diagnosing PLFS. He again used moving platform posturography (MPP) to investigate whiplash damage to the inner ear. He examined 48 whiplash patients referred to a centre for the management of chronic pain. Finding twelve with PLFS, he treated seven with tympanotomy (cutting of the eardrum) and repair of a fistula. He writes of these cases, "The aural, visual and autonomic symptoms along with the protracted illness behaviour have an understandable physiological basis and therefore can be more efficiently treated." He comments: "Nine out of ten whiplash patients will respond to routine care; the tenth will require extraordinary management."[22]

Chester's findings were used to give yet another lesson in the media's continuing education program to the public on the multifaceted and deleterious effects of whiplash. The *Executive Health Report*, under the title "Whiplash Injuries: New Hope for Whiplash Victims," gave extensive exposure to Chester's work:

In an 8 mph rear-end accident, your head can be whipped by a force of up to 5 g – or 160 feet per second – within one-quarter of a second. Even at low speeds, such vast acceleration forces can cause significant injuries … Many whiplash victims show no obvious neck injury or neurologic damage, yet complain of discomfort for years. Now a clinical study by John B. Chester, MD Salem Hospital, Oregon, sheds new light on the whiplash syndrome. In 48 whiplash patients he examined, over half had damaged inner ear structures. Apparently the oscillation forces of the car collision caused the hitherto undetected injury. Faulty inner ear functioning can result in disorders including poor muscle control of balance and erect posture.[23]

The public gets well educated on whiplash and while the articles by ENT surgeons are persuasive on the surface, from a scientific point of view they are all fundamentally flawed. All but one study failed to use control subjects. Van de Calseyde and his colleagues were the exception, but they added the control group by happenstance and not by design. Lacking controls, the authors blithely interpreted their positive test results as indicative of vestibular injury. Both Toglia and Grimm, finding equal numbers of positive test results in their head-injury and whiplash patients, even concluded that acceleration/deceleration forces of whiplash are as potent a cause of damage within the skull as is direct head injury. Grimm and his colleagues naïvely inquire: "Who would have believed that such injuries can arise from whiplash alone?" Of course, the answer to their rhetorical question is, "No one." Their test results failed to demonstrate injury in either group of patients. Their method is analogous to finding that 30 per cent of head-injured and whiplash patients have blue eyes and then being surprised that whiplash, like head injury, causes blue eyes. Medical practice is cunning when it comes to demonstrating disease, although too often its logic is surprisingly unsophisticated.

The authors of these studies unconscionably juggle apples and oranges. Every one of them equates the effects of whiplash in humans to the horrible injuries found in animal-simulated whiplash. Pang does the usual fear-mongering about whiplash. Augmenting the horrors of animal whiplash, he describes the Tom and Jerry version of whiplash: "a sudden and forceful flexion of the neck, followed, in some instances, by several less violent oscillations of the neck and alternating flexion and extension."

How is it that the treatments these practitioners recommend for dizziness were all effective yet they all predicated the dizziness on totally different pathologies? Compere and Woods, by decompression of the subclavian artery, cured 92 per cent of their patients; Hinoki and his colleagues, with their lumbar corsets, cured 80 per cent; Fitz-Ritson, using standard chiropractic treatments, cured 90 per cent; and Grimm, by repairing fistulas, achieved a 70 per cent good-to-excellent result. Too many explanations produce too much success. It doesn't make sense.

Most of the symptoms that humans experience do not indicate that anything is physically wrong that needs putting right; they have such symptoms for a multiplicity of other reasons. Winning a personal injury suit is often one of them. Even allowing for the natural tendency of doctors to inflate their cure rates, there is no reason to doubt that most of the patients' dizziness did remit. But not, I expect, for the reasons claimed by the practitioners. With their various investigations and treatments, these practitioners *scientifically* authenticated the presence of an injury. The claimant was then assured of compensation. With this uncertainty removed, he was free to recover. Of course, the more radical the treatment the alleged injury required, the more effectively the treatment fulfilled its purpose and the greater the recovery was likely to be. *If he needed surgery on the artery to the brain, most certainly he must have been seriously injured.* Woods, with his major neck surgery, did best; he cured 92 per cent of 227 patients. However, the fact that a doctor thinks a treatment works is not proof that it works in the way he thinks it does.

The concern with the objective validation of injury is of no incidental occurrence. Medico-legal considerations perfuse these articles. All the practitioners equated their positive test results with objective evidence of injury. All the authors took pains to point out that their objective findings confirm that the claimant was neither a malingerer nor a neurotic.[24] Some of the authors make the converse observation; claimants with negative test results were either fraudulent or neurotic. For instance, Compere reported that the 22 per cent of patients with normal nystagmogram (i.e., with no evidence of physical injury) "gave evidence [during their assessments] of severe emotional disturbance."

The ENG *scientifically* separated the sheep from the goats – the truly injured from the neurotics and malingerers. By its ability to do so, the ENT surgeons' ENG far surpassed any psychiatrist in diagnostic acumen. It also did more than print out nystagmograms: it printed out money as well. With its aid, surgeons lucratively certified thousands of whiplash claimants as authentically injured. The courts, always suckers for scientific gobbledygook, with due solemnity accepted the surgeons' spurious reports. (If you don't believe me perhaps you will after you have read the chapter on junk science.)

Another issue lurks between the covers of the ENT surgeons' reports. What about the confirmation of the fistulas' presence by surgery? A fistula is either there or not there. Or is it? The middle ear, besides being very small and surgically somewhat inaccessible, has much in common with a dank subterranean cavern. Mucosal sweat drapes the walls and, even when the inner ear is not leaking, it often looks as if it is – everything is wet. Perhaps only a miniscule troglodyte exploring these ruby chasms could be certain, but *interest determines perception,* and it is apparently easy, especially with the blind eye of faith, to see fistulas when they are not there. Faith leads many people astray!

John J. Shea, an ENT surgeon from Memphis, reports that during the course of thirty-nine years of surgical practice and more than 36,000 otological operations he has never seen one such fistula. He sets about debunking the fistula myth:

I believe that the modern interest in spontaneous perilymph fistula began in the minds of a small group of "true believers" who expanded this belief into a cottage industry of locating and closing "leaks," with the decline in the number of operations for otosclerosis and chronic otitis media. In my opinion, the myth of spontaneous perilymph fistula has become a "cancer" eating the credibility of otolaryngology. This myth has become so accepted that one is in danger of being sued for not exploring for spontaneous perilymph fistula, even when the patient has only the meagerest signs and symptoms, if he or she later gets into the care of one of the "true believers." ... I simply do *not* believe the reported sightings of spontaneous perilymph fistula, just as I do not believe the reported sightings of flying saucers.[25]

Dizziness, tinnitus, and deafness are the three primary signs of inner ear disease (as anyone with Menière's disease well knows), but the reverse is anything but true. These three exceedingly common symptoms are only occasionally associated with any demonstrable physical pathology.

Kurt Kroenke from Health Sciences, Bethesda, a leading expert on dizziness, calculates that in the United States, ten million visits to physicians are made each year on its account. "Next to fatigue, dizziness may be the most common non-pain physical complaint seen in primary care, yet like fatigue, dizziness remains a diagnostic and therapeutic gadfly."[26] Kroenke and his colleagues found a higher lifetime prevalence of psychiatric disorders in patients with dizziness than in matched controls. They estimated that psychiatric disorders were a primary or contributory cause of dizziness in 40 per cent of dizzy patients.[27]

Tinnitus is common. "Epidemiological studies suggest that up to 18 per cent of the adult population may experience a significant degree of tinnitus," but the buzzing often becomes bothersome only in situations of psycho-social distress. Tinnitus can loom large in a depressed person's life, but relatively seldom can any actual physical cause for it be found.[28]

Many people have hearing loss, commonly from middle ear infections of childhood, or inner ear damage induced by occupational or recreational noise. A recent study in Britain of 500 randomly selected conscripts for military service showed that 14 per cent had hearing loss, and all these conscripts were relatively healthy young men.[29] Hearing loss, especially for high tones, increases with age.

The ENT surgeons took these three ubiquitous symptoms, and, on the pretext that they can indicate brain or inner ear damage, turned them into money. Whiplash dizziness and tinnitus are indeed in the head, but only in the way that the rest of the world understands it. John Norris, a Toronto neurologist, is unequivocal: "Tinnitus, deafness and nystagmus rarely if ever occur in whiplash; the dizziness is a vague subjective disturbance seen in anxiety states or depression, and is not true vertigo. The main symptoms of whiplash, headache, sensitivity to light and noise, fatigue and impotence, are shared by patients with depression and not trauma."[30]

We are all adept at deceiving ourselves. How conscious were the surgeons of their ploy? Rubin, for one, sought to absolve the surgeon from any responsibility for the court decisions. He writes:

As an expert witness, the physician should not be cast in the role of bias towards either plaintiff or defendant. As in all other situations, the physician should merely report the facts based upon the objective, completely unbiased evaluation ... ENG recordings are absolutely essential as part of the complete work-up for such patients ... After the evaluation, the physician can state that the findings are consistent with the accident and with the patient's complaints. It is up to the judge or jury to decide on the veracity of the patient's history in relation to the accident."[31]

The judge or jury, having no reason to question the reliability of the ENG and no knowledge of how common dizziness is in the population at large, understandably assumes whiplash is the culprit. The plaintiff has his complaints authenticated, the lawyer wins his case, the ENT surgeon earns his fee (and with an easy conscience), and whiplash is confirmed to the world at large as a cause of yet another physical injury.

Perhaps you think I have portrayed ENT surgeons as too knife-happy, but we have already seen that maxillofacial surgeons operate on healthy TM joints, and that orthopaedic and neurosurgeons repair innocuous prolapsed intervertebral discs. There is no reason to think ENT surgeons any better than their surgical confreres; in fact, there is reason to suspect the opposite.

Again, it has to do with the story of tonsillectomy. Not only did tonsillectomy generally fail to do what it was supposed to do but it was an operation that induced a high rate of psychological disturbance; and it also had a substantial mortality.[32] The British Ministry of Health's *Inpatient Inquiry for 1962* scrutinized tonsillectomy and found its mortality to be 13 per 18,356 operations.[33] In the United States, mortality from tonsillectomy was even higher. For every 1,000 American children who had their tonsils out, one child died and 16 were made seriously ill.[34]

Although there were well-recognized indications for tonsillectomy, these indications were mostly ignored and the operation performed on the basis of other criteria. The American Child Health Association neatly demonstrated this disregard of the selection criteria. The association surveyed 1000 11-year-old children from the municipal schools of New York City. They found that 61 per cent had already had their tonsils removed; the remaining 39 per cent of the children were referred to physicians for assessment as to the advisability of tonsillectomy. The physicians recommended tonsillectomy for 45 per cent of the children and rejected the rest. The rejected children were referred to another group of physicians, who selected 46 per cent of them for tonsillectomy. The rejected 55 per cent were in turn sent to yet another group of physicians who selected 44 per cent of them. After three examinations, only 65 children (6.5%) remained for whom tonsillectomy had not been recommended. The experiment was discontinued because there were no more school physicians left to examine the children.[35]

In the case of tonsillectomy, the decision to operate seems to have been made on a percentage rather than a clinical basis. Against this background of rote decision-making, I do not suppose that the questionable indications for whiplash surgery were a problem. Surgeons like to operate, and almost certainly the victims of whiplash were eager to be operated on. I do not mean to single out surgeons for special censure. Traditionally, in medical practice, we all carve out our own niche by which we seek to make our livelihood. Sometimes our patients benefit and sometimes they don't, but in the case of the surgeon, the carving out of a niche inevitably involves the carving up of the patient as well. Is this really any worse than having one's mind messed up by inappropriate psychotherapy?

A.J.E.M. Fischer and his colleagues, ENT surgeons at St Jans Hospital in Weert, Holland, thoughtfully and thoroughly reviewed the otological findings after whiplash injury. With their understated comment, they deserve the last word: "The methodology of most of the reported studies is far from perfect."[36]

10

Whiplash: Head Injury or Legal Headache?

There are two sorts of recovery: legal and medical;
the one occurs at the expense of the other.
– An insightful lawyer

We have all been willing witnesses to the marriage of psychology and the law;
we have all been wilfully blind to the dreadful offspring they have spawned.
– Margaret A. Hagen[1]

In the 1950s, when Aspirin was still a standard cure for headaches, Americans consumed more than forty tons of it every day, an adequate testimony to how common headaches are.[2] Headaches that occur following rear-end collisions are attributed to whiplash, and whiplash headache has grown into a big topic – the book *Whiplash and Related Headaches* is over 1000 pages long.[3] It is true that whiplash can cause headache, but, as days turn into weeks and weeks into months, other causes of headache become more likely. At least a dozen explanations have been put forward for the persistence of whiplash headache, but the very number of these explanations calls their validity into question.[4]

Anyway, I will spare the reader the murky politics of whiplash cephalalgia and deal instead with the huge legal headache caused by post-concussion syndrome. This syndrome may be a complication of severe head injury but it is much more common after small bangs on the head and after whiplash.[5] Its symptoms include headaches, memory problems, fatigue, anxiety, irritability, concentration difficulties, and a labile mood – symptoms that last for months or even years.

Numerous authors report that brain damage is a frequent complication of minor collisions.[6] Other investigators have compared closed-head injury patients to whiplash victims and found that their head-injury symptoms are identical.[7] Victims and their lawyers often attribute post-concussion syndrome to brain damage.[8] But is that attribution accurate?

Ommaya and others produced gross haemorrhage and severe brain damage by inducing whiplash in monkeys.[9] When a collision is sufficiently forceful, humans occasionally sustain similar brain injury.

Indeed, Ommaya himself described two such cases: one, a 62-year-old physician who, while waiting at a stop light, was unexpectedly rear-ended by a fully loaded 10,000 lb truck travelling at about 30 mph; the other, a middle-aged woman who drove into an immovable barrier. Over the next few days, both the physician and the woman developed signs of bleeding under the covering membranes of the brain (subdural hematoma). The physician's condition was relieved by surgery and he returned to work five months after his accident. The woman died.

These patients and the animals in the whiplash simulation experiments sustained brain injury because of the magnitude of the forces acting on their brains. There was nothing mysterious about the intracranial pathology in these two human victims. Both developed the classical signs of an intracranial bleed that even a third-year medical student could be expected to diagnose. But do post-concussion syndrome claimants involved in minor collisions also have brain damage? Do they perhaps have "traumatic brain injury"? The exemplary case of Mr Smith and Mrs Jones may cast light on the question.

Mr Smith is driving home from the office. He is wondering whether his wife will have cooked him supper after the mean things he said to her at breakfast. Mrs Jones, his neighbour, on her way back from a visit to her doctor to replenish her weekly supply of pills, turns into her driveway but forgets to signal. Mr Smith knows that Mrs Jones never signals but he is thinking about roast beef and distractedly runs into the back of her car. Mrs Jones and her car both seem okay, but Mrs Jones goes to law. She claims that she was a well and happy woman before the collision but that now she has a constant headache, her memory has gone, she cannot concentrate, and she is so totally exhausted that she cannot do her housework, let alone go to work. Some people think that Mrs Jones's brain was well pickled before the accident, but did the collision damage her brain? Are all her numerous symptoms now due to traumatic brain injury?

It is not possible to refute categorically that the collision caused damage to Mrs Jones's brain. Plaintiff lawyers tend to think in terms of – "If it can happen, then why not?" In contrast, competent physicians think in terms of probabilities – "How likely is it that brain damage occurred?" To approach these questions some background information about head injury and the various issues involved will be helpful.

There are two categories of head injury: penetrating and closed. In the first, a bullet or sharp object penetrates the skull and injures the brain. Such injuries are not our concern. Closed-head injuries are caused either by a direct blunt blow to the head or by an acceleration/deceleration force. They vary in severity from minor (mild) to very severe, with degrees of severity in between. Clinicians usually use one of two classification systems to establish the probable severity of the head injury – the one based on the length and depth of the resulting coma (Glasgow Coma Scale), and the other based on the duration of post-traumatic amnesia.

Post-traumatic amnesia (PTA) is the loss of memory for the events surrounding the head injury, consisting of the period of coma (if there was any), a period immediately before the injury, and the period after it, which more or less coincides with the duration of the post head-injury confusional state. A PTA of 5 to 60 minutes pigeonholes the closed-head injury as mild, while a PTA of more than one month puts the head injury into the category of very severe.[10]

According to the Glasgow Coma Scale, roughly speaking, the head injury is considered minor if the coma lasts twenty minutes or less, and very severe if it lasts six hours or more.[11] In either classification system the presence of a focal brain injury, demonstrated either by localizing neurological signs or by brain imaging, makes the head injury by definition severe.

Over the last few years an additional category "mild head trauma" has crept into general use. A diagnosis of mild head trauma needs no loss of consciousness or PTA. Usually it is a lawyer who makes this diagnosis and it may be followed by prolonged and severe symptoms. The degree of severity of a head injury does not necessarily correspond to the extent of its objective recovery, but the levels of severity do provide useful guidelines. About 30 per cent of severe-head-injury survivors make a good recovery while 70 per cent continue to have problems of varying degrees.[12] Everyone involved in a case of severe-closed-head injury is likely to accept the authenticity of ongoing difficulties, and compensation will be awarded accordingly. The prognosis for the lesser degrees of closed-head injury, on the other hand, provides endless grounds for legal quibble.

Medical opinion has traditionally held that minor head injury is seldom associated with permanent brain damage, and its symptoms resolve within three or six months. However, it has been recognized that recovery from minor head injury is often delayed when the injury is compensable or if the patient has a previous history of neurosis.[13]

All this changed in the 1970s, when some psychologists transformed themselves into neuropsychologists. They devised and used tests to assess the cognitive functions and abilities of patients with severe head injury. These psychometric tests revealed a reduced capacity of cognition, attention, and memory, even in some patients whom the clinicians considered to have made a full recovery. The neuropsychologists' findings usefully provided a physical explanation for why some severely head-injured patients have difficulty in returning to the demands of their pre-accident lives.

Encouraged by their success, neuropsychologists extended their assessments to patients with minor closed-head injuries and then to patients with mild head trauma. They soon ferreted out an array of deficits and confidently attributed them to previously unrecognised brain damage. They loudly proclaimed that the extent of brain damage in the milder degrees of closed head-injury had been vastly underrated.[14]

Neuropsychologists, along with the other healthcare practitioners who provide rehabilitation services for patients with severe closed-head injury, lobbied for funds to provide their services to these minor-head-injured patients as well. Their cause was strongly supported by many journal articles espousing a structural-damage explanation of post-concussion syndrome.[15] Steven Mandel, chief of neurology at Mount Sinai Hospital, Philadelphia, in his "Minor Head Injury May Not Be 'Minor,' " can act as spokesperson for this emergent viewpoint.

Minor head injury is a major health problem, one that is often not recognized by the patient's family and employer. Because litigation frequently follows injury, the validity of the patient's complaints comes under question ...

Postconcussion syndrome develops in 50 per cent of patients with minor head injury. Its major features are headache, dizziness, and neuropsychological defects. Fatigue, impaired concentration, poor memory (especially short-term memory), enhanced irritability, emotional instability, intolerance to noise, loss of libido, and the presence of depression or mania are also characteristic findings ...

Injury to the left side of the brain, such as the left frontal lobe, causes difficulty with verbal processing, judgement, problem solving, and verbal memory. With injury to the right side of the brain comes an indifference reaction, unwarranted optimism, insensitivity to others, loss of perspective, and inappropriate self-criticism.[16]

Mandel reports that each year 320,000 people in the United States seek medical attention for minor head injury. He describes it as "an organic disease having objective abnormalities that necessitate early neurologic testing and treatment to prevent serious complications." (Even if there were going to be serious complications, it is difficult to fathom exactly what neurological tests or treatment would prevent them.) Such testing does, however, provide a lot more work for the profession!

From the early days of whiplash, healthcare practitioners have tried to link whiplash symptoms to brain injury. Shapiro and Torres, neurologists from the University of Minnesota, noting that 62 per cent of whiplash victims are reported to have suffered a loss of consciousness, looked for evidence of whiplash brain damage. They studied 47 consecutive whiplash claimants, none of whom had a prolonged period of unconsciousness – though some reported a momentary loss of consciousness lasting for a matter of seconds (certainly not long enough to put them anywhere near the category of even minor head injury).

They found that 45 per cent of their patients had moderate or marked abnormalities in the EEG at some time during the period of their study. Another 30 per cent had mild to minimal changes. They concluded: "In view of the present study and the high incidence of abnormalities in the EEG, it is possible that in some patients, at least, the apparent psychoneurotic symptoms are organically determined and are symptomatic of underlying brain injury … If EEGs are not obtained, no evidence will be forthcoming of the changes going on in the brain. In many instances the doctor will be deprived of this valuable information."[17] (The information is certainly valuable insomuch as the doctor can charge a great deal for it in a medico-legal report).

Other specialists had taken up the search for brain damage in post-concussion syndrome. Radiologists used CT and MRI scans but failed to find anything. It was against this background of failure that the neuropsychologists' success was so spectacular. Healthcare practitioners are competitive. The neuropsychologists were the new kids on the block and, with their sensitive tests that could demonstrate brain damage in minor head injury, they quickly won their spurs.[18] They had succeeded where others had failed; they had legitimized post-concussion syndrome as a physically based condition and, in doing so, had legitimized themselves as well.

Whiplash plaintiff lawyers were naturally delighted with the neuropsychologists' test results. The lawyer for Mrs Jones, the pill-popping woman who was rear-ended by the distracted Mr Smith, is no exception. Although no brain damage showed up on extensive physical investigations, psychometric tests performed two years after the accident have revealed problems with attention and memory, and some unexpectedly low scores. Since Mrs Smith was seen jumping out of her car immediately after the accident, she clearly did not lose consciousness; however, it is claimed she had some PTA. She reports having lost all memories of the accident, her first memory being some thirty minutes later when she was reviving herself with a stiff whisky.

Armed with this evidence of brain damage and a sheaf of journal articles tucked under his arm, Mrs Jones's lawyer has little difficulty in convincing a judge and jury that his client suffered brain damage in the collision. The award is large. Mrs Jones claims recompense for lost earnings and payment for the domestic service needed to help clean the house and prepare meals. Since she has lost her libido, her husband also requires compensation – for the loss of his wife's companionship.

Did Mrs Jones really sustain brain damage in the accident? In North America over the last two decades or so, plaintiff whiplash attorneys and burgeoning numbers of healthcare practitioners have developed the rehabilitation of minor head injury into a thriving multibillion-dollar industry; whiplash accident victims are an important source of its raw material. Many whiplash plaintiffs, even following the smallest of rear-end collisions, claim brain damage; and many psychiatrists, neurologists, psychologists, and rehabilitation specialists validate the presence of traumatic brain injury. Such allegations are easy to make but difficult to refute. Nevertheless, there is little hard evidence to support such claims and many good reasons to suspect they are false.

Gay and Abbott reported that 31 of their 50 whiplash patients had "historical or symptomatic evidence of cerebral concussion." It is this figure of 62 per cent that Shapiro and Torres quote as a reason to suspect whiplash brain injury. But did these patients really suffer loss of consciousness? In Gay and Abbott's account: "These patients suffered a momentary lapse of consciousness (from seconds to one-half hour). They describe a blinding or explosive sensation in the head at the time of the crash. Some recovered consciousness after the car was driven ahead several hundred feet by the impact, and sometimes the car was still in motion when they recovered consciousness. Immediately after the accident they had the sensation of being bewildered, stunned, dazed, or dull. Headache usually developed within a few minutes or hours."[19]

Certainly any patient with a half-hour lapse of consciousness (especially if it is confirmed by a witness at the accident scene) has had a *bona fide* minor closed-head injury, but what about Gay and Abbott's other "concussed" patients? Most of them did not, in fact, lose consciousness or even memory for the accident event. There is an old medical adage: "A concussed man does not know the blow that felled him." The Gay and Abbott patients remember their blow because "they describe a blinding or explosive sensation in the head at the time of the crash." They do not have any PTA because they remember both the blow and what they felt like immediately after the accident; they reported the "sensation of being bewildered, stunned, dazed, or dull."

Seldom indeed do present-day whiplash claimants have a loss of consciousness confirmed by a witness at the accident scene, though many lay claim to such a loss, along with amnesia for the accident – an amnesia that may take on a life of its own and increase in length over the months and years with the telling.

Like other people in relatively minor traffic accidents, whiplash victims swap addresses and insurance information. Mrs Jones, for instance, not only hopped out of her car immediately after Mr Smith had run into her back bumper but her level of cerebral functioning was such that she was able to leave Mr Smith in no doubt that he was responsible for the accident.

Most authors of whiplash studies make no mention of either loss of consciousness or PTA, so there is little reliable information as to how commonly these two conditions occur in whiplash. However, Richard Mayou and his psychiatric colleagues at Oxford University are an exception.[20] They studied post-traumatic stress disorder in relation to road accidents (see chapter 15); they were looking for the presence of intrusive memories of the accident and therefore paid particular attention to their patients' recall of the accident event.

A group of 74 "whiplash injury victims" consecutively examined at the Radcliffe emergency department in Oxford were their subjects. Thirty-seven per cent appear to have remembered the accident only too clearly, for they reported "horrific" intrusive memories of it. Another 62 per cent reported "not frightening" intrusive memories of the accident, and 3 per cent reported no intrusive memories. The authors do not make clear whether the 3 per cent reported "no intrusive memories" because they did not experience their memories as intrusive or because they had amnesia for the accident. I suspect it is the former but, even assuming that the 3 per cent of patients had amnesia for the accident, the investigation still demonstrates that amnesia in whiplash is unusual.

The brain is our most precious organ, and it is reasonable to have concerns that it may have suffered subtle but undetectable damage. A plaintiff lawyer may point out that loss of consciousness and PTA are only arbitrary conventions used by physicians to estimate the probable extent of brain damage induced by head injury. The possibility exists that traumatic brain damage may occur without either the loss of consciousness or PTA. While again it is impossible to prove the lawyer wrong, certain evidence makes this suggestion unlikely.

The parts of the brain most vulnerable to whiplash are the tracts of white matter that run the length of the brain. Strong acceleration/deceleration forces can shear the neural axons that comprise these tracts of white matter, causing "diffuse axonal injury" or DAI. DAI is associated with a general loss of brain function. Does such an injury occur in rear-end collisions?

Thomas Gennarelli and his neurosurgery team from the Universities of Pennsylvania and Glasgow studied this injury.[21] Using whiplash simulation, they subjected 45 monkeys to acceleration forces varying both in intensity and direction; they sacrificed the monkeys and looked for DIA. They found DIA only in those monkeys whose coma had lasted for more than fifteen minutes. They commented that the DAI in their experimental animals was identical to that seen in humans after a severe head injury. It is reasonable to deduce from this study that with short periods of coma no detectable injury occurs in the human brain.

Monkeys are not humans, and perhaps lesions other than DIA also impair brain function. However, some telling evidence that human whiplash is an unlikely cause of brain damage comes again from demolition derby drivers. The effects of brain injury are cumulative. Professional boxers, especially after a lifetime of losing in the ring, get punch drunk; they develop boxer's dementia. If whiplash causes brain damage, then the brains of derby drivers are also subjected to repeated trauma since as I have already mentioned, on average each driver is involved in about 500 severe collisions during his crashing career. These drivers show no evidence of brain injury.[22] Sceptics may suspect that the victims of whiplash, with their litany of complaints, are soft in the head, but all brains are of similar consistency, so it is difficult to see why one small collision should cause brain damage in one person when 500 large collisions do not cause it in another.

Nevertheless, gigantic efforts are made to demonstrate the presence of brain injury in whiplashed humans. No one can accuse healthcare practitioners of laggardness in putting the advances of science to profitable use. Here are the results of post-concussion studies using the two most recently available brain investigation techniques.

Single Photon Emission Computed Tomography (SPECT) imaging is a sophisticated (and extremely expensive) technique that monitors changes in blood flow to the various areas of the brain. Nils Varney and his colleagues from Iowa City used SPECT imaging to investigate the brains of mild head-injury patients.[23] They selected 14 mild-head-injury patients who were reported to have had an excellent work record before their head injury but afterwards showed "indecisiveness, absent-mindedness, poor planning and inflexibility," and had been unemployed for at least five years. The authors call them the "miserable minority" of mild-head-injury patients.

Two of the 14 patients had sustained their head injury in a whiplash accident and both reported a PTA of ten minutes. The other 12 patients had blunt direct head injuries with a mean PTA of 5.7 minutes. In most cases any loss of consciousness was self-reported.

The CT and MRI scans, and most of the cognitive tests on the 12 patients, were normal. The investigators chose five controls matched for age from among the hospital staff, "selected expressly because they had vocational success and no history of head injury or mental disorder to complicate the interpretation of their SPECT scans." The authors found some of the minor-head injury subjects had reduced blood flow in certain areas of the brain; the controls showed no such abnormality.[24]

What do these impressive results mean? As with most whiplash and minor-head-injury studies, the study is riddled with problems. Although the investigators report that their fourteen subjects had "well-established premorbid adult histories of responsible employment of five-years' duration" they also note that the neuropsychological test results showed that five subjects had "developmental dyslexia," a disorder strongly associated with adjustment disorders. All the subjects were selected precisely because they were the "miserable minority" of minor-head-injury patients, while the controls were selected precisely because they were psychiatrically well. Again, the researchers were comparing apples and oranges and attributing the differences to injury.

The SPECT results obtained from the minor-head-injury patients were virtually identical to those obtained in SPECT studies of depressed patients.[25] Since the investigators had deliberately selected depressed head-injury patients, their results are not surprising. However, in keeping with this genre of study, the investigators attributed the abnormal findings not to depression but to brain injury. They write: "For the patients in this study, SPECT evaluation has resulted in reclassification of their symptoms from 'psychiatric/neurotic' to 'neuropsychological'; the result of head trauma ... Thus the SPECT can be used to identify and reclassify behavioural problems as being the result of head trauma and thus enable patients to receive head trauma rehabilitation interventions." In other words some insurance company will have to pay the healthcare practitioners for providing "head trauma rehabilitation." It will not be cheap.

Although SPECT had spawned an abundance of published reports, well-controlled trials are singularly lacking. The 1996 Report of the Therapeutics and Technology Assessment Subcommittee of the American Academy of Neurology, an unofficial watchdog of scientific rectitude, states: "The scientific literature does not now support the routine use of SPECT for evaluation of patients with closed head injury or postconcussion syndrome."[26] Notwithstanding the academy's admonition, Bicik, Radanov and other members of the Swiss group of investigators with the record number of whiplash publications, citing the

"the enormous economic implication" of whiplash brain injury, used SPECT scans to examine the brains of whiplash claimants. They too found the changes characteristic of depression, though they did comment on the connection with depression.[27]

Despite Shapiro and Torres's original claim to have found abnormal brain waves following whiplash, no investigators since 1960 have replicated their findings; but hope springs eternal in the plaintiff whiplash lawyer's breast. There is now a revved-up version of the EEG – the qEEG – which entails computed analysis of the brain waves. The technique, also known as brain mapping, is complicated, and the legal rather than the medical profession are its experts. The American Academy of Neurology advises that the qEEG has very limited use, "cerebrovascular disease being the one area in which these tests may fill occasional specific needs."[28] Needless to say, despite this stated limitation, the qEEG is now widely used in the investigation of alleged whiplash brain damage.

Brains are easily damaged, and I would be among the first to be po-faced about boxing and to insist that cyclists wear helmets. Nevertheless, although personal injury litigation lawyers would often have us believe to the contrary, the evidence is that brains are quite resilient (see appendix 3). There is no evidence to support the supposition that a minor head injury causes permanent brain damage. In a minor head injury there is (by definition) a loss of consciousness, which is, at least, objective evidence of brain involvement, while in alleged whiplash even such confirmation is (with rare exceptions) lacking.

Whiplash experts repeatedly allude to the injurious effects on the brain of the "g" forces created by small collisions, but there is ample reason to doubt the legitimacy of such pessimism (or optimism if you are with the plaintiff's bar). Murrey E. Allen and his colleagues from Simon Fraser University, in British Columbia studied the acceleration/deceleration perturbations of the head in subjects involved in the normal activities of daily living. Eight volunteers were fitted with helmets to which were attached tri-planar accelerometers. These accelerometers precisely measure the acceleration/deceleration forces acting on the head from all directions. The volunteers then performed thirteen common activities of daily living.

Plopping backward into a chair had the maximum effect. It produced a peak acceleration of 10.1 g (about twice the force involved in the average rear-end collision). The authors comment that the perturbations of the brain caused by the activities of daily living resemble the jostling of the brain that occurs in low-velocity whiplash accidents. The authors conclude: "With no-damage accidents, one can reassure an accident victim who has otherwise been frightened by rumours of horror and mystery that sometimes follow the MVA whiplash scenario."[29]

Compared to the paucity of evidence to support underlying brain damage as an explanation for a whiplash induced post-concussion syndrome, there is much evidence to support a psycho-social explanation for it. Post-concussion syndrome develops much more frequently after a minor head injury and after mild head trauma, than after severe head injury (see chapter 16). Stand on your head or do whatever acrobatics you like, it is difficult to explain this inverse correlation in terms of brain damage, but this inverse correlation is characteristic of psycho-socially induced illness.

Lees-Haley and Brown and other investigators have demonstrated the high rate of so-called post-concussion syndrome symptoms in non-head-injury patients and an even higher rate in non-head-injured personal injury litigants.[30] Here again are some of their prevalence figures for "head injury" symptoms in non-head-injured personal injury litigants: headache 88 per cent; irritability 77 per cent; sleeping problems 92 per cent; chronic fatigue 79 per cent; concentration difficulties 78 per cent, and memory problems 53 per cent. These non-head-injury litigants had no reason to think that they had anything wrong with their brains and neither had they anything to gain by reporting these symptoms. In contrast, whiplash litigants, having been told they have sustained brain damage, are more likely both to fear they have something wrong with their brains and to wish to exploit head-injury symptoms – two factors guaranteed to increase the reporting of such symptoms.

Whiplash claimants once in contact with the head-injury rehabilitation system soon learn all about brain damage and the symptoms that go with it. Watched kettles may never boil but watched symptoms soon start to bubble, and every anxious or angry allegedly head-injured litigant will conclude that his everyday symptoms – headaches, irritability, sleeping problems, chronic fatigue, concentration difficulties, and sieve-like memory – are caused by brain injury.

As an astute reader, you will have perceived that the post-concussion syndrome has all the makings of a fashionable illness, an illness which, of course, it has now become. Its sufferers often fondly call it "TBI" (traumatic brain injury) to emphasize the physical nature of the condition. With TBI, as with other fashionable illnesses, many of a patient's difficulties pre-exist the accident that has become their alleged cause. Needless to say, such information is carefully suppressed both by the patient and his lawyer.[31]

Sir Aubrey Lewis, the august psychiatrist at the Maudsley Hospital in London, neatly demonstrated in 1942 the presence of these pre-accident difficulties in post-concussion patients. He compared the past records of patients with post-concussional syndrome admitted to hospital to the past records of a group of patients admitted for neurosis but with no history of head injury. He found no significant difference in the pre-accident histories of these two groups of patients. Lewis concluded: "The striking thing is that the longstanding, relatively intractable, post-concussional syndrome is apt to occur in much the same person as develops a psychiatric syndrome in other circumstances without any brain injury at all."[32]

Once mild head injury (TBI/traumatic brain injury/post-concussion syndrome) became linked to whiplash, lawyers and head-injury rehabilitation experts lovingly nurtured this association so that it blossomed. The American College of Rehabilitation Medicine (always on the lookout for people to rehabilitate) confers the term "mild traumatic brain injury" on anyone who claims to have felt "dazed" or "stunned" from a whiplash accident – a diagnosis that leaves room for all whiplash patients to suffer from it.[33]

In Ontario, TBI received an unexpected boost when the provincial government, in a hurried attempt to curtail the rising costs of auto insurance, rewrote the Auto Insurance Act. The new Act established an injury threshold that had to be reached before an MVA claimant could sue for damages (see chapter 18). This threshold was a "permanent, serious impairment of an important bodily function caused by an injury which [was] physical in nature." No longer was it going to be possible to sue for aches and pains, or for depression and anxiety attributable to small injuries like whiplash.

Catastrophe! This new Act was a calamity to personal injury litigation lawyers and to healthcare practitioners in the rehabilitation industry. How could they possibly demonstrate that an undemonstrable neck injury had caused "a permanent, serious and physical impairment of an important bodily function"? The Act was a terrible threat to their incomes; something had to be done. The brain was the obvious solution. The brain performs "an important bodily function" and psychometric tests reveal an injury.

In October 1992, Rehabilitation Management Inc. chose Toronto as the location for the first major worldwide conference on minor head injury. Marilyn Dunlop, the health reporter for the (Toronto) Star heralded the conference: "Every year 50,000 Canadians suffer head injuries, primarily as a result of traffic accidents or falls. But it is estimated that at least twice that number go undiagnosed; the conference organizers say [the conference] is designed to make physicians more aware of hidden brain injuries and how to help."

The conference came up to expectations. Whiplash plaintiffs by the thousands were soon diagnosed as having TBI, and "Head-injury Rehabilitation Centres" became one of Ontario's fastest growing industries. These centres, colloquially known as "head-injury factories," mushroomed everywhere. Lawyers owned some of the centres and employed the neuropsychologists and other healthcare practitioners who worked in them.[34] Making the diagnosis of "hidden TBI" was a walkover. Canadian automobile insurers had gone from paying $200 million for rehabilitation services in 1990 to $1 billion by 1999, four-fifths of this sum going to Ontario entrepreneurs.[35] If doctors did as well at making their patients better as our medico-legal system does in making its clients worse, medicine would be a great profession.

The cognitive rehabilitation of the genuinely head-injured patient is hard work often requiring much professional care and dedication. It is much easier to rehabilitate head-injury claimants who do not have anything wrong with their brains. Whiplash claimants are ideal. Neuropsychological tests can be relied upon to demonstrate a brain injury, thus making large numbers of candidates with perfectly intact brains available for cognitive rehabilitation.

Not only are whiplash claimants ideal for head-injury rehabilitation centres; these centres are also ideal for the whiplash claimants. Group therapy is their favoured mode of treatment and, while group therapy can provide excellent mutual support for group members who are struggling to recover from a shared incapacity, it can also, and perhaps even more effectively, provide support for people who want to stay sick.[36] The sessions are seminars on head-injury symptomatology; the whiplashed are provided with in-depth discussions on the symptoms with which head-injury victims are expected to contend.

The whiplash claimants learn their lessons well. "A collision with a forensic neuropsychologist can be dangerous."[37] In fact, such a collision is often more far-reaching in its injurious effects than was the original accident. I have assessed some of their graduates who could not even remember where and when they were born, or the name of their spouse – the kind of memories that are the last to go in a profound dementia.

Two sets of investigators have studied the problem of cognitive brain damage in whiplash claimants. Ann Taylor and her colleagues from the University Health Network in Toronto provide an example of a study with an excellently designed methodology, while experts of the Swiss whiplash team provide an example of how not to conduct such a study.

Taylor and her colleagues psychometrically assessed fifteen consecutively referred whiplash patients with longstanding *head-injury* symptoms.[38] They compared their test results to the results obtained from patients in two control groups. One control group consisted of patients with chronic pain in whom there was no history of head injury, the patients being matched to the patients in the whiplash group for age, IQ, duration and intensity of symptoms. The second control group consisted of consecutively referred moderately to severely head-injured patients in whom the length of coma varied from three hours to three days. These *bona fide* head-injured patients, like the whiplash patients, had been referred for medico-legal assessment.

All the whiplash patients in Taylor's study had been symptomatic for at least four years. None had suffered any loss of consciousness or had been retained in hospital. They had been able to get out of their vehicle independently and conduct formalities with the police. All the patients complained of memory problems and other brain injury symptoms, and all had been awarded the diagnosis of *traumatic brain injury*.

In their battery of psychometric tests, the investigators included two tests of attention that are extremely sensitive to the effects of brain injury. All three groups of patients had low scores on these two tests, the mean scores of each group being about equal. Clearly, these tests that are customarily used to demonstrate brain damage are not specific to actual brain injury. In regard to their psycho-social level of functioning, the patients in both the whiplash and chronic pain groups had more complaints of physical and emotional dysfunction than did the patients in the *bona fide* head-injury group. More of the patients in the *bona fide* group had resumed their former occupation than had the patients in the whiplash and chronic pain groups.

The Taylor study nicely illustrates that the whiplash claimants with alleged head-injury have much more in common with chronic pain patients (see chapter 11) than with *bona fide* head-injury patients. The patients with genuine brain damage had fewer symptoms and claimed less disability.

Bogdan Radanov and other colleagues from the Department of Psychiatry at the University of Bern in Switzerland had previously reported a high incidence of cognitive impairment in whiplash claimants.[39] Such a finding has far-reaching medico-legal implications. These Swiss whiplash investigators sought to elucidate the association of whiplash and brain injury.[40] To this end they obtained 30 whiplash claimants (23 women and 7 men) with various long-lasting post-concussion symptoms referred for neuro-orthopaedic examination. None of the claimants had lost consciousness.[41] The mean time-interval between the accident and examination was 27 months. "None of the patients admitted to having current treatment with medication ... Prior to injury all patients felt fit for work and pursued their profes-

Headache	87
Dizziness	83
Tiredness	77
Poor concentration	73
Irritability	63
Blurred vision	57
Sleep disturbance	50
Forgetfulness	50
Sensitivity to noise	43
Anxiety	20
Sensitivity to light	37
Loss of control	16
Cervical pain	10

Fig. 10–1   Putting the blame on whiplash.
Incidence of head-injury type symptoms in whiplash claimants with no objective evidence of any head injury, percentages.

sions," but following their accident the patients were unable to work and were in receipt of generous disability payments from the Swiss insurance system. [42]

The Swiss investigators assessed the level of cognitive functioning by three means: the CFQ (Cognitive Failure Questionnaire: a self-assessment test), the Number Connection Test (consisting of numbered circles from 1 to 90 placed randomly on a sheet of paper which the patient is required to connect consecutively as quickly as possible), and the PASAT (Paced Auditory Serial Addition Task: a test of divided attention.) While a tape supplies an ongoing series of single digit numbers, the patient must mentally add up the numbers and provide the answers to the psychometrist. The psychometrist rates the speed and accuracy with which the task is learned and performed. The test results have been standardized using large numbers of normal people. If the patient is slow or inaccurate then something is assumed to be wrong with his brain; i.e., damage from a head injury. The results are shown in Figure 10–1.

The Swiss investigators found that the patients had high scores on the CFQ and significantly low scores on the PASAT. (Both results indicate cognitive difficulties.) They comment on the PASAT results: "The impaired divided attention in patients suffering from [post-concussion syndrome] suggested that whiplash could lead to neuropsychological sequelae in a considerable number of injured patients. This is remarkable because relevant head injury might have occurred in only a few of the investigated patients. The impaired divided attention might help explain the cognitive complaints of patients suffering from [post-concussion syndrome]. By trying to sustain attention and overcoming the problem, the patient may become fatigued and irritable, and headache can develop."[43]

The psychiatrists' attribution of fatigue and other symptoms of psychological distress to brain damage is guaranteed to delight both their somatizing patients and the referring lawyers, but as an explanation for the presence of such symptoms it is wrong. The authors note that it is "remarkable" that so many of the patients had head-injury symptoms when so few of them seem to have had a head injury. It is not remarkable at all. There is a perfectly adequate explanation for the findings.

No head injury is required to explain the presence of their patients' symptoms since these symptoms are frequently found in anxious and depressed people. Eugene Bleuler, the great Swiss psychiatrist, also described these very same symptoms more than half a century ago as the symptoms of neurasthenia.[44] And Lees-Haley and Brown found the same incidence of symptoms (in fact a little higher) in non-head-injury litigants.[45] In good whiplash tradition, the Swiss investigators had used no control group.

Psychometric tests show abnormal results in head-injured patients, but they show similar results in many non-head injured people as well. In addition, psychometric tests are *notoriously unspecific* for head injury.[46] Depression, anxiety, drug use and abuse, alcohol abuse, low IQ, somatic problems, and even pregnancy all are associated with abnormal results.[47] In fact, these other conditions are demonstrably a much more potent source of abnormal test results than is minor head injury.

The subject's attitude towards these tests is crucial. The tests are standardized on subjects committed to doing their best. Without an effort on the subject's part the test results are totally unreliable. The tests require considerable effort – they are a headache to do – and the personal injury litigant has no incentive to score well. Psychologist Julie Suhr and her colleagues from Iowa College demonstrated in 1997 that head-injured subjects who were identified as "probable malingerers" perform more poorly on these tests than persons with similar or even more severe head injuries, but who were not identified as malingerers.[48]

Financial disincentives also produce poor test results.[49] Pankratz and Binder, psychologists from the Oregon Health Sciences University, in reviewing these tests have estimated that approximately 20 per cent to 60 per cent of patients with mild head injury and financial disincentives demonstrate improbably poor performances on these kinds of tests.[50]

Of course, litigants, psychologists, physicians and lawyers sometimes deliberately use psychometric tests dishonestly, but honest professionals can also be misled by such test results. Psychometric tests appear so *scientific* that it is easy to equate them with x-rays and accept their results as infallible. Until a few years ago I naïvely did so myself. I abruptly learned better. I had assessed a middle-aged business executive with a multi-million-dollar claim for head injury. One sunny day, while driving his Audi on a country road with the sun in his eyes, he had had a head-on collision. He claimed to have been unconscious for at least half an hour and following his recovery he reported the symptoms of a severe post-concussion syndrome, the most distressing feature of which was an inability to perform at work at anywhere near his former level of achievement.

His lawyer had sent him for two neuropsychological assessments and the defence lawyer ordered another assessment. All three assessments gave much the same results. His IQ was average, at around 100, and the MMPI showed a wide spread of psychological dysfunction. Something was amiss. This man was an MBA graduate from Harvard who, before the accident, had had a successful career as an executive in a large corporation; his test scores should have been well above average. There was some suspicion that heavy alcohol use contributed to his poor performance but, as did the other expert witnesses, I accepted that his reduced mental capacity resulted from brain damage consequent upon a severe head injury.

Then, at least for the defence attorney and the insurance company, a miracle occurred. The case, having dragged on for years, was soon to be heard in court. In anticipation of his being free to work again, the plaintiff had applied for, and successfully obtained, an executive sales position in a multinational corporation. He had advised the corporation president of the upcoming trial stating that he could not take up his new appointment until the trial was over. Under the circumstances, the president requested that a neuropsychologist of the corporation's choosing should also assess the plaintiff's level of functioning to ensure his capacity to perform his new duties. By chance, the defence lawyer heard of this fourth assessment and subpoenaed the results. The businessman had an IQ of 142 and a normal MMPI, though with a somewhat high reading on the psychopathy scale. The president was delighted with the test results. His new executive was exceptionally bright and, since sales people with raised psychopathy scores on the MMPI tend to do well in their careers, his new executive of sales was well matched for the job. I lost my innocence about the reliability of neuropsychological test results.

In a more formal demonstration of the unreliability of these tests, Larry Bernard, a neuropsychologist at Loyola Marymount University,

Los Angeles, randomly divided student volunteers into two groups.[51] The students in one group were asked to respond to the tests as if they had been head-injured in a traffic accident, and the other group served as controls. Each volunteer was neuropsychologically assessed for over two hours. The volunteers in the group mimicking head injury scored significantly lower than did the control group.

Bernard reasonably concludes: "Neuropsychological memory tests are vulnerable to faked deficits." He also found that the volunteers simulating head injury endorsed more symptoms than did the controls, and the simulating students automatically attributed the overwhelming majority of these symptoms to their alleged head injury. Bernard observes: "The process of personal litigation affects patient behaviour in ways that serve to undermine the validity of psychological assessment procedures, increasing the number of false positive findings which resemble neuropsychological impairment or brain damage."

Henry Berry, the Toronto neurologist who studied demolition derby drivers, also studied pseudodementia occurring in the context of accident litigation. Some of the alleged dementias were attributed to whiplash.[52] Pseudodementia is a condition in which the patient exhibits all the symptoms of dementia, but has no actual brain damage or disease to account for it. Berry selected a group of 30 patients with pseudodementia whose mean age was 39 years. They had each been involved in a motor vehicle accident for which they claimed compensation. For the most part, these patients had had no loss of consciousness. The average length of their illness was 45 months.

Misinterpretation of neuropsychological test results formed the basis for a misdiagnosis of brain damage in 27 of these 30 patients. Berry described how these patients revealed their pseudodementia:

They differed from the brain-damaged patient in that their intellectual difficulties had either not changed from the outset or had worsened. This was in striking contrast to the usual time course of gradual improvement from the immediate post-accident state to a stable level of disability. They differed also in that some of their disabilities were of a type seen only with the severest brain injury and after a coma of days or weeks. They differed in that their difficulties were selective, unusually severe, with preservation of other intellectual functions, and their interview behaviour was usually out of keeping with their symptoms and professed disability. Although the majority of patients did have a family physician somewhere in the background, their [legal] counsel had often effectively assumed control of their management.

Psychological tests to demonstrate malingering are now available.[53] In one such test the patient is presented with a series of questions in which he can choose one of two possible answers – one right and the other wrong. The questions are so easy that even severely brain-damaged patients have little difficulty in selecting the right one. A subject who has genuine difficulty with the test and is guessing the answers is right half the time; his score averages out at 50 per cent. A patient who knows the answers but opts for wrong ones in order to make himself appear brain-damaged scores significantly less than 50 per cent. Although these tests are reliable and easy to administer, few neuropsychologists choose to use them.[54]

Frank Kenny is both an excellent neuropsychologist and an excellent friend. He was one of the first neuropsychologists in Ontario to use tests for malingering in the neuropsychological evaluation of head-injury claimants. Here is one of his case histories in which these tests were diagnostically helpful.

The claimant in question I shall call "the Surfer." In his late 30s, the Surfer was the owner of a small coffee shop that had not prospered. One afternoon, while the municipality was repairing the road close to his shop, the Surfer reported to the local hospital that he had stepped into the hole in the municipality's sidewalk and was hurt. The ER doctor could find nothing wrong and sent him home.

Some hours later the Surfer's wife brought him back. She reported that on returning home from work she had found him in a state of confusion. On the second visit he did not appear cognizant of his surroundings and was unable to communicate in any sensible way with the medical staff. He was found to have a right hemiparesis (weakness of the right side of the body) which became progressively more obvious during his stay in the ER. Although there was no trauma about the head and face, and despite the fact that earlier he had given a lucid account of the incident, a head injury was diagnosed. He was admitted to hospital.

The doctors investigated him with every means at their disposal but could find no explanation for the hemiparesis. Neuropsychological assessment showed a "profound impairment" in virtually every cognitive system. He performed in the manner of an advanced Alzheimer's patient. Since nothing could be done, he was sent home to the care of his wife.

The Surfer retained a lawyer to sue the city. Because of the impending lawsuit, he was intensively investigated over the next four years. In his six-inch-thick file he had six neurological and four neurosurgical consultations, along with opinions from multiple rehabilitation experts, physiatrists, psychiatrists, and psychologists. He attended the Workers' Compensation Board Hospital Rehabilitation Program for many months but without improvement. Repeat neuropsychological assessment showed a pattern of deterioration. The examiners agreed the dementia was consequent upon traumatic brain injury, though they disagreed about the exact nature of the injury.

The defence lawyer referred the Surfer to Kenny for a defence neuropsychological examination. The Surfer walked with an impaired gait, taking several minutes to negotiate his way from the waiting area to Kenny's office. He wore a plastic sling and described his arm as having been totally useless for the previous five years. At first communication was difficult, but his speech improved sufficiently over the course of the interview for him to provide a long list of complaints.

On the psychometric tests he again performed in the manner of a patient with advanced dementia, most of his scores being at the first percentile or lower (out of 100 randomly selected people he would be placed at the very bottom). Noting the marked inconsistency between the Surfer's ability to provide a history and his inability to perform on the psychometric tests, Kenny added two tests to assess for feigned impairment. Both were strongly positive. All the previous examiners had accepted the Surfer's complaints and test results at face value.

Suspicious of the Surfer's impairment, Kenny tried to observe him leaving the building: while he had entered Kenny's office inordinately slowly, on leaving he vanished almost instantaneously. Kenny reported a diagnosis of *probable malingering*; the insurance company arranged for surveillance.

Two months later the defence lawyer's assistant brought over some photographs. He wanted Kenny to certify that the man in them was the same man who had attended his office. The photographs had been taken four weeks earlier from the shore of a lake 50 miles north of Toronto. The Surfer had been windsurfing around the beach area for a good part of a day and the entire episode was videotaped. Presumably he felt confident that no detective would follow him out of the city. He was mistaken. Fraud charges are seldom pressed in such situations and in this case no charge was laid, but the man dropped his suit against the municipality and agreed never again to bring forward such a claim.

It is unusual for spurious head-injury claims to be so dramatically refuted; most bogus head-injury claims slip by unexposed. Many claims for brain damage attributed to whiplash are allowed, but real whiplash brain damage must be exceptionally rare. Shapiro, Teasell, and Steenhaus are from the group of whiplash experts at the University of Western Ontario. In their writings this group strongly supports physical damage as the explanation for ongoing whiplash symptoms. However, in a recent review of mild traumatic brain injury these authors report that there is "little or no evidence for enduring brain injury after whiplash."[55] If even these friends of whiplash do not think whiplash causes persistent brain injury, then it almost certainly does not. Nevertheless, the absence of any such injury has not hindered the investigation and rehabilitation of whiplash head injury from becoming a multibillion-dollar industry!

Mrs Jones, the woman whom Mr Smith absent-mindedly rear-ended, claimed brain damage. In order to have Mr Smith pay for her damaged brain, Mrs Jones must show in civil court that the odds of his having damaged her brain are greater than 50:50 – 51 to 49 will win her the jackpot. I doubt though, if many competent clinicians would put the chances of Mr Smith having damaged Mrs Jones's brain at any more than 1 in 500. The burden of proof lies with the claimant, and civil courts, proud of their scales of justice, painstakingly weigh out the balance of probabilities. Not many betting junkies would be happy, on purely scientific grounds, with Mrs Jones's odds on winning, but she, along with most of the other Mrs Joneses of this world, won her case. How did she do it? Mrs Jones's lawyer referred her to a neuropsychologist who assessed her psychometrically. Mrs Jones's daily consumption of pills – often washed down with whisky – had slowed up her mental functions. She did not try hard on the psychometric tests; in fact, she even helped her case along a bit with a few wrong answers. She soon had a score of someone with dementia.

The neuropsychologist reported Mrs Jones's test results as compatible with severe brain damage. In personal injury litigation, anything that is compatible with an injury is caused by the accident; Mrs Jones was assumed to be *brain-injured*. After some expensive but futile attempts at brain injury rehabilitation, Mrs Jones's case came up for trial. In court, Mrs Jones cut a sorrowful figure, and the judge, commenting that the brain is a *sine qua non* of a human being, awarded her massive compensation. Her lawyer's bill was colossal and the neuropsychologist got paid well. Mrs Jones's "future did indeed come from behind." She left her tiresome husband with his incessant demands for sex, gave up her boring job at the department store, and retired to Florida.

Mr Smith did not have to pay for Mrs Jones's brain damage out of his own pocket; indeed he never even found out how the case ended. He did not care; his insurance company took care of everything – it is their profitable business to do so. Mrs Jones's brain injury was indeed a fairy story with a happy ending. The judge felt warm and benevolent; all the professionals involved in her case made good money; Mrs Jones enjoys the Florida winter, and Mr Jones, while appreciating his award for loss of matrimonial companionship, soon replaced his wife with a more amenable one. Thinking about roast beef can have unexpected consequences – although, not unexpectedly, everyone's auto insurance premiums inched up a fraction higher.

1 1

Accidents, Illness Behaviour,
and Chronic Pain

There is nothing like a little pain to take one's mind off one's problems.
– Snoopy

To think of a man as a machine does aid us in understanding
something about bodily function and about man's role in the universe,
but it does not follow that treating the body like a machine will heal it.
But medicine appropriated the idea as the premise for its practice.
– Rick J. Carlson[1]

Accidents most often happen because people make mistakes. An estimated 80 per cent of all accidents are due to human rather than machine error.[2] A World Health Organization study found that on average a driver commits one error every two miles.[3] Even people especially trained to be careful make mistakes. A study of hospital pharmacists showed that they made 1,371 errors in dispensing 9,846 prescriptions, an error rate of 12.5 per cent.[4] Community pharmacists do even worse. Investigators disguised as patients monitored 100 randomly selected community pharmacies; they detected 24 errors for every 100 prescriptions dispensed.[5]

Some people are constantly error-prone, while others are so only in particular circumstances: a raised blood alcohol, the consumption of tranquilizers, fatigue, anger, depression, boredom, excitement, psychological and social distress, male adolescence, and premenstrual tension being some of the more outstanding ones.[6]

Whether these errors cause accidents depends upon the situation. A housewife muddling the ingredients of a recipe ends up with a stodgy sponge cake, but a chemical engineer may end up with no factory. A plumber joining up the wrong pipes has hot water coming out of the cold tap, while a surgeon who mixes up pipes faces a huge lawsuit. Few of us have not driven absentmindedly through a red light and we perhaps owe it to our guardian angels that we are alive to tell the tale. Some of us, the Mister Magoos of this world, always seem to have accidents, while others seldom do.[7] Both industry and the insurance industry recognized the "accident habit" long before the medical profession took anything more than a passing interest in it.[8]

Human errors are responsible for untold numbers of deaths and injuries. In the United States, before World War II, 460 million man-days were lost to industry each year through accidental death and injury. There is nothing like war to make governments concerned about the health of their citizens. The National Safely Council estimated that had these accidents been prevented, when war was declared in December 1941, America would have had about double its instruments of war: 20 more battleships, 100 more destroyers, 9000 more bombers and 40,000 more tanks.[9] Personally, I am not much in favour of saving lives in industry so that more people can be killed in war, but such figures talk.

Relatively small numbers of people have relatively large numbers of accidents. Again under the influence of war, it was shown in a British munitions factory that 10 per cent of workers incurred 56 per cent of the accidents.[10] In a study of 1400 drivers in four large American industrial concerns, it was found that "a small number of drivers had multiple accidents whereas the majority had one or none." The accident-proneness of the multiple-accident drivers persisted over the years, often with diminishing intervals between their accidents; even when the accident-prone drivers were transferred to non-driving jobs they still had accidents.[11] One doctor dubbed these *born-to-crash* Mister Magoos as the "heartsink patients."[12]

Much of the medical profession's interest in accident-proneness started accidentally. Flanders Dunbar, a world authority on psychosomatic illness, along with a group of physicians at Columbia University Medical Center, decided to study the personalities of people who develop cardiovascular disease and diabetes.[13] To yield meaningful information, such studies require a control group, and the investigators chose as their control group the steady flow of patients admitted to the fracture ward. They made an unexpected discovery. It was not the heart and diabetes patients who had the interesting personalities and unusual premorbid histories; it was the fracture patients; they had had many previous accidents. Dunbar and his colleagues expanded their study to involve 1300 fracture and cardiac patients. Two-thirds of the fracture patients had had one or more previous accidents, while less than 1 per cent of the cardiac patients had had any accident at all.[14]

Errors are perhaps not the only cause of human-induced accidents. Several observers have suggested that people sometimes have accidents on purpose, even if unconsciously so. Freud, stringing some Greek words together, coined the term "traumatophilic diathesis" to denote the tendency some people have of *acting out* through accidents.[15] Alfred Adler, another big name in psychiatry, studied 130 workers with histories of repeated accidents, identifying in these accident-laden workers a "revengeful attitude" and a "longing to be pampered."[16] Dunbar and his colleagues described the case of a Roman Catholic penitent who avoided having to admit to the priest her use of contraceptives by unexpectedly breaking her hip on the way to confession.[17]

It is always difficult to know whether such anecdotal accounts by gifted and creative observers really reflect significant patterns in human behaviour, or if they are just eye-catching observations that illustrate the author's idiosyncratic perceptions of the human condition. Medicine is replete with so-called clinical impressions by charismatic physicians, which later are shown to have been disastrously wrong. Only well-designed epidemiological studies can provide reliable information about the connection of events to illnesses or accidents.[18] Such studies are expensive and difficult to perform; they are in short supply. However, the reasonably well-designed studies that have been undertaken suggest that some people have "accidents on purpose."

We have already seen that the consequences of accidents can be useful in all manner of ways, and since human beings are ingenious, it would not be out of character for us sometimes to deliberately instigate one to suit our purposes or at least put a fortuitous accident to profitable use.[19] The secretary slips on the office doormat and although she has no signs of injury, she insists that her hip is too sore for her to sit and type. Did the secretary fall on purpose? Is she really injured? Is she tired of having to bring the boss endless cups of coffee? It is difficult to know.

Making a minor injury work to one's advantage can be a challenge. Bodies are resilient and a minor injury soon heals. To ensure its usefulness, it is necessary to make a great to-do about the injury and ensure that its pain persists. Accident proneness and minor-injury enhancement are so entwined that I will deal with them together.

Being sick or injured is not just a question of going to the doctor and getting fixed up. Ill people behave in an assortment of ways. Cultural, ethnic, and family background, religious denomination, social class, personality, personal experience, and psycho-social circumstances all determine how a person responds to illness or injury.[20] Not surprisingly, sociologists find these diverse factors an irresistible subject for study and by the 1950s they had lots of interesting things to say about illness and behaviour.

In his classic study of reactions to pain, for example, Mark Zborowski found that Jewish and Italian Americans tend to respond emotionally and to exaggerate their pain experience, while the Irish and "old Americans" are more "stoical."[21] Talcott Parsons, professor of sociology at Harvard, and Henry Sigerist, professor of the history of medicine at Johns Hopkins Hospital, developed the concept of the "sick role" – the patterns of behaviour that people adopt when they are ill or hurt – or when they think they are.[22]

People who fear the dependency of illness often avoid doctors like the plague. At the other extreme are the patients who take to patient-hood naturally; they play the sick role with devotion and nurture every symptom with meticulous care. When not in hospital, they almost live in doctors' offices.

David Mechanic, a sociologist at the University of Wisconsin, pro-posed the now popular concept of "illness behaviour."[23] Mechanic defined this behaviour as "the ways in which given symptoms may be differentially perceived, evaluated and acted (or not acted) upon by different kinds of persons." He described the range of illness behav-iour as extending from "making light of symptoms, shrugging them off and avoiding seeking medical care," to "responding to the slightest twitches of pain or discomfort by quickly seeking medical care." When physicians talk about illness behaviour it is the "slightest-twitches" patients, the ones who pack their waiting rooms, that they have in mind. The "shrugging off" patients keep out of the physician's way. Out of sight, out of mind.

Such illness behaviour puts up the cost of health care, a problem that sociologists appropriately worry much about. Mechanic com-ments: "One of the prime functions of public health programs is to teach populations to accept, and behave in accordance with, the defi-nitions made by the medical profession." He is quite right. If patients behaved sensibly and went to the doctor when they should and, even more so, did not go when they should not, healthcare costs would go down overnight.[24]

While Mechanic clearly understands patient behaviour, he is less insightful about the behaviour of doctors. Doctors also vary in their ill-ness behaviour and some can be just as enthusiastic about illness as are their patients. To them even small injuries require a great deal of med-ical attention. They are delighted to have their patients tucked up safe-ly in bed, except of course, for a daily visit to the doctor. The right combination of patient and doctor can work wonders for a minor injury.

Most of us know only too well what pain is, but what do physicians think about it? If the pain from a minor injury is to be substantially prolonged, it is indispensable to have a doctor on-side. From a scientific point of view, pain is a subject that leaves much room for medical and legal controversy. Our traditional medical understanding of pain dates back to 1664, when René Descartes, philosopher and mathematician, proposed that pain, arising from "a diseased or broken body part," travels through "pain channels" to the brain.

The Cartesian pain model suited medicine's new mechanistic approach to the problems of the human body; physicians quickly adopted it. It was the doctor's task to discover the pain-provoking part and either to cure it or remove it. When cure or removal was impossible, the doctor dealt with the pain by escalating doses of analgesics. The injured victim whose complaints of pain continued could (and indeed still does) easily ensnare even sensible and responsible physicians into endless suppositions as to the cause of the pain and into prescribing astronomical amounts of opioid.

Three hundred and one years later, Melzack and Wall[25] refined the Descartes pain model by hypothesizing a conceptual "gate" in the spinal cord – an undoubted improvement on the Cartesian model since it better explains what we know about pain.[26] Pain impulses from pain receptors pass along nerve fibres to the gate in the spinal cord; if the gate is open the impulses pass on to the brain and into consciousness, but if the gate is closed, nothing happens – no pain is experienced. Various events close the gate. Nerve impulses from touch receptors close it. We all know that a knee banged on a coffee table hurts much less when given a good rub. Nerve impulses descending from the brain close it – a mechanism that allows hypnosis, emotion, and distraction to abolish pain perception. The pain of a sprained ankle is forgotten during a heated argument with the neighbour.

In any one second, over a million nerve impulses pass up the spinal cord to the brain; among them are the impulses from pain receptors, which, in a grumbling sort of way, fire off continuously. Fortunately, most of these impulses get lost in the crowd, but if anxious attention is focused on any part of the body, they get noticed. Pay attention to all the sensations from your thumb while you vigorously wiggle it around; it will soon hurt. All the neurophysiological mechanisms are in place for the pain of an anxious-victim-of-a-minor-accident to become chronic.

Acute pain is associated with injury, and healing with a decrease in pain intensity. Acute pain that persists becomes chronic pain. Pain authorities argue as to when this change occurs, some choosing six months, some three months; others, perhaps less arbitrarily, define chronic pain as any pain that persists longer than is normal for healing of the injured tissues involved.[27] Anyway, acute pain that persists becomes chronic, and it is the controversy over the nature of chronic pain that causes such medico-legal mayhem.

There are two sorts of chronic pain, and, although they are as different as a Starbucks and a McDonald's coffee, it is only in the last few years that they have been clearly differentiated from each other. Even today, many doctors and healthcare practitioners muddle them up, a muddle that has serious consequences both for the patient and for society, because, for its effective management, each sort of pain requires a diametrically opposite approach. Chronic pain, like acute pain, can indicate that something is wrong with a *body part:* tumours, inflammatory and degenerative diseases, various neurological conditions, and even, on occasion, injuries that fail to heal. Fortunately, this kind of chronic pain is usually amenable to relief by medical means, particularly through the wizardry of the pharmaceutical industry.

The chronic pain of a chronic pain syndrome (CPS) is entirely different. This pain is somatoform, and occurs, not from tissue injury, but in association with psycho-social distress. The CPS patient often conspicuously adopts the sick role along with all the concomitant illness behaviour. The pain of a patient with CPS seldom responds to analgesics, though patients often get hooked on the analgesics that their physicians prescribe in an attempt to stay the patient's complaints.

Chronic pain requires, if possible, treatment of its underlying cause, and appropriate pain control, whereas CPS requires an avoidance of medical intervention and the patient's restoration, if possible, to a more normal way of life. Treating a CPS patient as if the pain has a physical cause serves only to confirm the patient's conviction that his injury is unhealed and that he requires continued care. An injury victim who wishes to extend the consequences of a minor accident needs a practitioner who can be relied upon to muddle up these two kinds of chronic pain; such practitioners are a dime a dozen.

Patients with CPS usually complicate their diagnosis by simulating (unintentionally or otherwise) the signs of organic disease. Seldom, however, is it difficult to detect that they are doing so. CPS patients, especially males, are usually ham actors; they present to the doctor with glaringly obvious illness behaviour – grimaces, groans, holding of the breath, sighs, shifts of posture, and unrelenting complaints about their agony. Such a patient, like the Surfer, limps into the doctor's office, ostentatiously using a cane. On examination, inconsistencies are perceived in the degree of tenderness, weakness, and limitation of movements, and a claimed loss of sensation over areas of the body that makes neither anatomical nor physiological sense. These signs are in marked contrast to the more dubious physical signs that are invoked to support a diagnosis of underlying musculoskeletal damage. A doctor would have to be blind not to see the gross somatization entailed in the CPS patient's presentation, circumstances, and behaviour.[28]

Of course, doctors have good reason for not seeing. The patient expects the doctor to deliver an acceptable organic explanation for his pain, and any doctor who fails to find the expected pathology may well find an angry and threatening patient instead. Life is short and it is easier to live and let live. If the patient wants a physical explanation for his pain, then it is simple to concoct one; besides it is usually in the practitioner's interests to do so. Nevertheless, practitioners who treat CPS patients as if their pain were caused by persistent physical injury leave a trail of disabled patients in their wake.

While Hippocrates might not be happy with doctors who fail to distinguish between the pain of tissue damage and the pain of chronic pain syndrome, it has become politically incorrect to make the distinction. The International Association for the Study of Pain has 5800 members in over eighty countries. The association's definition of pain asserts: "Many people report pain in the absence of tissue damage or any likely pathophysiological cause; usually this happens for psychological reasons. There is usually no way to distinguish their experience from that due to tissue damage if we take the subjective report. If they regard the experience as pain and if they report it in the same ways as pain caused by tissue damage, it should be accepted as pain. This definition avoids tying pain to the stimulus."[29]

In other words, if someone says he has pain then the pain he has is real. Perhaps it is, and then perhaps it is not. Frequently a doctor asks, "On a scale of 1 to 10 (10 being the worst pain imaginable) how bad is your pain?" The CPS patient often gives an estimate of 10 or close to it. Now, I have never suffered serious injury, but the pain of even the small injuries incurred in everyday life seems intolerable; manifestly, such pain does not even approximate being the worst imaginable. I, for one, find it difficult to believe anyone can experience the worst pain imaginable while sitting quietly in a doctor's office. Certainly, there are excellent reasons for a doctor to acknowledge psychogenic pain, but that does not mean such pain should be accepted to be as real as a pain from an injury; to equate the two pains diminishes the significance of both.

David Bell, the Australian psychiatrist who reviewed the ravages of the Australian RSI epidemic, warns about the practical implications of turning the pain of CPS into real pain:

The failure to exercise responsible standards of diagnosis extends to the broad category of chronic pain without recognizable cause. Clearly, great difficulties attend the diagnosis of conditions, which are distinguished only by a subjective complaint, but they do not justify the current approach of assuming the pain [of chronic pain syndrome] is the equivalent of the real experience. The assumption has allowed many to ignore completely whether a complaint is unfounded. The failure helps to explain why pain without a recognisable cause has become a major burden for the healthcare services and compensation systems in developed nations ... Those who drew attention to the evidence of simulation or malingering for gain were stigmatised with derogatory terms such as "punitive," "authoritarian" and "extreme".[30][31]

Accepting the pain of CPS as the equivalent of pain from a tissue injury allows healthcare practitioners lucratively to prescribe unlimited treatments for a supposed injury, which perhaps explains the hostility directed at anyone who questions the propriety of conflating the two kinds of pain, and why the International Association for the Study of Pain seems so determined to equate the two.

It is difficult to make even a ballpark estimate of accidents that are deliberately engineered, or of minor accidents that are assiduously nurtured, but these numbers are high. Alexander Hirschfeld and Robert Behan, from Wayne State University, were, in the early 1960s, among the first to study accident-proneness and injury enhancement. Their subjects were 300 workers involved in industrial accidents, who were referred to them during the course of accident litigation. Hirschfeld and Behan took thorough psychiatric histories, and examined the events leading up to an accident and the role that physicians played in the subsequent evolution of the injury into chronicity and long-term disability.[32] They describe their findings in three *JAMA* articles, "The Accident Process":

Before the accident occurs there is a state of conflict and anxiety within the patient. As a result of this condition the worker finds a self-destructive, injury-producing act ... From this moment the patient reacts exactly as do other psychiatrically ill people, except for the character of his symptom. Instead of having a presenting complaint of anxiety, depression, or other classical psychiatric symptom, he has a physical disorder, a disorder which resulted from the accident ...[33]

Without this solution, financial and psycho-social bankruptcy faces them and the accident paradoxically represents both an emotional boon and a self-destructive psychological process. Such patients come to physicians because of their pain, but not for the purpose of getting cured ...[34] The symptom serves a purpose [and] the choice of the symptom is to hide the real problem ... Such patients run from doctor to doctor trying to get help they will not accept, because relief of the symptoms would refocus attention on real and too-painful conflict. They exhibit much hostility towards physicians with whom they never completely cooperate.[35]

Hostility provokes hostility. Hirschfeld and Behan comment that "to this witch's brew of hostility" is frequently added the physician's over-compensation for his anger at the patient who so frustrates his best therapeutic interventions. "Perhaps an extra x-ray, a myelogram, extra medication ... thus is born the multiple test procedure. Further, when the piqued anxious physician leans over backwards not to attack the patient in any way, he not only finds himself testing more and more in terms of laboratory procedures, but he tries new treatments. Perhaps a little traction will help. Perhaps another month of physiotherapy. And so is born the deleterious multiple somatic treatment which was shown to be so unsuccessful in the cases we reviewed."[36]

The degree of conscious intentionality underlying the production of somatoform symptoms is an ongoing debate. Hirschfeld and Behan found that many of their patients were well aware of the use to which they put their symptoms; some even had well-developed plans for a new business or a move to a better house once their case was won. Of the motives of the treating physicians, the authors were less certain: "Because we threw out all cases in which the doctors seemed consciously dishonest, we were left with those in which the physicians were ethical and well trained. Yet, predicated on insurance figures in our case histories, it is apparent that prolonged somatic therapy is financially rewarding to the physician. The average medical bill in these cases paid to the physician and his adjuvants was approximately the same amount as was paid to the claimant. We call attention to these figures in order to raise the question: Do physicians as well as patients also suffer the problem of unconsciously gaining from chronic illness?"[37]

Subsequent investigators of CPS consistently emphasize the same themes:

- The financial and social costs of the syndrome are enormous;
- The patient's problems antedate the designated cause of the pain;
- The pain persists for a variety of psycho-social reasons;
- Medical interventions do more harm than good;
- The lives of CPS patients revolve around pain;
- CPS patients provoke anger and distress in their caretakers.

Automobile accidents trail behind minor industrial accidents as a source of CPS, but whiplash is the second most common cause of accident-induced CPS. James Hodge, a psychiatrist from Ohio who first described this accident process in whiplash patients, suggested that the initial physical symptoms of whiplash were "captured" for psychological purposes upon which claimants then constructed and justified a new psychological equilibrium.[38] The healing time for most soft tissue structures of the neck is from a few days to a few weeks, which is about as long as whiplash neck pain lasts when uncomplicated by psycho-social and legal issues. However, thanks to whiplash's nefarious reputation, anyone involved in an auto collision who wants an illness has got one ready-made.

Hodge also found that whiplash patients who developed persistent symptoms have strong elements of hostility and dependency in their personalities. Many whiplash plaintiffs, like other CPS patients, use their pain as a camouflage for a legion of distressing difficulties. Orthopaedic surgeon David Florence, director of the chronic pain rehabilitation program at the Sister Kenny Institute in Minneapolis, also studied 300 patients with CPS. He reported that the most striking feature of these patients was that "they described their symptoms and behaved in a remarkably similar fashion." Florence found the physical and chiropractic treatments prescribed for them were ineffective. Indeed, some patients became psychologically addicted to them, showing signs of anxiety when the treatments were withdrawn. "Medication [with the exception of the antidepressants]" he wrote, "is the most devastating enhancer of the syndrome." While commenting that psychiatric treatment seems indicated, Florence found that "psychiatrists unfamiliar with these cases merely enhance symptoms with pills and standard psychotherapy, neither of which produces the desired behavioural change."[39]

Florence reported in addition that "a careful psychological examination, or even sufficient time spent with the patient," demonstrates that the real problems are psychological, social, economic and (in all probability) sexual. "CPS," he observed, "is most likely to originate among the 'worried well' – individuals who do not have significant physical problems but are actually programmed for any type of incident that will result in a reward system."

Florence also drew attention to long-entrenched patterns of self-defeating behaviour, which, under the debilitating effects of medical care, often progress to a state of angry "learned helplessness." CPS patients, he stressed, "are very demanding and often display anger, producing a panic-type reaction on the part of the treatment team. As these patients become more aggressive and belligerent, the errors of the reactive treatment by the medical team compound ... The greatest trap in treating the CPS patient is the inability of most physicians, in particular specialists, to perceive the difference between physical and psychological illness and to treat each in accordance ... By their logic and behaviour [CPS patients] have *literally manipulated and outsmarted the entire healthcare system to the degree that their treatment takes the largest single bite out of the health care dollar."*

Florence concludes that "[CPS] is not entirely within the realm of a physically treatable entity but rather a disease process existing at least partially in the patient's perception – an area that defies standard medical (most especially surgical) and psychiatric treatment." CPS patients may outsmart the entire healthcare system, but a substantial section of the system is content to be outsmarted. CPS patients bring in business.[40]

In a recent study, Jack Richman, medical director of a Canadian company specializing in medical evaluations, reviewed the medical evaluations of 3000 patients with chronic pain and other disabilities. In nearly half of these patients, he found evidence of the deliberate augmentation of difficulties. He also opines that many practitioners opt not to see this aspect of patient behaviour: "Society has held members of the healthcare profession in such high esteem that they have become unaccountable. A majority of healthcare workers continue to close their eyes to fraudulent behaviour, believing no one will challenge them. These manufacturers of disability need to be held accountable. They create illness in gullible populations and end up doing far more psychological harm than any accident ever could."[41]

Chronic pain syndrome is not all a one-sided battle. Some practitioners do what they can to reduce its disaster. The late John Bonica, a gifted anaesthetist, had good reasons to be interested in pain. He earned his way through medical school as the Masked Marvel, a professional wrestler, an occupation that left him with painful injuries requiring four spinal operations and countless hip and shoulder procedures. He was not impressed with the results.

Bonica became the director of a pain unit in Seattle in 1960. Believing that the standard medical care of chronic pain required reinforcement, he opened up the problems of chronic pain to the skills of many different disciplines. His unit, the Multidisciplinary Pain Center, became a Mecca for the treatment of chronic pain, and the University of Washington at Seattle became a world focus for the study of psycho-social aspects of chronic pain. The centre served as a model for the many multidisciplinary pain centres now established in other parts of the world.[42]

John Loeser, the present director of the centre, in an article co-authored with Michael Cousins, encapsulates the centre's views on chronic pain:

The preponderance of patients with chronic pain do not really have an identifiable aetiology. Physicians give these patients labels which fit the physicians' concepts of disease and human behaviour, but we really do not know the pathogenesis of most chronic states. Patients with chronic pain of unknown aetiology are often found to be depressed, deactivated and physically out of condition. The treatments they have received from a wide array of healthcare providers not only fail to lead to improvement but are often additional causes of chronic pain and disability. Inappropriate medications, poorly planned and executed surgical procedures, prescriptions for rest and inactivity, and the home and workplace environments are major factors in this type of chronic pain.[43]

The authors emphasize the array of environmental influences that are determinants of the continuing pain behaviours, determinants that very much include "the advice of attorneys in reference to the expectation of financial gain."

Wayne Katon, a distinguished psychiatrist associated with the centre, along with his colleagues investigated 37 patients admitted to the Seattle Center with CPS.[44] They found that the majority of patients had a history of one or more episodes of major depression and/or alcohol abuse before the onset of their chronic pain. The family histories revealed higher than expected incidences of a first-degree family member with chronic pain, mood disorder, or alcohol abuse. In other words, personal and family problems preceded the CPS rather than CPS being their cause as it is almost invariably claimed to be. Further studies on CPS from the Seattle Center and from teaching hospitals in England obtained almost identical data.[45]

Patients with CPS not only enmesh their own lives in pain, but they implicate the lives of others as well. Harvey Sanders, a pain expert from Vancouver, uses the mnemonic SHAFT for the characteristic of CPS patients:[46]

S   Sad
H   Hostile
A   Anxious
F   Frustrated
T   Tenacious

The mnemonic is particularly apt for institutions and individuals who, following a claimant's small mishap, suddenly find themselves held financially responsible for his entire life's suffering. They have been SHAFTed!

While the staff of multidisciplinary pain centres and other responsible healthcare practitioners struggle with the uphill battle to persuade CPS patients to get on with their lives and relinquish their pain and anger, our medico-legal system is intent on doing the opposite. It encourages patients to be overwhelmed by their pain and to stay sick and resentful. There are currently about 18 million lawsuits a year in the United States; chronic pain, along with the loss of consortium and life's pleasures, accounts for about 80 per cent of the awards arising from these lawsuits.[47] In the ever-fattening medico-legal briefs of minor accident victims, one medical report after another testifies that an injury is the cause of the litigant's ongoing pain.

The personal injury litigation lawyer lives off the awards granted to his clients. No judge is going to award substantial sums for an accident that has caused neither apparent injury nor any noticeable impact on the plaintiff's life. The lawyer, if he is to do well, must present his client as having previously lived an idyllic life that is now shattered by the accident and the unrelenting pain and suffering that it has caused. Of course, the plaintiff is delighted to have his problematic life presented in such terms. The accident messed up his life, not him.

The lawyer builds his case with diligence. He reminds his client that pains often worsen with time and informs him of the dangers of too early a settlement. He talks of the usefulness of a "pain diary" to ensure that no pains are overlooked.[48] He may suggest a change of family doctor, to one with a special interest in accident-induced pains who understands the need for rest and adequate amounts of painkillers. Some law firms have their own *in-house* family doctor while others have lists of practitioners who can be relied upon to support the plaintiff's pain. The plaintiff will be referred to specialists who, while meticulously leaving no diagnostic stone unturned in a search for hidden physical injuries, discreetly avoid mention of the patient's longstanding emotional and social problems.

Undoubtedly the specialists with their new high-tech investigations will find abnormalities. They will make alarming diagnoses and recommend time-consuming treatments. The large doses of analgesics and tranquilizers they prescribe make the patient somewhat soporific and forgetful.[49] With such excellent encouragement, the plaintiff is soon cultivating his pain and playing the sick role with aplomb.

Long rests on the settee, twice-weekly visits to the chiropractor, weekly visits for physiotherapy in the heated pool, and long waits for specialists' appointments make time pass quickly. In what seems like no time at all the magic number of two years off work is exceeded – magic because studies show that a person's chances of returning to work after two years' absence for chronic pain are virtually non-existent.[50] There will be no difficulty in obtaining reliable expert witnesses who will confidently testify to the dismal chances of the plaintiff ever again obtaining remunerative work. The plaintiff will require compensation for pain and suffering and, in addition, sufficient funds to replace the lost earnings for the rest of his life. The award is substantial – and so is the lawyer's one-third slice of it.

A quarter of a century ago, Hirschfeld and Behan calculated that healthcare practitioners receive about as much financial reward from chronic pain as do its sufferers. Twenty years later, Florence went even further: "Standard treatment of chronic pain literally supports the medical profession (and its allied services)."[51] The costs of CPS continue to rise and make their way into the pockets of physicians and other healthcare practitioners.

"Do physicians as well as patients also suffer the problem of unconsciously gaining from chronic illness?" was a reasonable question for Hirschfeld and Behan to ask in 1963. It is no longer even a question. Much more is now known about the causes of persistent pain that follows minor accidents. Practitioners have no reason to be unaware of the large role that their activities play in the perseveration of chronic pain and the induction of chronic disability. Practitioners who remain blind to the iatrogenic effects of their investigations and treatment opt to do so intentionally.

With patients, lawyers, physicians, and other healthcare practitioners all using pain for so much gain, CPS long remained a well-cared-for condition. Nevertheless sceptics had their doubts. An Ontario judge, said in respect to a woman who claimed disablement from a CPS attributed to a small whiplash accident: "The legal profession must … know that a personal injury action before a jury based on chronic pain syndrome is, to use the vernacular, 'a crap shoot.' "[52]

Just as CPS was starting to lose its shine, and more people were looking askance at a chronic condition for which no physical basis could be found, CPS was saved by the count. Fibromyalgia appeared. The pain of whiplash and the industrial low back was no longer just due to simple CPS, it was due to the mystical and mysterious fibromyalgia syndrome, a medical condition in which the ongoing pain requires no underlying injury to justify its presence. Whiplash sufferers developed fibromyalgia, a fatiguing condition that is perceived to be even more debilitating than CPS. Whiplash and other musculoskeletal pain received a new lease on life! So many whiplash plaintiffs now develop fibromyalgia that I have devoted the next two chapters to this remarkable condition.

12

Fibromyalgia: A Tender Point?

Fibromyalgia is a form of illness behaviour
magnified by the medical model of care.
– Nortin Hadler[1]

Both physicians and patients seeking a single cause
for an organic disease now have a convenient label with absolutely
no pathophysiologic meaning.
– John B. Winfield[2]

Fibrositis's rise from rags to riches is an illuminating story. Sir William
Gowers, a distinguished English physician, first introduced the term
"fibrositis" in 1904 to describe the hypothetical inflammatory changes
in the fibrous structure of lumbar muscles as the supposed cause of
backache.[3] In the same year, Ralph Stockman, an Edinburgh pathologist, described a group of patients with aching, stiffness, a readiness to
feel muscular fatigue, interference with free muscular movement, and
often a want of energy and vigour. He reported that biopsies from this
group of patients all showed inflammation of the fibrous intermuscu-
lar septa. He thus established fibrositis with its "itis" ending (implying
inflammation) as the popular explanation for our everyday muscle
aches and pains.[4]

The only problem with fibrositis as a disease concept is that no one
besides Stockman has ever found any evidence of inflammation in the
affected tissues. The name "fibrositis" sounded so good that it
remained a useful term for a condition for which nothing other than
the usual stock of home remedies was required. Fibrositis was an illness without stature.

In 1975 its fortunes changed. Hugh Smythe, a Toronto rheumatologist, reported the presence of specific tender points in fibrositic
patients and then, along with Harvey Moldofsky, a psychiatrist also
from Toronto, he reported that fibrositic patients have increased
alpha-rhythm (brain waves) in the non-REM (non-rapid-eye-movement)
phase of sleep.[5] These waves are recorded on the electroencephalogram (EEG). Normally, large slow delta waves are seen in this phase of

sleep, while the small rapid alpha waves occur in the waking state. The finding made sense. Fibrositic patients frequently complain of "unrefreshing sleep." If their brains were active at night, it was not surprising that these patients were tired in the morning.

With such scientific validation, fibrositis – a struggling nuisance complaint trying to make it as a *bona fide* clinical disorder – received the helping hand it needed. "Fibrositis" with its name changed to "fibromyalgia" (algia=pain), began its upward journey to renown.[6] It soon spread from the University of Toronto around the world and acquired some more symptoms, becoming "fibromyalgia syndrome." Kelley's *Textbook of Rheumatology*, the rheumatologist's bible, says of this new syndrome:

Fibromyalgia is more than a muscle pain syndrome, in that most patients have an array of other somatic complaints. Nearly all patients with fibromyalgia experience severe fatigue, poor sleep, and postexertional pain. Other symptoms include tension-type headache, cold intolerance, sicca symptoms [dry mucous membranes], unexplained bruising, fluid retention, chest pain, jaw pain, dyspnea [shortness of breath], dizziness, abdominal pain, parathesias [altered sensation of the skin] and low-grade depression and anxiety. Some symptoms relate to specific syndromes whose prevalence appear to be increased; these include irritable bowel syndrome, migraine, premenstrual syndrome, Raynaud's phenomenon, female urethral syndrome, and restless leg syndrome.[7]

How did fibromyalgia syndrome get tied up with whiplash? Moldofsky, the co-discoverer of alpha-delta sleep along with Paul Saskin, described eleven young women who, following traffic or work-related accidents, developed fibromyalgia although they had had no signs to confirm the presence of an actual physical injury.[8] Once written up in the literature, it was soon accepted that minor trauma caused post-traumatic fibromyalgia. Fibromyalgia syndrome became "post-traumatic fibromyalgia syndrome" (PTFS) and, in the case of collisions, it was whiplash that provided the minor trauma.

Some years later Moldofsky gave PTFS another boost to fame and popularity. Along with two colleagues he described seventeen cases of PTFS following minor motor vehicle accidents – accidents that were virtually non-events. The accident victims did not appear to have suffered any physical or psychological trauma:

Structural damage or injury was usually absent. The event was not enough to alter the patients' physical ability to continue work or return to work the following day. The accident caused little initial worry or distress and symptoms were reported as minor. Pain was recalled as mild, slightly annoying, somewhat discomforting and all patients remained conscious after the accident ...

All the patients showed – in some as long as twelve years after the accident
– persistent disturbed sleep characterized by light unrefreshing sleep, chronic
fatigue, diffuse musculoskeletal pain. Tender points were present ...

[They] were unable to sustain any form of employment, unable independently to run a household or bring up children ... They [had] to make special
arrangements to allow continued running of household or caring for children
(e.g., by compensatory adaptation by spouse, by some extra support from
social network, by purchase of labour-saving devices, or by employment of
some paid assistance with general duties such as cleaning ...)

[They] were rated as having restricted social participation or having impov-
erished social relationships such that they had difficulty in sustaining relations
with friends, neighbours, and colleagues ... Overall, they remained self-suffi-
cient only by virtue of appreciable support from or dependence on financial
or material aid from other people or the community.[9]

With its ability to invest a minor accident with the legitimacy of a *debilitating illness*, fibromyalgia could hardly help but do well. Whiplash
lawyers clamoured to have their clients' symptoms validated by *the
objective findings of an abnormal sleep* EEG. An epidemic of PTFS ensued.
Whiplash plaintiffs, if not disabled by alleged head injury symptoms,
became disabled by PTFS. Many plaintiffs, playing it safe, became disabled by both.

"In North America, Europe and Australia payments for injury-related fibromylagia and disability increased dramatically."[10] In Australia
"kangaroo paw," the RSI epidemic of fibromyalgia, led to the near col-
lapse of Australia's disability and workers' compensation system.[11] In
Europe, Norway was the country the hardest hit – fibromyalgia
became the most common cause of disability, with nearly 11 per cent
of Norwegians having the illness.[12]

Fibromyalgia is now rampant in North America, where two million
men and four million women claim to have it; 5.8 per cent of females
aged from 40 to 60 years are estimated to be its victims.[13] Fibromyalgia
has become an extremely expensive illness, yet its militant supporters
are concerned that only a mere 11 per cent of American fibromyalgia
patients are able to draw disability payments for it.[14]

Fibromylagia generates much public interest.[15] A recent Internet
browse of an on-line bookseller's list of titles showed seventy-seven
books with "fibromyalgia" in the title. Of the 200 or so health topics
available in the new Consumer Health Information Service at the
Toronto Public Library, fibromyalgia is the most sought-after subject.[16]
When it comes to learning about fibromyalgia there is no shortage of
autodidacts.

Not only was the public enthusiastic about fibromyalgia; so were

rheumatologists. Over the past two decades or so, new drugs for osteo-
and rheumatoid arthritis, two painful scourges of mankind, have so
simplified the treatment of arthritis that family physicians rather than
rheumatologists can now provide much of its appropriate care. For
healthcare practitioners, true treatment breakthroughs have a down-
side – fewer patients need care. For rheumatologists, fibromyalgia's
arrival was providential, and fibromyalgia has become the most common disorder treated in rheumatological practice.[17] Professor Edward
Shorter, the Toronto medical historian, observes: "Rheumatologists
often say they long for the odd case of arthritis midst the torrent of
fibromyalgia sufferers."[18] No doubt Shorter is correct, especially as
fibromyalgics tend to spread around their pain; but without these discontented fibromyalgics, the rheumatologists' waiting rooms would be
empty.

The popularity of an illness does not actually turn it into one.
"Tender points" and the sleep EEG established fibromyalgia as a disease; but both these abnormal findings are of dubious significance.
Alpha-delta sleep is a completely non-specific finding. While it is
found only in about one-third of fibromyalgics, it is also found in association with other common conditions and also in up to 15 per cent
of healthy subjects.[19] The validity of tender points is also a very tender
point indeed with fibromyalgia's supporters.

A tender point in this context is a specific location on the body
which, when pressed by the finger or thumb of the examiner, is reported by the patient to be painful. The presence of tender points is far
from being an objective sign of disease, however. The examiner has to
use subjective judgment as to how hard to press, and the patient has
to evaluate subjectively when the pressure becomes painful. Attempts
have been made to replace the examiner's finger or thumb with a
dolorimeter (an instrument adapted from the one used by the Egg
Marketing Board to test the fragility of egg shells by delivering a measured amount of pressure), but they have been unsuccessful.
Frederick Wolfe, a patriarch in the world of fibromyalgia, reports that
the dolorimeter provides a less effective way of making the diagnosis
of fibromyalgia.[20] The fact that an *objective* dolorimeter performs less
well than an examiner's finger seems to illustrate the degree to which
a rheumatologist's subjectivity is involved in the detection of tender
points. There is no reason to suppose that a patient's subjectivity is any
less involved.

Then there is the problem of the location of the tender point sites
and how many sites have to be tender to substantiate its diagnosis.
Even Wolfe and Muhammad Yunus, (another leading fibromyalgia
pundit) could not agree. Yunus judged that two tender points, in the

presence of other characteristic symptoms, were sufficient to make the diagnosis, while Wolfe considered high counts of tender points were necessary and some rheumatologists have suggested that as many as sixty-five tender points are needed for the diagnosis.[21]

Uncertainty about tender points was harming fibromyalgia's reputation. A report from the American College of Rheumatology (ACR) expressed concern: "Among some investigators, fibromyalgia may be thought of as a psychological disorder or, perhaps, as local myofascial pain syndrome. This disarray in construct has led to a blurring of the margins of the disorder and to the consequent idea that fibromyalgia means something different to every observer."[22] If rheumatologists were going to keep their newly acquired – albeit somewhat fractious – part of their professional domain, then they had to settle their differences about the tender points. Fibromyalgia had to be established as a *bona fide* illness.

In 1990 Wolfe, Yunus, and twenty-two other rheumatologists from the ACR collaborated to establish the criteria for its diagnosis. Their consensus, known as the "Copenhagen Declaration," provided the diagnostic criteria for fibromyalgia. Somewhat arbitrarily (at least from the point of view of those outside the college), the rheumatologists set a level of eleven tender points out of eighteen specific tender point sites as a requirement for its diagnosis. Two years later fibromyalgia received its official recognition by the World Health Organization.[23]

With its Copenhagen Declaration, the College of Rheumatology took pains to point out that its criteria were for classification and research purposes only, a proviso that has not discouraged courts all over the Western world from carefully adding up tender points and awarding compensation packages on the results of their arithmetic.[24] Apparently also, an unwritten understanding from Washington DC directs that disability payments will be granted when a claimant is tender at thirteen or more tender point sites but at no control sites.[25]

Following the publication of the ACR criteria for the diagnosis of fibromyalgia, the problem of tender points remained as confusing as ever. Two Australian rheumatologists pointed out that the ACR had defined fibromyalgia by circularity: fibromyalgia is said to cause pain and tender points, and because there are tender points, fibromyalgia is the diagnosis. Separate groups of investigators from Finland, the United States, and Australia also found problems with its diagnosis when they compared groups of fibromyalgia patients with control groups.

These investigators all found the same thing: while fibromyalgic patients were tender at many tender-point sites, they were tender at many other places as well.[26] Their findings amounted to the fact that

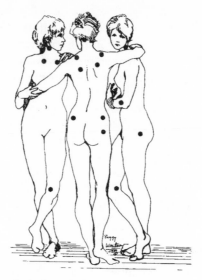

Fig. 12–1   The rheumatologists' new beauty spots?
The American College of Rheumatology's 18 tender point sites.

fibromyalgics have a painful response to pressure wherever the exam-iner chooses to prod. The traditional concept of fibromyalgia as a con-dition having tender points at specific locations was breaking down.[27]

Just as with other alleged results of whiplash, though claims for a physical basis for fibromyalgia abound, no hard evidence has ever been forthcoming to support these claims.[28] All laboratory investiga-tions have proved negative.[29] Besides the lack of objective evidence of illness, many of fibromyalgia's symptoms are clearly somatoform. Any self-respecting neurotic has them all in his symptom repertoire.[30]

The essential symptoms of fibromyalgia are muscular pains com-bined with fatigue. While aches, pains, and fatigue can be distressing, do they constitute an actual disease or even a syndrome?[31] Such symp-toms are extremely common and their presence in a severe form may well just reflect the extreme end of a normal continuum. The extent to which any one member of a *population* experiences such symptoms varies according to the normal *(Gaussian)* distribution curve. At one end of this bell-shaped curve are a few people who never seem to ache and at the other end are a few people who are perpetually wracked with pain, but most people are somewhere in between – having a few aches and pains each day. It is the same with fatigue; a few people are never tired – they party all night and go to work next day full of pep. At the opposite end of the continuum are people who are exhausted from the time they wake up to the moment they go to sleep. Most of us are somewhere in the middle; we are a bit tired some of the time.

It is, of course, tempting for the middle majority to consider people who are bright and chirpy after the all-night party as *abnormal*, and tempting for people who are constantly exhausted to regard themselves as *abnormal*, though probably, neither are justified in doing so. This kind of variation of normal is how Nature, in her infinite wisdom, arranges things. However, superimposed on a normal distribution curve are the *abnormal* or *ill*. Bone secondaries from the spread of cancer may make a person ache all over, or thyroid insufficiency may cause overwhelming exhaustion. These two diseases are not variants of normal. Of course, the $64,000 question is: Are fibromyalgics at the extreme end of a normal distribution curve or are they afflicted with a genuine physical illness? The evidence favours the former.

Straightforward psychological tension, from whatever cause, is itself a common cause of aches, pains, and fatigue. In the 1950s the Mayo Clinic coined the term *tension myalgia* for this form of muscle ache.[32] A less straightforward relationship to psychological tension is the conversion of psycho-social distress into somatoform symptoms, and many authors have pointed out the importance of the conversion mechanisms in the production of fibromyalgic symptoms.[33] John Sarno, the New York physiatrist who condemns the concept of structural damage as an explanation of chronic pain, studied 100 consecutive patients presenting with neck, back, and shoulder pain. He found a frequent association of fibromyalgic-type symptoms with prior somatoform symptoms such as nervous stomach, tension headache, spastic colon, and palpitations.[34] All these symptoms are the very ones that beset the anxious and distressed.

The psychological difficulties that fibromyalgics have were shown in an unexpected way. Two Canadian radiologists used the MRI to examine the radiological characteristics of the tender points. They found that the tender points appeared normal but not the fibromyalgics: they were claustrophobic. Being put in the MRI scanner is a bit like being laid prematurely in a coffin and having the lid nailed down with a pile driver. Understandably, many patients are discomfited by the experience and about 8 per cent become panicky. The fibromyalgic patients became much more so. "Most of the patients required a lot of reassurance, greatly prolonging the scanning time. Scanning had to be completely discontinued in 4 of the 18 patients (22%) because they were too frightened to stay in the machine."[35] Fibromyalgia is an unlikely cause of claustrophobia, which suggests that fibromyalgics either run at high levels of anxiety or that they are unable or unwilling to contain normal levels of anxiety. Fibromyalgia does not seem to be a straightforward physical illness. Indeed its symptoms are so similar to those of chronic fatigue syndrome, ME, and neuromyasthenia that it is impossible to pry them apart.[36] Fibromyalgia has become a fashionable illness.

Who gets fibromyalgia? Clinicians and epidemiologists disagree. Doctors in clinical practice diagnose fibromylagia eight to ten times more frequently in women than in men, the affected women being mostly between 40 and 50 years old.[37] Two Finnish epidemiologists examined the data for the Mini-Finland Health Survey, using material collected between 1977 and 1980 before fibromyalgia had become fashionable. In this mini-health survey over 7000 representative Finns aged 30 and above were asked questions relating to fibrositis symptoms: "hurt all over," painful body sites, general fatigue, poor sleep, and gastrointestinal problems. The epidemiologists examined the subjects who reported moderate to severe levels of symptoms for tender points. They found the prevalence of fibrositis was low, less than one per cent of the population. Women had it only twice as frequently as men, and its peak age group was between 55 and 64 years of age. Its prevalence was inversely related to class. There were in fact no cases of fibrositis in people with high school education or above. In addition, the presence of fibrositis was associated with a high risk of having a mental disorder.

The Finnish authors report that they had no success in identifying fibrositis as an independent syndrome. In concluding their study they debunk the mythology surrounding it: "[Fibrositis] resembles a constellation of stars: its components are real enough but the pattern is in the mind of the beholder. That the ancient Greeks gave a group of stars the name of a mythical being is not enough to suppose that the constellation has any actual meaning, much less the attributes of the creature."[38] Again, rather than curing diseases, medicine is manufacturing new ones.

Fibromyalgics are similar to other patients with a chronic pain syndrome in that their pain seems to substitute for all sorts of other difficulties. Smythe himself noted that fibromyalgics often have a particular type of personality: "[They] tend to be perfectionist, demanding of themselves and others, and effective in their areas of activity. Unlike the classic victims of civilized tension, they dislike the effects of tranquilizers and use drugs and alcohol sparingly. Their vices are their virtues carried to excess."[39]

Fibromyalgia, in common with other fashionable illnesses, is a condition with many subjective complaints but few, if any, objective signs to substantiate the presence of illness. Besides this lack of supporting evidence of illness, fibromyalgic patients paint themselves worse off than they appear to be. A Dutch study, for example, examined patients with three different rheumatological conditions: ankylosing spondylitis (a painful inflammatory condition in which the spinal column becomes completely rigid), rheumatoid arthritis, and fibromyalgia. They compared the measures of functional disability made by the patients about themselves to the clinical observations made by the clinical staff, all experienced at rating disability.

There was close agreement between the assessment made by the ankylosing patients and their clinical observers, less close agreement with the rheumatoid patients, and for the fibromyalgic patients there was little agreement at all. This discrepancy is statistically highly significant. The fibromyalgic patients saw themselves as far more disabled than did the clinical observers who rated them.[40]

If self-estimates of disability are accepted as the criteria for disability, then fibromyalgics are extremely disabled. A study from the University of Washington, Seattle, ranked patients in various disease categories according to the patients' own estimates of disability. Patients with histories of cardiac arrest, myocardial infarct, angina, kidney failure on dialysis, and oxygen-dependent chronic obstructive lung disease all rated themselves less disabled than did the fibromyalgics. The only patients who rated themselves as more disabled were patients in the end stages of Lou Gehrig's disease.[41]

The adage "People who do not feel pain seldom think the pain is real" reflects our somewhat diminished capacity for empathy. Nevertheless, in a situation in which fibromyalgics' subjective perceptions are accessible to confirmation, their perceptions were found incorrect. A frequent refrain of fibromyalgic patients is that their pain predictably worsens with changes in the weather.[42] To determine the *realness* of their climate sensitivity, a team of Dutch rheumatologists asked their self-styled weather-sensitive fibromyalgic patients to keep a pain and symptom diary. They then compared the level of pain reported by the patients with meteorological data. There was no correlation whatsoever between the patients' level of reported pain and any weather changes. The team's conclusion was: "Fibromyalgic patients prefer to relate their symptoms to external causes rather than to an internal state of mind."[43]

Fibromyalgia is catching. Angela Mailis and two colleagues from the University Health Network in Toronto, report the case history of a family who developed symptoms following a minor car accident involving parents and their four children. The government health records show that the children were seen by a paediatrician the day of the accident but had no further medical contacts until the family had consulted a lawyer five months post-accident. After their consultation, the visits to doctors escalated. All the family members had similar multi-system complaints. Seven years after the accident, Harold Merskey, the psychiatrist member of the whiplash experts from University of Western Ontario, examined the family and diagnosed all six members as having fibromyalgia.

Nine years after the accident, the case came to court. The family was seeking three million dollars in damages. Perhaps because of the competence of the expert witnesses for the defence, the case collapsed half way through the trial and the family was awarded only $50,000.[44] *There is honour even among thieves;* lawyers certainly take care of their own. Even in cases totally without merit, the settlement always seems sufficient to cover the plaintiff lawyer's expenses and fee. The plaintiff can be left destitute.

From a medical point of view, fibromyalgia would be a pointless condition if it had no treatment. Treatments for it abound. Some American neurosurgeons, claiming that the squeezing of the brain by a too-tight skull is its cause, will, for $30,000, drill and snip away the back of the fibromyalgic's skull.[45] Perhaps wisely, with orthodox medicine offering this kind of treatment, many fibromyalgics regard the medical profession as far too obtuse and ham-handed to handle a disease as subtle as fibromyalgia. They are high consumers of alternative interventions. In fact, however, both orthodox and alternative practitioners have little success.

Fibromyalgics appear to do equally badly with both kinds of care. Rheumatologists from McGill University in Montreal divided 82 fibromyalgic patients into two groups. In one group were 33 fibromyalgics who had used non-physician treatments in the prior six months; in the other were 49 fibromyalgics who had not. The patients were rated on various scales for "disease severity." The rheumatologists found that the patients in both groups reported similar pain and functional impairment.[46]

Medicine is seldom simple. Fibromyalgia has a painful-muscle cousin, "the myofascial pain syndrome" (MPS), which, like fibromyalgia, is difficult to tie down as an illness entity and manages to cause about as much diagnostic confusion. Like fibromyalgia, MPS frequently complicates minor injuries and its physical signs are uncertain. In place of tender points, MPS has as its hallmark "trigger points," taut bands in muscles that, when pressed, cause shooting pains and local twitches. MPS is the elder of these disease cousins, having had its beginnings in 1942 with the publication of a paper by Janet Travell, an internist in Washington, DC.[47] Travell later joined forces with David Simons, a Californian physiatrist, to write a two-volume tome on MPS, *Myofascial Pain and Dysfunction: The Trigger Point*

Manual. Their book quickly won a prominent place in accident litigation.[48]

Thomas Bohr, a neurologist from Loma Linda who is sceptical about fibromyalgia, is equally sceptical of MPS. He describes *The Trigger Point Manual* as "a 'veritable bible' among many physiatrists, as well as some neurologists, anaesthesiologists, chiropractors, and dentists." Bohr notes that "the strange characteristics of this unusual work" have mostly gone unchallenged by orthodox practitioners, and that its "critics are susceptible to the charge by believers that they simply do not have the training, the expertise, or palpative 'feel' to make the diagnosis. They lack the 'magic finger of faith.'"[49]

Tender points make the diagnosis of fibromyalgia, and trigger points the diagnosis of MPS, but in practice even the specialists have difficulty using either to diagnose fibromyalgia or MPS. In a contest of Leviathans, four leading fibromyalgia experts were paired against four leading MPS experts. These diagnostic champions, by the use of tender points and trigger points, were to demonstrate their prowess in assigning various musculo-skeletal pain patients and controls to the appropriate diagnostic groups. The subjects of this medical jousting match were divided into three groups: patients previously diagnosed with fibromyalgia; patients diagnosed with MPS; and healthy subjects. The experts, *blinded* to the diagnosis, looked for tender points, trigger points, and taut muscle bands.

Problems soon arose. In the training sessions that preceded the contest, the uninitiated rheumatologists could not master the techniques required for an MPS examination; the rheumatologists therefore confined themselves to tender points. Some of the MPS experts were unable to examine for trigger points and taut bands in the fifteen minutes allotted to each subject; they restricted themselves only to eight right-sided muscles.

The results were a fiasco. The contestants agreed at least that the subjects in the two patient groups had more muscle tenderness than did the controls. When averaged out, the rheumatologists found 15.2 tender points per fibromyalgic patient, 11 per MPS patient, and 2 tender points in each healthy control. The MPS experts did even more poorly. They only found taut bands and local twitch responses in about half the MPS patients, about the same number that they found in the fibromyalgic patients; they also found these taut bands and local twitch responses in many healthy controls.[50] If the experts cannot distinguish between the MPS patients and the healthy controls in these rather ideal conditions, it seems unlikely that Dr Joe Doe in the hurly-burly of a medical practice will succeed in separating MPS and fibromyalgia into two disease entities. (Other investigators have confirmed the similarities of the two conditions, including similar sleep disturbances.)[51]

Fibromyalgia was again blurring at the edges and the tender point confusion was worse than ever. In June 1994 a synod of rheumatologists from around the world convened in Vancouver to clear up the controversial issues of fibromyalgia. The-number-of-angels-on-a-head-of-a-pin arguments are always divisive, and the number of tender points it takes to make a diagnosis of fibromyalgia is no different. However, under the pontifical eye of Professor Wolfe, they sought consensus. Two years later the Vancouver Fibromyalgia Consensus Group promulgated its report.[52]

The report reviewed the many problems attendant upon fibromyalgia and its tender points, and in so doing created consensus in most non-rheumatologists' minds that the syndrome or disease concept of fibromyalgia should be quietly left to die. However, true to the nature of such groups, the Vancouver Consensus Group confirmed the 1990 American College of Rheumatology's diagnostic criteria for fibromyalgia, and even added some more of its own: "Patients who have fewer than the required number of tender points may also be diagnosed as having fibromyalgia providing they have widespread pain and many of the characteristics of the syndrome ... Tenderness at sites not specified by the ACR criteria does not exclude the diagnosis."

The Vancouver Fibromyalgia Consensus Group deliberated on whether the diagnosis of fibromyalgia "could be 'falsely' manipulated by a claimant," and noted that "[this problem] has not been addressed by any investigation."[53] Although Wolfe remains steadfastly loyal to fibromyalgia, he redeems himself by being meticulously forthright about fibromyalgia's many failings. He records that he "has seen and is convinced that both the tender point count and dolorimetry score can be manipulated by a patient." He also makes it clear that fibromyalgia, when used in a legal and compensation situation, has a different meaning: "Almost nothing is known about [its] diagnostic validity and reliability in the compensation setting."[54]

Even rheumatologists seem to be losing faith in tender points. A study from Britain's Arthritis and Rheumatism Council Epidemiological Research Unit found that "tender points are a measure of general distress" and that "fibromyalgia does not seem to exist as a distinct entity."[55] Hadler, the distinguished rheumatologist from North Carolina, thinks there has been too much mathematics: "Thanks to tender points fibromyalgia has been elevated to the status of Boolean algebra"; and he suggests that "the patient with fibromyalgia can be better served if the tender points are ignored or better yet, not even demonstrated."[56]

PTFS is a *cash-cow* both for rheumatologists and personal-injury litigation lawyers.[57] T.J. Romano, one of the rheumatologists who helped develop the ACR criteria for the diagnosis of fibromyalgia, reports on 14 of his own patients whom he treated for PTFS; all but two had been involved in auto accidents.[58] All complained of fatigue, painful muscles and joints, and non-restorative sleep. "In addition, they reported inability to work or perform activities of daily living such as shopping, running the sweeper, doing laundry, washing dishes, and lifting, without precipitating a flare-up of their generalized painful condition."[59]

Romano's patients all received either a cash settlement or an award from a civil court, the amounts ranging from $45,000 to $300,000. He reports that following settlement 9 of the 14 patients (64%) continued to attend his office for ongoing treatment of PTFS. Romano suggests that such a percentage of litigants returning for further treatment is evidence that "patients who meet the strict fibromylagia criteria are not malingering." What about the 36 per cent of patients who did not continue treatment after settlement? Did settlement cure them?

The trauma considered necessary to be the cause of PTFS became progressively more trivial, until even the memory of trauma was enough to cause it. Even "remote and unverifiable events such as supposed childhood abuse recalled afterwards have been deemed to cause it."[60] Wolfe provides a list of minor events to which PTFS has been attributed and for which lawsuits have been filed: "Operating an office copying machine, sexual harassment, an automobile accident at less than 2 mph and, in one instance, the threat of trauma."[61]

The symptoms of PTFS are essentially the same as those of fibromyalgia except that they are more severe. PTFS patients were found to have higher rates of loss of employment (70%) and reduced physical activity (45%) than did patients with primary fibromylagia.[62] There is no acceptable evidence to support that fibromyalgia is caused by severe physical injury let alone by the questionable stress of minor collisions. Nevertheless, lawyers and plaintiff expert witnesses confidently attribute fibromyalgia to these non-events.

Twenty years ago when *traumatic fibrositis* was hardly more than a gleam in a lawyer's eye, Lawrence Weinberger, a rheumatologist from Ventura, California, soundly deprecated its concept:

Though it has been useful to physicians as a facile explanation for persistent and baffling complaints, "traumatic myofibrositis" [PTFS] appears to be an example of how a rheumatic malady, by the arbitrary insertion of a modifying adjective, is converted into an acceptable consequence of trauma. Such heedless wordsmithing not only leads to wide medical legal and economic consequences, it inevitably invites disbelief ... It seems apparent that traumatic fibromyositis [PTFS] should be regarded as one of the many medical myths making up the folklore of trauma and therefore should be discarded as a serious clinical entity.[63]

Time proved Weinberger right. Even the members of the Vancouver Consensus Group, staunch believers in fibromyalgia, recommend the elimination of the term *post-traumatic fibromyalgia*.[64] But new illnesses, while easy to create, are more difficult to terminate. PTFS received the warmest of welcomes on its emergence from Pandora's box, but, having spread around the world, its mischief is not easily contained. PTFS still gives lawyers a contentious issue about which they can litigate; healthcare practitioners an illness which they can endlessly treat and never cure; and patients an illness for which they can claim both sympathy and compensation. For all sorts of people, PTFS is a perfect illness, though, as an illness, it has a lot wrong with it.

Some physicians are contrite over how the profession has let this so-called disease flourish and cause so much havoc. With varying degrees of self-reproach, a number of physicians have written their *mea culpas*. Simon Carette, professor of medicine at Laval University, Quebec, and a leading Canadian rheumatologist, writes: "We physicians have taken an entity that existed for centuries, given it a new name, created a major health issue by elevating it in importance, researching it and suggesting it now deserves disability coverage. We have created a monster and now it is up to us to make amends."[65]

Chan Gunn, a physiatrist from the Pain Center in Seattle, asks, *"What have we created?* Fibromyalgia has recently become a popular diagnosis, and many doctors now apply the ACR criteria for the classification of fibromyalgia. Regrettably, this has brought hopeless despair to countless individuals ... Far from being a distinctive condition, fibromyalgia merely describes the most extreme and extensive of mundane aches and pains that we all have, in various degrees, at one time or another."[66] Gunn's statement is perhaps a somewhat questionable confession of responsibility, because he then goes on to extol the virtues of myofascial pain syndrome, a diagnosis that is no more tenable than that of fibromyalgia and causes just as much disability.

Wolfe and the Vancouver Fibromyalgia Consensus Group, while not conceding that fibromyalgia has been a mistake, recommend more studies: "The insurance industry must play an important role in sponsoring research in the area of assessments, treatments and outcome of work and disability-related fibromyalgia."[67] Such sponsorship will, of course, entail large research grants to rheumatologists. Rheumatologists may be feeling guilty for having foisted fibromyalgia upon the world, but it does not take a psychiatrist to point out that their guilt hardly goes even skin deep. They are still at the stage of seeing it as someone else's responsibility to put it right.

In contrast, Hadler takes a more vigorous stance:

Dr Wolfe cannot bring himself to abandon the fibromyalgia construct ... For the long-beleaguered believers in fibromyalgia, whether physicians, alternative health professionals, or patients, the [ARC] criteria were an epiphany ... Growing numbers of North Americans are labelled as having fibromyalgia and are drawn into "medicalization and dependency" ... We rheumatologists have devoted our lives to helping people cope with chronic musculoskeletal disorders. We know that coping requires avoiding the magnification of symptoms ... [Fibromyalgia] fosters a life of somatizing. When it comes to disability determination, anyone who has to prove he or she is ill will be rendered more ill in the proving. When a physician participates in the process, it becomes worse than counterproductive, it becomes iatrogenic.[68]

Rather than encouraging fibromyalgic patients to perceive themselves as sick, Hadler sees the physician's calling as "championing their patients' quest for whatever place in the sun is their birthright."

Perhaps in the end common sense may prevail in the legal system, and fibromyalgia will be perceived as the medical myth that it is. Two recent Canadian judgments have called into question the medical legitimacy of this condition. Mr Justice Donald, a Vancouver judge, in 1993 found: "Fibromyalgia is not a disease entity. It is the name applied to a constellation of symptoms, the most prominent feature of which is chronic pain. The origin of the pain is unknown. The manifestations of the syndrome in any person must be understood in the light of that person's background and psychological make-up."[69]

More strikingly, Mme Justice Rawlins, judge on the Queen's Bench of Alberta, captured journalists' attention with a thoughtful judgment. The case encapsulates many of the medico-legal problems surrounding a typical case of whiplash-induced fibromyalgia and the ways in which courts handle these issues. Since thousands of similar cases are processed by the legal system every year, I will use the information contained in Mme Justice Rawlins's judgment to illuminate these types of cases. Her judgment deserves a chapter of its own.

13

Fibromyalgia:
A Case in Point

I would be loath to speak ill of any person who I do not know deserves it,
but I am afraid he is an attorney.

– Samuel Johnson

The case heard before Mme Justice Rawlins was a run-of-the-mill
whiplash suit.[1] The injury sustained by the plaintiff appears to have
been small, yet its effects are alleged to have lasted nearly a decade.
The plaintiff had a typical pre- and post-accident whiplash history, and
many specialists got in on the act. What is unusual about the trial is the
care and thoughtfulness with which Mme Justice Rawlins considered
the case. In her ninety-five-page judgment she quoted the findings and
opinions of the various expert witnesses, and of course provided her
own opinion as well.

I have extracted relevant material from her judgment to illustrate
how medical arguments about whiplash and fibromyalgia unfold in
court. The case provides a bird's eye view of lawyers and doctors at
work.

The plaintiff, Mrs M, a registered nurse with three children, was
aged 41 at the time of the collision and had been married for twenty
years. The accident happened on the TransCanada Highway near
Medicine Hat on 1 July 1985, nine years prior to the court hearing. Mr
M was driving his wife and their four-year-old daughter to British
Columbia on the first day of their two-week summer vacation. Mrs M
was in the front passenger seat and their daughter was seated between
them, all three wearing lap belts.

The defendant, driving a truck, merged from the road shoulder into
the driving lane but failed to signal. Mr M applied neither the brakes
nor the horn but attempted to pass. The passenger-side door of the
Ms' car was hit and both vehicles pulled onto the shoulder of the road.
Neither Mr M nor his daughter suffered injury. Mrs M reports no
direct injury but remembers little about the accident except that she
felt shaken up. Four hours later she developed a severe headache, and
that evening and the next day had severe pain in the right side of the

neck and right shoulder. She took hot baths and Aspirin, but reports that these measures failed to help. The next day, the family rented another car and continued on their holiday. During the vacation Mrs M suffered intermittent pain down the right arm and across the back of her neck but did not seek medical attention.

On their return two weeks later, the family had clocked over 3000 km on the rental car. Mrs M consulted her family physician but he did not prescribe anything because the Tylenol she was taking appeared to be working well. Mrs M went to work on 22 July but, because her headache was severe, she left and did not return to work until nine months later. Over the balance of the summer of 1985, Mrs M's symptoms progressively worsened and extended to other parts of her body.

Mrs M reported that before the accident apart from some headaches her health had been good. She said of her marriage: "We had fun, worked, played, and laughed together." Their various social activities included "dancing, camping, vacationing in their motor home, cabin, and boat, and they had a busy social life." Mrs M "was considered an excellent housewife, completing all the usual tasks of vacuuming floors, cupboards, meals and washing by herself with min-imal assistance from her husband."

The pre-accident medical records told a somewhat different story. She had, for instance, indicated to various specialists that she was aller-gic to "practically everything." In the years following the accident, Mrs M consulted her family physician over 100 times. He either "referred her to various specialists and caregivers, or was aware of her involve-ment with them, including physiotherapists, a chiropractor, rheuma-tologists, a neurosurgeon, a radiologist, physiatrists [rehabilitation experts], neurologist[s], an orthopaedic surgeon, an orthodontist, and an acupuncturist."

Her medications included Robaxisal and Parafon Forte II (muscle-relaxing analgesics), Flexeril (a muscle relaxant and tranquilizer), Dolobid (a nonsteroidal anti-inflammatory analgesic), Extra Strength Tylenol, Naprosyn (an anti-inflammatory), Reglan (to prevent vomit-ing in migraine), Sibelium (an anti-migraine drug), Cytotec and Sulcrate (drugs used to avoid gastric problems when using anti-inflam-matory medication), as well as amitriptyline and Prozac (antidepres-sants). It was particularly noted that the two antidepressants were pre-scribed *not* for depression but to improve her sleep pattern. Mrs M, perhaps not surprisingly, reported that all these medicines made her so forgetful that she had to keep a diary of her day-to-day activities. She recorded her various pains for virtually the entire nine-year period leading up to the trial.

The practitioners she consulted made sundry diagnoses. In the latter part of July 1985, the chiropractor diagnosed hyperflexion extension injury to the cervical spine with posterior joint fixation. He manipulated her neck but failed to relieve her symptoms. The orthopaedic surgeon found everything normal except for neck tenderness and some reduction of flexion and left-sided rotation.

In September Mrs M saw Dr Verdejo, a rheumatologist. He noted that there were times since the accident when Mrs M had been without symptoms. He found a full range of motion of both active and passive neck movements. His only finding was mild tenderness of the shoulder muscles. He assessed that her "neck pain was of a functional nature" (i.e., not having any organic basis) and that her symptoms were mostly "in keeping with the so-called fibrositis syndrome, secondary to muscular spasm."

Dr Verdejo saw her symptoms as a reaction to stress: "We call it somatization ... Stress becomes obvious to the individual in the form of pain." He explained that "not being able to find an explanation for her symptoms [did] nothing more than aggravate her complaints as a self-pitying mechanism." He suggested stopping [passive] physiotherapy in favour of a more active back education program, and stopping all drugs other than Tylenol and amitriptyline.

In December that year she saw a neurologist on account of her headaches. He found everything normal except for minimally impaired neck movements and the fact that she was "slightly obese." He diagnosed "chronic cervical sprain and anticipated that she would be well enough to resume normal activities in a month or two."

By April 1986 Mrs M still had pain. Her doctor referred her to a second neurologist, who found that despite some muscle tenderness she had a full range of neck and shoulder movements. Mrs M was gaining weight and the neurologist emphasized that if the pain was to go away she should increase her physical activity. In July, a third neurologist examined her and found her essentially normal. Her family physician discussed with her the possibility of her staying off work for the rest of the summer.

In September she was examined by a physiatrist (rehabilitation expert) who observed "soreness and stiffness of her right neck, with pain radiating down the right arm to the index and middle fingers, aching discomfort of the left arm, facial numbness, and discomfort to the inner left leg." He determined that "there [was] likely craniovertebral dysfunction with involvement of the cervical plexus." (What the physiatrist meant by "craniovertebral dysfunction with involvement of the cervical plexus" is anybody's guess.) In November, the physiatrist suggested that Mrs M see an otolaryngologist to exclude any altered breathing habits, a dental surgeon to exclude temporo-mandibular joint disorder, and an allergist to exclude allergy as a cause of her headaches.

Nerve conduction studies done in early December showed no evidence of peripheral neuropathy or root lesions. At the end of December her doctor noted that she was feeling generally better and had only minimal tenderness in her neck muscles. She was again working full time. In July 1987 the family physician recorded that acupuncture was helping her, but by September it had stopped doing so. Her doctor sent her to a rehabilitation specialist who found a good range of neck movements but some pain present at the extremes of movements. He had a long discussion with her about the importance of doing daily neck exercises.

In December 1987, Dr G, an orthodontist, reported that Mrs M's hyper-extension/hyper-flexion injury of the neck had "caused a displacement of the jaw joint disc assembly leading to vascular damage to the ligament," and that she had TMJ disorder. He fitted a TMJ splint that she wore at nights up to the time of the trial. By July 1988, Mrs M's pains were so bad that they interfered with her performance at work. Her doctor recommended that she be given home services to help her undertake household chores.

In August 1988, Dr Verdejo (the rheumatologist) examined her for a second time. He found everything normal except for diffuse tenderness along the spine, not confined to the fibromyalgic tender point sites. As he saw it, the whole picture was closely related to "underlying depression, chronically abnormal sleep pattern and aggravation of all the symptoms by stress." He commented: "She has been treated with physiotherapy, basically with TLC [tender loving care] and although she was referred to the back program and advised to lose weight, *neither suggestion has been followed* and, in fact, she has put on further weight ... I have made certain that she understands that a proper exercise routine is most important to treat some of the causes of pain – in this case, neck, and back strain – in spite of her fatigue towards the end of the day. Most importantly, [she should] seriously consider developing other interests in regard to her job which has become frustrating to her. She should perhaps take a leave of absence of a year or two with the view to taking some training to keep up her motivation."

In September 1988, Mrs M had chest pains and was admitted to a coronary care unit for nine days. No heart abnormality was found but she did not return to work. In November she saw another neurologist on account of blurred vision. He found no abnormality. However, she was hospitalized in December for a coronary angiogram. Everything was again found to be normal. Mrs M returned to work.

In February 1989 her severe chest pain returned and was readmitted to hospital. Her heart was fine but she was found to have gallstones. By now, Mrs M's supervisor was losing patience because of all her sickness, and a personality clash arose between them. Mrs M obtained a doctor's certificate stating that she was able to work without restriction, and returned to work in May. Fifteen days later, Dr Verdejo observed that her job frustration and lack of motivation were aggravating her symptoms. "[Her] problem will not improve by just staying at home or taking anti-inflammatory medication." He suggested she take a year's leave of absence "to improve her motivation and direct her energies in a different field."

Dr Austin, an orthopaedic surgeon, examined Mrs M in August 1989 as an expert witness on her behalf. He found she had "vague and doubtful tenderness in various areas of the back" but that everything was normal. He could find no disability that he could "relate to the shaking up she sustained in the accident."

In September Mrs M (presumably at Dr Verdejo's suggestion) enrolled in the Faculty of Education, completing one course in the winter session of 1998. In January 1990, she enrolled in three university classes, two in psychology and the other in health, but after the first month, finding that she could not carry the books or materials required for presentations and that the workload was too heavy, she withdrew from all three courses. She obtained two part-time nursing jobs on "an as-needed" basis. In February her family physician noted she was feeling better and was working part-time as an occupational health nurse.

In response to the plaintiff's counsel's inquiries, Dr Verdejo wrote two letters. (Her lawyers were no doubt concerned that Dr Verdejo had attributed so few of her symptoms to the accident.) Dr Verdejo stuck to his guns: "From my point of view, based on previous examinations, although the patient has stated that she has pain on pressure of any part of her body or pretty well any soft tissue of her body, no anatomical abnormalities have ever been found to consider her disabled in any way. You will understand that the definition of pain is purely subjective and there is no way that a physician – or anyone else, for that matter – can debate its severity."

Dr Verdejo wrote a second letter in March 1990:

[Such local factors referred to in my letter are] mechanical instability of the neck and lower back due to poor posture, to being overweight, lack of proper muscle tone, to some extent stress in those areas related to normal use, including bending, standing, walking; aggravating factors such as fatigue, tension, immobility; the personality traits of some individuals which make them demanding of themselves; precipitating stress, such as an accident, but also unhappy situations related to dissatisfaction with job or employer and consequently secondary gain with the purpose of avoiding or by-passing stressful situations which may worsen the syndrome and, not uncommonly, nomogenic [lawyer engendered] factors, and frequently underlying depression or anxiety.

In July, Mrs M stopped taking amitriptyline (the antidepressant prescribed to improve her sleep pattern), but by September, because her symptoms had returned, she recommenced the antidepressant. She also had some gynaecological surgery and developed "tendonitis" (RSI), neither of which was attributed to the accident.

In July of the same year, Dr Gross, a physiatrist, examined Mrs M as an expert witness on her behalf. He found a reduction in the range of motion of the cervical spine that constituted "a permanent partial disability in the order of 2 per cent to 3 per cent." He agreed that the plaintiff's symptoms were "of a psychoneurotic nature which may respond to psychological counselling." He believed that the plaintiff could continue in an occupation that entailed minimal stress and responsibility, since "it appears as though these are the situations that have caused her the most degree of difficulty."

In February 1991, Dr Sibley examined Mrs M as an expert rheumatologist on her behalf. Except for slight reduction of neck movement and right-sided pain, he found everything normal, but he was concerned by her lack of physical activity. In June Mrs M complained of "swollen feet and whole body swelling." She was feeling bloated, gassy, and nauseated, and had abdominal pains. (Her doctor noted that "A lot of people might feel they have swelling in their bodies but it does not necessarily mean they are swelling.") He attributed the symptoms to her having again stopped amitriptyline. She had gastro-intestinal x-rays, all of which were normal.

Mrs M's migraine was again investigated in July 1991. Her doctor prescribed Prozac (an antidepressant drug that is sometimes used in the prevention of migraine). Within a few weeks Mrs M had lost twenty pounds. (This was an impressive response in view of Mrs M's intractable weight problem. She had weighed 138 lb when the accident occurred, but afterwards "ballooned" up to 204 lb; despite subsidized Weight Watchers, Nutri/System, and many exhortations from her caregivers to lose weight.)

In October Mrs M was examined by Dr Trachsel, a rehabilitation specialist who sees many people for "fibromyalgia, myofascial pain or soft-tissue injuries." Dr Trachsel, acting as an expert witness on Mrs M's behalf, noted that Mrs M "moved around easily," did not have "evidence of any pain symptomatology," and had "a full range of movements of the neck and spine." However, she found Mrs M had myofascial trigger points in her neck muscles, and, as other examiners had done, recommended a regular exercise program.

Dr Sibley re-examined Mrs M in October 1993. He found her worse than when he had seen her three years previously. "She seemed to have more problems with headaches, neck pain, and diffuse back pain ... She was having more difficulties with many aspects of her life ... She said she has difficulty with housework and carrying heavy pots and pans, trouble with dressing, trouble with using toilet paper and pro-longed driving, and particularly backing up. She said she was still able to vacation, but avoided using the boat at the cottage if the water was rough because of increased neck pain. She had resumed physiothera-py in the spring of 1993, which consisted of heat, ultrasound and mas-sage, and just recently started a general home exercise program con-sisting of a range of motion exercises for the neck."

Later in October, Dr Gross re-examined her. He, like Dr Sibley, had examined her some three years previously, but Dr Gross found her improved. "[She can] pick and choose her shifts and she is putting in less than 40 hours per week." She "no longer requires psychological counselling."

Dr Glenn McCain, rheumatologist expert on her behalf, examined Mrs M a month later. Dr McCain was previously affiliated with the whiplash experts at the University of Western Ontario, but was now head of a private clinic in North Carolina specializing in the treatment of patients with fibromyalgia. *Unlike any of the other examiners,* Dr McCain found Mrs M was tender at all eighteen of the ACR designated tender point sites (only eleven such tender points are required to meet the ACR criteria for the diagnosis of fibromyalgia). He reported that the plaintiff's clinical course over the preceding eight years was typical of severe fibromyalgia. He found subjective and objective evi-dence for a diagnosis of this syndrome.

Dr Keith Pearce, a psychiatrist expert for the defendant, examined Mrs M in January 1994. Her chief complaint at that time was headache, and while Dr Pearce accepted that some of her headaches may be due to whiplash, he noted that she gave a family history of headaches and she herself "had suffered headaches prior to the acci-dent usually as a delayed response to certain allergens." Dr Pearce learned that following her accident Mrs M had begun to use a feather pillow. He pointed out that feathers are a common antigen, but Mrs M denied she had ever been allergic to feathers.

Dr Pearce obtained "a very clear and definite impression that 'in no uncertain terms' [Mrs M] did not like her job and that perhaps she was stressed and not satisfied with her marriage." Dr Pearce

asked Mrs M to complete several psychological instruments including the MMPI-2.[2]

When her case came to trial, Mrs M still had intermittent pain in the
left hip and arm, numbness in the outer aspect of her left leg from her
hip to her knee, and numbness in her right arm from her shoulder to
her fingers. She occasionally slept in a recliner chair and suffered
from irritable bowels accompanied by severe headaches. "Her sexual
life [was] very bad, largely as a result of her ongoing pain and depression ... She continue[d] to have periods of general unhappiness and
anxiety as well as a quick temper ... She [said] she [was] unable to perform all of her pre-accident household duties and could not perform
the heavy housework including cleaning walls, cupboards, vacuuming
carpets, and washing, waxing, and stripping floors."

Various witnesses, including a labour economist, an actuary, and an
economic consultant, gave evidence at Mrs M's trial. Ten physicians
gave evidence about Mrs M's symptoms and fibromyalgia, and the
effect of pain upon her life. As is apparent from their comments, there
was little agreement, even among her own expert witnesses, about the
presence or absence of straightforward physical signs such as limitation of neck movements, let alone the presence or absence of tender
points and trigger points. I have selected the various points of view
that Mme Justice Rawlins documents in her report to demonstrate
how medical discord over fibromyalgia is played out in court.

Much was said about trigger points and tender points. Dr Trachsel
carefully explained to the court how to differentiate between the two.
Dr Pearce, on the other hand, considered tender points and triggers
points to be much the same. Dr Pearce then reviewed the various
painful muscle syndromes and the problem inherent in their
diagnosis. Dr Pearce found no trigger or tender points, in contrast
to Dr McCain who found them all. Again, Dr Trachsel did
not find any tender points and stressed that "tender points don't
disappear."

There were the usual horse and cart arguments about Mrs M's distress and the accident. Dr McCain "sees many patients in his clinics
that have a temporal relationship between trauma and the onset of
fibromyalgia symptoms." All his clinic patients complete the MMPI
(Minnesota Multiphasic Personality Inventory). Dr McCain noted that
the profile of the typical fibromyalgic on the MMPI scales forms an
inverted "V". He added: "They have high scores on the scales for hysteria, depression and hypochondriasis." Dr McCain reported that
"[Mrs M's] emotional and mental status were a direct result of her
pain and not the cause of it," but did not elaborate why he came to
that conclusion.

In contrast, Dr Austin, the orthopaedic surgeon for the defendant, perceived Mrs M's emotional and mental state as the cause rather than the result of her symptoms: "The nature of her complaints suggests these are of an emotional nature, based on tension of psychological causes and have persisted and extended to include most parts of her body." He deemed her symptoms to be of a psychoneurotic nature that needed no treatment but could well respond to psychological counselling.

Dr Pearce was of a similar opinion. He presented extensive information on the evolution of fibromyalgia and the fashionable illnesses, quoting freely from Professor Shorter's book *From Paralysis to Fatigue* (see chapter 4). Dr Pearce commented on the ubiquitous and perennial nature of hysterical conversion – the tendency of hysterics to convert psycho-social stress into acceptable physical symptoms: "Hysteria has been present with mankind for hundreds of years, and what is interesting about hysteria is that while the basic syndrome seems not to change with the ages, the manner in which it presents undoubtedly does. For example, in medieval times, there is no doubt at all that the unfortunates who were diagnosed as witches were, in fact, hysterics. If you go back that early, there is a book called *Malleus Malifarium*[3], written by two monks, [Sprenger and Kramer], which purports to instruct you on how to identify witches; and one of the interesting things about it is that it tells you how to look for tender spots. In other words, in hysterics it is very common to find localized areas which, as the result of suggestion, are either hypo or hyperaesthetic."

Dr Pearce maintained that Mrs M had a "hysterical personality and [had] been experiencing considerable social stress long before the motor vehicle accident. He did not believe that the motor vehicle accident caused any of her problems, other than minor whiplash, but it was pivotal to her 'as a scapegoat for an ongoing process that was already there.'"

Mme Justice Rawlins's judgment goes on to report that Dr Pearce disagreed with Dr McCain's opinion that Mrs M would have enjoyed excellent health but for the motor vehicle accident. He was of the view that "the plaintiff was heading for trouble irrespective of the accident and sooner or later some event in her life would have occurred that would have allowed this condition to manifest itself through symptoms."

Dr Clarke, an anaesthetist and an expert in the management of chronic pain, testified for the defendant. He had examined Mrs M's records but did not examine Mrs M. Dr Clarke agreed that it was common for patients to keep pain diaries, but said of hers: "It would be extraordinary for somebody to keep a diary of such detail and for such a long period of time ... After 20 years or more of seeing chronic pain patients, I have seen a lot of pain diaries and I have had a lot of extremely obsessional patients who will [record] the most minute detail, but nothing to compare with this. And it has made me wonder why it is being kept.

Judicial points: Mme Justice Rawlins found that Mr M "could have taken certain reasonable steps to avoid the accident such as braking or sounding the horn," and he was therefore "contributorily negligent to the extent of 15 per cent." She was not impressed by the plaintiff's car having been a "write-off." "Much was said about the fact that the plaintiff's car was 'totalled,' presumably in an attempt to heighten the severity of the accident. Given the fact that the plaintiff's car was a 1977 Cadillac, I would expect that the repair work to the passenger door and front fender would have exceeded the value of the car."

The judge took note of the fact that Mrs M's body [neck] may have been turned somewhat to avoid the accident in an attempt to shield her daughter, but found: "The injuries causally related to the accident were minor and the damages reflect that she would have lingering effects for approximately 6 to 8 months after ... Clearly the pain that the plaintiff suffers and did suffer was real; of that I have no doubt, and that pain was accepted by all of the medical experts called except to the extent there was a concern that malingering may have developed in the later stages."

Mme Justice Rawlins remarked that a "host of medical experts called by the plaintiff" attributed Mrs M's pain to the accident, though she named four other expert witnesses who disagreed. She noted that Dr Sibley did not dispute the diagnosis of fibromyalgia, but gave the impression that such a diagnosis would not necessarily help Mrs M. The judge "found Dr Verdejo's experience and comments on fibromyalgia to be by far more helpful than any other rheumatologist or physician called by the plaintiff." She pointed out that Dr McCain had admitted there was no known cause of fibromyalgia, adding, "I assume he meant no physical cause."

Mme Justice Rawlins observed that one of the plaintiff's requests for compensation was US$20,000 to attend Dr McCain's clinic for the treatment of fibromyalgia, even though there is evidence that no treatment works. The judge also took note that Dr McCain was one of the rheumatologists involved in the development of the American College of Rheumatology's criteria for the diagnosis of fibromyalgia. She discounted his evidence on the grounds that "he may have a personal and perhaps financial interest in perpetuating the existence of this condition." Dr Austin considered specifically the possibility of fibromyalgia, but "found that her pain emanated from her 'bony prominences' and not from any accepted tender spots."

Mme Justice Rawlins said of Mrs M's complaints of pain: "It is interesting to note that fibromyalgia or chronic pain syndrome, as it is often called, had been the subject of litigation only in the recent past. It is as if all previous motor vehicle accident plaintiffs were fortunate enough never to have contracted this apparently debilitating condition whereas many recent plaintiffs have done. It is a late 1980s/1990s condition that some courts have welcomed as a new medical condition worthy of extensive damages. I attribute these decisions to the nature of the evidence presented, which was predominantly from rheumatologists."

Mme Justice Rawlins quotes other judgments on fibromyalgia, and provides a page of detailed legal argument of causation and responsibility, arguments that entail such phrases as "avoid the ultimate risk of non-persuasion," legalese that ordinary mortals cannot understand. She then renders her judgment:

The evidence here convinces me that the medical profession itself would not say that fibromyalgia, on the balance of probabilities, exists, much less [is] causally related to a motor vehicle accident. I am satisfied that fibromyalgia has become a court-driven ailment that has mushroomed into big business for plaintiffs, particularly in British Columbia and Saskatchewan ... The evidence in this case satisfies me that the symptoms diagnosed as fibromyalgia are a relabelling of a condition by rheumatologists that has been with mankind for hundreds of years and represents a personality disorder. This particular disorder is often found in individuals who will not or cannot cope with everyday stresses of life and convert this inability into acceptable physical symptoms to avoid dealing with reality.

Implausibility points: Mme Justice Rawlins was concerned with the plaintiff's credibility: "The plaintiff's life before that accident had not been an easy one. She was uprooted several times with her husband's employment, sometimes to centres where the population was less than ten people. The pay was often very poor ... There were periods of unemployment for her husband and her career as a nurse was intermittent at best ... [She worked with] patients who are totally disabled and count upon nursing assistance to do everything. According to some of the medical specialists, it could be considered one of the most difficult and demanding jobs as a Registered Nurse." She continued to express reservations about the veracity of Mrs M's statements: "The plaintiff's own evidence I found somewhat lacking and I did not believe her when she said her job and the obvious events in her life that would normally be considered stressful were not. Her evidence was not consistent with circumstances; I simply did not believe her in those areas where it was relevant."

The judge raised further doubts: "Although Mrs M on more than one occasion told the court she does not have an allergy to feathers, she reported the contrary on hospital admission forms submitted at the trial ... In addition to having some concerns about her credibility, I find there is a real possibility that she could have been allergic to the feathers all along, which may have contributed to or caused some of her symptoms."

Weighty points: The judge was critical of Mrs M's lack of effort to improve her situation: "The plaintiff was overweight and out of shape at the time of the accident. Her lifestyle choices resulted in her obesity and de-conditioning, the effect of which severely affected her well-being ... [Mrs M] failed to mitigate the damages by consistently failing to follow prescribed treatment or lifestyle changes that were within her control, particularly weight loss and exercise programs ... I do not accept her evidence, or that of her experts, that she did everything she could. I find that she did not."

Sticking points: In regard to Mrs M's work, Mme Justice Rawlins questioned Mrs M's motives: "I would have to agree with Dr Austin, who noted that every time the plaintiff attempted to return to work her symptoms appeared to worsen. The plaintiff said she loved her work, but I have serious doubts about her veracity, given her extended absences from work and her vague complaints of pain. I would have thought someone who loved their job would have made many more attempts to return to it than she did. In fact, not surprisingly, her job was in jeopardy because of these absences and she was, in a sense, forced to return when she did to preserve her employment." The judge said of Mrs M's home situation: "It does not appear from the evidence that her children helped her much during this period of her incapacity, nor did her husband. In fact, his evidence indicated that he was aware how difficult it was for her to do tasks, but it appears he did very little to pick up the slack."

Additional points: Mme Justice Rawlins did not accept the extent to which Mrs M claimed the accident had interfered with the completion of these tasks, for the simple reason that the arithmetic for her pre-accident workweek did not add up: "Mrs M said she spent 25 to 30 hours per week devoted to cleaning and managing [her] house. Considering she worked 8 to 10 hours at her job, probably spent 1 to 3 hours getting dressed, having breakfast and getting to work and 8 to 10 hours sleeping, she has already used 17 to 23 hours of a day without anything devoted to her household. Additionally, she said that she and her husband socialized a lot, 'dancing and partying and visiting and entertaining,' went to their cabin 2½ hours away at weekends, and spent a lot of time with their children doing their activities prior to the accident." The judge found that Mrs M's "capacity to do household services directly related to the accident was diminished by one to three hours [per week] for a period of six to eight months.

Brownie points: Mme Justice Rawlins found that "of all the experts who gave evidence at the trial" Dr Pearce was "the most lucid, knowledgeable and believable." She "detected no objective bias on his part to 'colour' the evidence one way or the other." Mme Justice Rawlins noted "the Minnesota Multiphasic Personality Inventory (MMPI) has been around since 1935. It has been translated into over 100 languages; it is universally used and often presented as evidence in court. Although the Court has been careful in not placing too much reliance on the results, in this case, however, Dr Pearce went to some distance to explain the improvements in the MMPI, most notably MMPI-2 and how objective it had become. The computer now scores and interprets the test, and compiles a personality profile."

Acknowledging her reservations about such tests, the judge continued: "One would have thought the results would have been relatively general without too much specificity, somewhat like horoscopes because of the impersonal approach to the patient's personality and symptomatic behaviour. Such was not the case here ... The results were quite interesting, considering what I learned about the plaintiff during the course of the trial."

Although her observations were couched in general terms, Mme Justice Rawlins considered the MMPI report to have remarkably described the plaintiff. She provided extracts from the report: "

[Mrs M's] profile presents a rather mixed pattern of symptoms in which somatic reactivity under stress is a primary difficulty. The client presents a picture of physical problems and a reduced level of psychological functioning. Her physical complaints may be vague, may have appeared suddenly after a period of stress, and may not be traceable to actual organic changes. She may be manifesting fatigue, vague pain, weakness or unexplained periods of dizziness. She may view herself as highly virtuous and show a "Pollyannaish" attitude towards life ... Individuals with similar profiles tend to be somewhat passive – dependent and demanding in interpersonal relationships. She may attempt to control others by complaining of physical symptoms. She is likely to experience low sexual drive and may have problems in her marriage because of this ... Her physical complaints are likely to be used to gain attention from her spouse. Physical complaints may also be employed to avoid sexual relations ... [She] will probably be resistant to mental health treatment, since she has little psychological insight and seeks medical explanations for her disorder. She is probably defensive and reluctant to engage in self-exploration. In addition, she seems to experience little anxiety over her situation and may have little motivation to change her behaviour.

Biting points: The judge "had difficulty in accepting that Mrs M suffered from TMJ disorder to start with, but more importantly that this condition, if she does suffer from it, was caused by the accident."[4]

Award points: The judge awarded Mrs M $25,000 in non-pecuniary damages and $800 for loss of household services, the estimated cost of the service that Mrs M was unable to do for the eight months following her accident. Mme Justice Rawlins denied Mrs M's request for $2,000 for the future maintenance of a TMJ splint, and US$20,000 (to attend Dr McCain's clinic).

MY DISCUSSION POINTS: I am amazed that Mrs M did not know the location of the tender point sites. Newspapers and magazines regularly publish charts showing their location.[5] In Ontario fibromyalgic plaintiffs all seem well acquainted with these charts so I am left wondering if the lawyers in Alberta are more honest than in Ontario or just less competent at coaxing their clients on how to be convincing fibromyalgics.

Mrs M's case is of general interest because she demonstrates so many of the typical features of the fibromyalgic patient. The accident was minor with few or no physical findings to explain the presence of pain. In the weeks, months, and years succeeding the accident, her symptoms and even the signs of injury, as demonstrated by some of her examiners, steadily worsened. Mrs M idealizes her pre-accident existence and bemoans her post-accident state. While nothing relieved her pain, Mrs M continues to subject herself to various useless and some potentially dangerous treatments.[6] At the same time Mrs M managed to avoid most of the prescribed activities that more realistically might have helped her.

Whiplash vantage point: With little hard scientific evidence to support it and considerable epidemiological information to refute it, courts have accepted the belief that whiplash is a likely cause of six months or so of disabling pain. Mme Justice Rawlins, while being quite sceptical of many of Mrs M's claims, accepted without question Mrs M's claim that whiplash pain diminished her "capacity to do household tasks for a period of six to eight months." Such legal precedent virtually guarantees that whiplash plaintiffs (and their lawyers) are entitled to receive some compensation for at least a half-year's incapacity. The whiplash plaintiff's problem is not whether or not he will receive compensation; it is just how much he can manage to get.

MMPI score points: Mme Justice Rawlins wondered about the MMPI's lack of specificity, suspecting that its impersonal approach to a person's personality and symptomatic behaviour would be somewhat akin to horoscopes. However, she was impressed at the uncanny way the results reflected Mrs M's personality. Yet Mme Justice Rawlins was right, these MMPI results are like horoscopes because they nicely fit so many plaintiffs in Mrs M's situation. The personality profile that the MMPI describes belongs to many young and middle-aged women who opt to become long-term whiplash victims. Just as horoscopes fit almost everyone's romantic and financial aspirations, so these MMPI results can be relied upon to fit the personality profiles of most female whiplash claimants.

Whiplash plaintiffs are often both angry and unhappy. Like Mrs M, they usually perform the lion's share of the household and family chores, for which they receive little appreciation or support. They often lack both the psychological understanding and the inner resources necessary to change the discomfort of their lives. They tend to deny their psychological distress and worry about physical symptoms instead.

Erotic points: Fibromyalgics, as do patients with other fashionable illnesses, often function poorly in adult sexual relationships. They are relieved to have the excuse to avoid any sexual obligations. "Fibromyalgia" is a near-perfect permanent "Not tonight, Dear, I have a headache" escape. In contrast, chronic pain from a clearly identifiable physical cause is seldom used as a reason to avoid sexual contact. In fact, sex is often welcomed as a diversion from the misery of such discomfort. For someone who dislikes sex, it is perhaps doubly gratifying to receive compensation for not doing something that he does not want to do anyway.

Missing the point: Dr McCain reported that Mrs M's MMPI results reveal the typical profile of the fibromyalgic patient. While he was right about the typical profile, he was wrong about what he called an inverted "V". The V is not inverted and it is called a "conversion V" – the characteristic MMPI finding in patients with fibromyalgia and, indeed, with other fashionable illnesses.

Dr McCain allowed that he was no expert on the MMPI, so his getting the V upside down is excusable. However, he then reported that fibromyalgics typically have high scores on the hysteria (conversion), depression, and hypochondriasis scales, a mistake which shows that he missed the whole point about the psychological findings in fibromyalgia. Fibromyalgics, while showing the features of depression, deny any depressed feelings. They have a *high* score for hypochondriacal concerns, a *low* score for depression and a *high* score for conversion (somatoform) symptoms, a pattern which, when represented graphically on the MMPI scoring sheet, forms the typical V configuration that gives the *classical conversion* V its name.

In failing to understand this mechanism, a physician is likely to regard all a patient's symptoms as having an organic basis. It is the physicians' attempt to find and treat the hypothetical injuries that soon brings the costs of doing so up to $20,000.

Crooked points? Dr Pearce noted that while "secondary gain" (the financial or personal advantages that accrue to a person through illness) are at first usually unconscious, they may not remain so. "If this process is prolonged, eventually, the patient begins to help it along a bit. In other words, he consciously appears to be a little more disabled than he really is or whatever the situation happens to be and, under the circumstances, as the secondary gain becomes less unconscious and conscious elements begin to enter, we get into the realm of faking [illness] or malingering."

Dr Pearce takes the traditional psychiatric stance that patients like Mrs M start off as honest but, on discovering that their symptoms have uses, then give them a helping hand. Is this perception correct? Most people know that whiplash is an acceptable cause of disability, and many seem to exploit an alleged injury as soon as bumper touches bumper.

The "P" word and power points: Mrs M worked long hours at a demanding and often unrewarding job. She was the main caregiver to an unappreciative and unsupportive family. She had a constant struggle with her weight. The family frequently moved locations and there were worries about her husband's employment. All things considered, Mrs M had understandable reasons to be anxious, tired, and depressed, but like many patients with fibromyalgia she was reluctant to see herself in these terms.

I do not mean this to be a plug for psychiatry, but the determined avoidance of a psychiatric diagnosis is oddly paradoxical. Competent and well-functioning people get episodes of depression, a condition that is now recognized to have a physical basis in altered brain chemistry. In contrast, fibromyalgics are perceived as troubled people who do not function well and whose *illness*, despite much research, has not been "reassuringly" shown to have a physical basis.

Mrs M was, in fact, treated with amitriptyline and Prozac, antidepressants prescribed, not for depression, but to "improve her sleeping pattern and for the prevention of migraine." Perhaps her doctor surreptitiously used such a pretext to prescribe them as a way of persuading Mrs M to take them. Certainly, the antidepressants seem to have helped. Her symptoms became worse on two occasions when she reduced the dose of amitriptyline, and within a few weeks of starting Prozac she had lost twenty pounds and was reported to be feeling better. However, this roundabout way of prescribing antidepressants is far from ideal since it makes it difficult for the physician to fine-tune the required dose. Avoiding the dreaded "P" word perhaps comes at a cost!

Pointless work and pointless years: Much professional time is invested in personal injury trials. The length of Mrs M's trial is not stated in Mme Justice Rawlins's report, but trials move slowly and the processing of such a large number of expert witnesses probably took several weeks, if not months. Like many judges, Mme Justice Rawlins struggled nobly with difficult medical material, but to what avail? Judgments do not produce a constructive solution to the management of the widespread problem of chronic pain syndrome, and the plaintiffs rarely benefit from the trials.

It took nearly ten years for Mrs M's case to come to court, during which time her life was on hold. To protect their claims for damages, the Mrs Ms of this world are locked into *invalidism* from which they often never recover. The judge awarded Mrs M $25,800 in compensation for her alleged injuries. In her judgment, Mme Justice Rawlins did not mention the legal costs. If Mrs M was not awarded these costs, all her financial award and much more – will have been used up in the payment of her legal fees. Fibromyalgia is good for the professionals, but questionable for the plaintiff!

14

Whiplash: An Eye to the Main Chance?

It is more important to know what sort of a patient has a disease
than what sort of a disease the patient has.

– Sir William Osler

Sometimes everything goes wrong – three collisions all in the same
week. Faced with this kind of expensive misfortune, which of us has
not been tempted to attribute the broken headlight, the dented fender, and the bent bumper all to the same accident, the one covered by
insurance? The body shop owner might think it odd that a small accident should have damaged both sides of the car at the same time, but
what does he care? He might even suggest it! He will get generously
paid and, without insurance coverage, the car owner would probably
just stay with the dents. In this way, human bodies and car bodies are
similar. All the pre-accident damaged and malfunctioning parts get
lumped in with damage caused by the accident. Again like body shop
owners, healthcare practitioners are on the lookout for work – and
often again like body shop owners, about double their charges when
an insurance company pays.[1]

In the early days of whiplash, when various medical specialists were
dividing up its spoils, eye doctors were no exception. In a twinkling of
an eye they found that whiplash caused all manner of eye problems.
The year after the publication of Gay and Abbott's original article,
Braaf and Rosner listed twelve ways in which whiplash affects the eye.[2]
Since then, ophthalmologists writing in medical journals have added
even more.

However, despite this list of twelve eye whiplash injuries, the ophthalmologists' articles – and numerous plaintiff claims of whiplash eye
injury – whiplash-induced eye problems are in fact rare. North
American courts began to find ophthalmologists' claims preposterous,
so there was no longer any point in making them and claims of
whiplash eye damage dwindled in North America. Whiplash eye damage journal articles also trailed off. Except for two recent entries from
the United Kingdom, the last MedLine entry for articles on whiplash
eye damage dates back to 1970 and was from Japan.

The disappearance of whiplash eye damage articles and the reduction in whiplash eye damage claims does not mean, however, that whiplash lawyers have removed ophthalmologists from their whiplash referral lists. As part of their *fishing expeditions* for whiplash-attributable injuries, lawyers still arrange consultations with compliant ophthalmologists. I often found one, two, or even three eye doctor reports in the medico-legal briefs of whiplash plaintiffs.

I have seen no reports in which an ophthalmologist attributes any actual eye problem to the accident, but the absence of such attribution is seldom apparent to the reader. The doctor writes in this vein: "Following the accident the patient complained of pain in the eyes and blurred vision. On testing, his vision is reduced to 20/80 in the left eye and 20/60 in the right." Naturally, most people conclude that the accident caused a visual problem; they fail to realize that the patient, like many of us, is short-sighted and was so long before the accident. Besides this small legal ploy, such doctor visits serve another purpose. Along with all the other arranged visits to specialists, they help delay the plaintiff's return to work, small but critical steps towards the induction of remunerative chronicity.

Following a pattern that by now will be familiar to the reader, the whiplash eye articles provide an instructive overview of how the relatively uncommon and usually trivial eye manifestations of whiplash were elaborated into a subject of conspicuous medico-legal concern. This review makes another convincing vignette on how quickly healthcare practitioners can turn a sow's ear of ordinary good health into a silk purse of diagnosis and treatment.

Ophthalmologists are not noted for being in the forefront of medicine, but Myron Middleton, an American ophthalmologist, published the first whiplash article only two years after the publication of the Gay and Abbott article. He promised great things both for lawyers and his colleagues: "The pupil of the eye and its associated structures can provide many valuable clues in diagnosing residual trauma from whiplash injuries ... Patients with whiplash injuries frequently present vague visual complaints. It is sometimes difficult for them to describe these complaints. They say they have 'blurred vision,' or 'objects seem to recede,' or 'I seem to lose my focus.'" Middleton described the neuroanatomical pathways involved in the control of the pupil and suggested ways by which whiplash brain injury may interrupt these neural circuits and so explain the eye findings.[3]

The last paragraph in Middleton's article was guaranteed to arouse the cupidity of whiplash lawyers: "Perhaps in the not too distant future, pupillography may become a common procedure in the office, as common as Roentgenography [the x-ray] is today. With a more refined technique, we will be less inclined to consider complaints as functional because we cannot satisfactorily prove them to be organic. When it is realized that, in addition to the legion of eye signs caused by head injury, we have those resulting from whiplash injury, the ophthalmic evaluation of patients becomes very important." The last line translated into lay language means many more jobs for ophthalmologists!

Then in 1959 Geraldine Knight from Seattle, Washington, presented a paper on whiplash to the annual meeting of the American Association of Orthoptic Technicians. (Orthoptics means "straight eyes.") Why were these technicians interested in whiplash? On moving the gaze from something in the distance to something close by, the eyes converge, the pupils contract and the lenses accommodate. These changes maintain binocular vision and serve to keep the visual image sharp. In some people this process is out of balance; the person squints or, more commonly, has a tendency to squint – a *latent squint* which the body corrects by increasing the tension in the appropriate small external muscles of the eye. It used to be believed that this extra tension, especially in children, caused headache.[4]

Orthoptics seeks to correct this imbalance through eye exercises, a technique that is still used but much less so than when Knight wrote her article. As a small boy, my friends and I would do our daily eye exercises – trying to keep in focus the end of a trombone-like gadget in front of our eyes. Like piano teachers, orthopticians were on the lookout for pupils to whom to teach their eye-straightening exercises. Knight had discovered that whiplash sufferers required them.

Knight began her article in traditional whiplash style; "How often have you heard the patient who has been a victim of a head injury or whip-lash injury described as 'neurotic' or 'malingering'? His symptoms are vague and disconnected and frequently related to obscure visual problems." Knight found that whiplash symptoms were caused by a loss of convergence. She searched the literature but could find little information about head injury and such loss.[5] Then she found a paper by A.C. Cross, in which he described his wide experience with terrible injuries from World War II – a perfect comparison for whiplash injury!" Cross had written: "Most cases show equal defect of the two functions (convergence and accommodation) but occasionally either may be deficient separately. Spontaneous recovery occurs in some of these patients but the process is hastened, and in other cases brought about, by orthoptic treatment. The rapidity with which cure may occur under treatment is an indication of the absence of organic cause and of the functional [physiological] nature of the defect."

Knight tried orthoptics on her whiplash patients, the majority of which had been in rear-end collisions. "When this great force strikes, the head is lashed forward and then backward. The result of this whip-like action on the neck may range in severity from only temporary stiffness to permanent disability or even death." Knight wrote her article five years after Gay and Abbott had popularized whiplash, yet whiplash enthusiasts, although frequently referring to the "great force" of whiplash, and all that it can do, had not yet noticed that Gay and Abbott had got the action of whiplash the wrong way round.

Knight examined thirty whiplash patients and in the majority of them observed "a notable loss of convergence [as] the one common symptom." Most of her patients rapidly responded to simple convergence training: "An average of six treatments at the clinic and conscientious home exercises relieved the symptoms." No doubt Knight was a popular speaker with orthopticians; she had provided them with an ever-replenishing supply of orthoptic pupils.

Harry Horwich and David Kasner, ophthalmologists from Coral Gables, Florida, opened their 1962 article with background material on the medico-legal reputation of whiplash injury. "In the minds of many, the term 'whiplash' has become opprobrious. This is to be expected when a medical syndrome of increasing incidence has become a magic password outside medical circles. Plaintiffs' attorneys have seized upon whiplash injuries as a dramatic and effective means of obtaining large settlements in the presence of nebulous medical findings. The net result of the popularization has been reluctance on the part of some doctors to use this term, in direct ratio to the eagerness of attorneys to make capital of the syndrome."[6]

Horwich and Kasner, having appeared to hold a balanced view in this controversial issue, set out to establish a physical basis for ocular whiplash complaints. They then argued that such complaints, "while often ascribed to neurosis or malingering," are a legitimate consequence of whiplash-induced brain injury – an injury revealed by loss of convergence and accommodation. Knight had only found loss of convergence, but these ophthalmologists found that accommodation had gone as well. The nerve cells that control eye movements are located in the brainstem, so this is where the ophthalmologists located their brain injury.

There was one snag. A doctor tests for convergence and accommodation by asking the patient to watch his finger as he moves it closer to the patient's nose. It requires some effort on the part of the patient to keep his eyes focused on the approaching finger, and whiplash plaintiffs are certainly not over-zealous in making such efforts. Horwich and Kasner expressed their concern: "Naturally, when a patient involved in an accident giving rise to litigation complains of difficulty in focusing, we regard him with some measure of suspicion. We have all seen patients who obviously have not been trying to focus at near, and we are powerless to tell how hard he is trying, unless we can outwit him."

To outwit the apathetic patient the authors used prisms. This strategy worked poorly and the ophthalmologists had to admit that they were "at the mercy of the patient's volition and motivation."[7] Despite their misgivings, however, the authors still attributed the sluggishness of convergence and accommodation that they elicited to whiplash brain damage.

Treatment always works best when there is nothing wrong in the first place. In the same way that ENT surgeons reported that nystagmus (which they mistook as pathological) responded well to treatment, Horwich and Kasner reported success in treating weakness of convergence and accommodation: "Fortunately, this condition is self-limited, and responds readily to treatment. In the average case symptoms are present for only two to six months, and only rarely do symptoms persist over two years ... General treatment consists of cervical traction, orthopaedic collars, diathermy of the neck skeletal muscles, relaxants and [painkillers]. In about two per cent of whiplash injuries operation is required for treatment of an injured cervical disc." Rather reassuringly, Horwich and Kasner were not too keen on the knife: "In all fairness to the patients we treat, we must acknowledge that their anxiety, tension, nervousness, and even hostility is real. They may not be justified, but the symptoms disturb the patients, and as doctors we must not scoff at them. Reassurance, patience, kindness, and understanding are more important in our armamentarium than the scalpel and the tongs."

Herbert Wiesinger and DuPont Guerry III, ophthalmologists from the Medical College of Virginia, the same year confirmed the finding of "impairment of convergence and accommodation," and did even better than Horwich and Kasner. Besides finding that 7 out of 10 whiplash patients had a complete or partial weakness of accommodation and convergence, they also found a similar weakness of the external muscles that move the eye, which they hypothesized was caused by small haemorrhages and areas of softening in the brainstem – the part of the brain that controls eye movements.[8]

Weisinger and Guerry support their supposition of whiplash-induced brainstem damage by references to horrific examples of human whiplash in the medical literature, most of which did not actually exist. They did not refer to the whiplash animal studies because these had not yet been published. The authors end up with the completely erroneous statement: "The frequent association of contusion of the brain with whiplash injury was stressed also by Gay and Abbott." Gay and Abbott in their famous article did *not* stress "the frequent association of contusion of the brain with whiplash injury." In fact, they did not even mention the word "contusion." In reviewing their own series of ten whiplash patients, Weisinger and Guerry seemed equally ready to embellish their findings, ascribing unimpressive symptoms to whiplash injury. The more serious injuries they described were almost certainly caused by trauma other than whiplash.

By the time William Gibson, from the University of Florida College of Medicine, wrote *The Eye and Whiplash Injuries* in 1968, the results of the whiplash animal studies had been published. Gibson adds a description of these studies to the mostly mythical human whiplash catastrophes:[9] "The belief is widely held that these are 'simple sprains' which will resolve with time and resolution of the attendant litigation. Most physicians and defence lawyers imply that complaining patients are either neurotic or malingerers who are presenting a case of litigation neurosis. In the cases with demonstrable findings it is remarkable how seldom there are complaints of associated injuries." Gibson was again using a simple clinical test to separate the sheep from the goats: the truly injured from the neurotics and the frauds.

He illustrated his point with reference to ten of his own cases. In three cases, brain injury was validated by the presence of "paralysis of accommodation and conversion;" these patients had few complaints. In the other seven there was no demonstrable injury; these patients had many complaints. Of the seven *goats* without confirmatory evidence of brain injury, Gibson wrote: "Three were proven malingerers who described the same visual field at two meters as at one meter and who expressed their colour fields the same as white. The four remaining cases had multiple subjective symptoms but none that could be objectively demonstrated in relation to ocular function." He concluded his study with the hope that his paper would prevent "injustice to the many victims of rear-end collisions who, as a result, have real disabilities." In painting the sheep very white and the goats very black, Gibson turned himself into an excellent arbiter of which whiplash plaintiffs deserved compensation and which did not. Both plaintiff and defence lawyers would have need of his services.

Two years later Donald Fite, an ophthalmologist from Florida, after citing catastrophic reports of both animal and human whiplash and the "growing evidence that significant damage occurs to the central nervous system," quoted Ommaya's advice: "Patients with whiplash injury that persists beyond 24 hours [should] be managed the same way as closed-head injury patients."[10] Since it is estimated that well over a million Americans sustain a whiplash injury each year, and since every would-be-whiplash claimant, and even the odd non-claimant is likely to have symptoms that last more than 24 hours, this advice, if followed, would bring battalions of patients under intensive medical care.[11] Again, *more jobs for the boys!*

In "Ocular Manifestations of Whiplash Injury," P.D. Roca from the Rochester Medical School complained that the symptoms of whiplash eye damage are customarily attributed to "psychoneurosis" and "psychic inadequacies."[12] He presented fifteen cases to prove otherwise. I beg to differ. Some of his cases were not even automobile injuries, such as a man who twisted his neck when slipping in a shower and developed unequal sized pupils, or a zoo attendant who was charged by a North American elk that struck him on the head, rendering him unconscious for twenty minutes. "Even insignificant attempts to move his head or neck or use his eyes produced severe headaches. He had marked photophobia (claiming he could not read), dizziness and unsteadiness of gait." X-rays showed a chip fracture of part of a neck vertebra. Roca commented: "Until it was realized that this patient had suffered a whiplash in addition to concussion his case was somewhat baffling." Actually if these symptoms *had* been due to whiplash they would have been baffling, but as they were due to a blow on the head they were not. If the zoo attendant had been struck on the backside he might indeed have sustained the most genuine rear-end whiplash injury ever recorded in medical literature, but the irascible elk hit him on the head and not the bum.

Several patients whose cases Roca details were actually in collisions but appear to have suffered a direct head injury rather than whiplash, which again is a legitimate cause of eye injury. However, even the genuine whiplash-type injuries are of doubtful significance, such as the example of a 40-year-old executive who complained of inability to read, light sensitivity, and headaches following a minor collision one week earlier. He was found to have developed "presbyopia," a hardening of lens that is common in forty-year-olds. It is a safe bet that the insurance company paid for the glasses he would have needed without the accident.

And some, like the proverbial old lady who kicks the cat and fractures her osteoporotic hip, were injuries waiting to happen. Take the 70-year-old "retired paediatrician who sustained a typical whiplash with moderate concussion in a car crash, for instance. The afternoon of the accident, he suddenly noticed floaters in his right visual field." He was found to have bilateral detachment of the vitreous in both eyes. Examination of the eye also showed extensive degenerative changes in the back of the eye of the kind associated with severe short-sightedness. Roca is no doubt correct: "The whiplash injury sustained apparently intensified this patient's pre-existing ocular degenerative changes," but this certainly does not incriminate whiplash as a significant cause of eye injury.

As far as whiplash eye injuries go, Roca's fifteen cases were not worth a hill of beans, yet on the strength of these injuries he theorized: "Small amounts of subarachnoid haemorrhage can produce severe headache and a markedly stiff neck, two of the cardinal symptoms of whiplash victims." He again quoted Ommaya's self-serving *jobs for the boys* advice that whiplash patients whose symptoms persist for more than 24 hours should be treated as for head injury.

Johns Hopkins Hospital, Baltimore, is distinguished for the excellence of its medical care, but even there whiplash was given a raw deal. James Kelley and his colleagues from Johns Hopkins entitle their article "Whiplash Maculopathy."[13] (The macula is a small spot on the retina at the position of maximum visual acuity.) The authors describe this maculopathy as a condition in which there is "a history of immediate mild reduction of central visual acuity in one or both eyes." The injury is associated with discernible but minute and subtle changes in the macula. The authors present three cases.

A 32-year-old woman was a passenger in a forcibly rear-ended car. Both cars were severely damaged but she suffered no direct bodily injury. She noticed hazy vision in both eyes and was found to have characteristic retinal changes. Within two weeks her visual acuity had returned to normal.

A 15-year-old boy braked too suddenly and went over the handlebars of his motorcycle. "His helmet prevented any direct injury to either head or eyes, but there was sharp flexion of the neck … The next day, while at school, the boy became aware of blurred vision, particularly in his left eye." The characteristic retinal changes were observed and his vision returned to normal within two weeks.

A 50-year-old woman was found to have the characteristic retinal changes on routine examination. She gave a history of having been in a severe car accident two years previously, after which she reported that her vision was slightly blurry for a month.

While the transitory damage to the macula is no doubt a genuine injury, by labelling the condition "whiplash maculopathy," the authors saddle whiplash for injuries it did not cause. In no way did the 15-year-old who went over the handlebars have a whiplash injury. And who knows whether the woman in the severe car accident had a direct or acceleration/deceleration injury? The Johns Hopkins ophthalmologists may have been unfair to whiplash, but they, unlike most other whiplash authors, indicate that the effects of the whiplash eye injury are short-lived.

Until the days of Mrs Thatcher, private medical practice in United Kingdom was minimal so there was little reason for British ophthalmologists to have an interest in whiplash. When private practice began to flourish in Britain, whiplash patients were soon in demand. Ophthalmologist John Burke and his colleagues studied 39 consecutive patients presenting with whiplash injury in the emergency department. They assessed these patients within one week of the accident, six weeks later, and, where clinically indicated, up to three months after the accident. They found that 10 (26%) of the 39 patients "had ocular symptoms and signs which developed shortly after the accident;" six (15%) had decreased convergence and accommodation; two (5%) had weakness of the superior oblique muscle (one of the external muscles of the eye); and one (2.5%) had bilateral vitreous detachments.

Only one patient of the ten who were found to have "ocular symptoms and signs" actually seems to have complained of an eye problem, the eye symptoms and signs in the other nine patients having been uncovered by the ophthalmologists' direct questions and examination. The single patient who spontaneously complained of eye symptoms was a 31-year-old woman with bilateral vitreous detachment who had had spots in her visual fields within thirty minutes of the accident. The patients mostly did well, and the authors conclude: "Oculomotor abnormalities following whiplash injuries are generally mild, have a good prognosis, and would appear from this study to be commoner than hitherto expected."[14]

This statement probably sounds innocent enough to the uninitiated, but it is not. England is at least three decades behind the United States in building up its whiplash industry and its doctors and lawyers are still at the stage of generating enthusiasm for whiplash. A study showing the frequent association of eye problems and whiplash would quickly induce every English plaintiff whiplash lawyer to refer their whiplash clients to an ophthalmologist.

You may well wonder why a lawyer would bother to do so since the ocular manifestations of whiplash (if they actually exist) are reportedly mild with a good prognosis. Any ocular problem caused by whiplash will be long gone by the time the case comes to court. Although the manifestations may be mild and transient, however, the finding that 15 per cent of consecutive unselected whiplash patients presenting at an emergency department have decreased convergence and accommodation has far-reaching implications – implications that brain damage frequently occurs in whiplash injury.

In their article, Burke and his team discuss whiplash's potential to become chronic even after the litigation has settled. They dwell on the probability of brain damage. They quote the work of the previous whiplash investigators who reported weakness of convergence and accommodation and cited brainstem damage as its cause. They quote Wickstrom's animal whiplash studies, in which 32 per cent of the primates were found to have such damage. Building their case, the authors continue: "The majority of patients will improve to their own satisfaction with the passage of time and learn to live with their intermittent residual discomforts. However, about 12 per cent are left with discomfort of sufficient severity to interfere with their capacity to enjoy themselves in their leisure even after litigation claims have been settled." In conclusion, these English ophthalmologists subtly tip the scales: "We believe that many minor visual symptoms after whiplash injuries have an explainable ophthalmic basis and a good prognosis but, if persistent, merit referral for ophthalmic evaluation and appropriate treatment."

The "explainable ophthalmic basis" is the brainstem damage. No court is going to pay out big money for transient and symptomless ocular problems, but, at least in the public's imagination, *brain damage* is a different matter. Whiplash litigants could now comfortably attribute all their psychological problems to the accident. They cannot concentrate, their memory has gone, they are constantly irritable and fatigued, and their personality has changed (always for the worse) ... the effects of brain injury, of course!

Plaintiff neuropsychologists routinely assess whiplash litigants for evidence of altered brain function. They attribute any deviations from normal (which are exceedingly common) to whiplash-induced brain injury. The supposition that 15 per cent of run-of-the-mill whiplash patients have brain damage makes psychologists' claims appear less fanciful and, of course, much more difficult to refute. Compensation for brain damage can run into hundreds or thousands – even millions.

Burke and his colleagues' article is sloppy science. As justification for their study, these authors note that "whiplash is a common occurrence" but that there is a "dearth of information outlining the frequency of such complication among the whiplash population at large." However, has their study added anything to the world's whiplash literature? Knight, Horwich and Kasner, and Wiesinger and Guerry all reported finding a high incidence of convergence and accommodation difficulties in whiplash patients. There is no reason to believe that ophthalmologists have become better observers of reduced convergence and accommodation in the intervening thirty years, or that they have become any more or any less honest in the reporting of their findings. Which of all these investigators, if any, is correct? There are at least two reasons why it is impossible to know.

The first reason is that whiplash is not a homogeneous condition. A collision with severe damage to vehicles and obvious injury to the occupants is different from a collision in which there is no vehicle damage and no observable injury – and the only reason for a hospital visit is to document the accident's occurrence for future litigation. None of the studies gives any indication of the level of severity of the collisions in which their subjects were involved.

The second reason is the problem of reliably identifying a *decrease of convergence and accommodation*. People differ in the flexibility of their bodies, and of their eyes no less so. It is a clinical judgment call to say when such a decrease of convergence and accommodation is present. The only certain way to determine the reliability of such observations is to use control subjects matched for age and gender, and have observers blinded to the status of the subjects and controls they examine.

The failure to use a control group leads to medico-legal mayhem. ENT surgeons with nystagmus, dentists with TMJ intra-articular disc displacement, orthopaedic surgeons with bulging intervertebral cervical discs, physiatrists with trigger points, and rheumatologists with alpha-delta sleep all looked for abnormal findings in whiplash victims and all found them. It was only much later, when control subjects were included, that ordinary healthy people were also found to have an equal share of supposed *abnormalities*.

British eye doctors have behaved badly! In the 1950s, when American eye doctors published their findings of reduced accommodation and convergence in whiplash patients, medical science was unsophisticated about the pitfalls inherent in such prevalence studies. Medical science is no longer unsophisticated. British medical education is excellent and it is hard to believe these eye doctors, publishing in the 1990s, did not know better.

The eye doctors failed at epidemiology but what about their neurological diagnoses? How reliable is their contention that a decrease in accommodation and convergence indicates brain damage? Their colleagues, the neurologists, are wont to say, "The only use that ophthalmologists have for the brain is to stop the eyeballs from falling into the skull" – a snide remark, but perhaps it's true. Ophthalmologists show little understanding of the organ that lies behind their area of interest. The brainstem, in which they suppose the damage to be located, is a vast pathway of vital neural activity. It is hard to envisage any damage in this area of the brain that would not immediately be made apparent by all manner of other things going wrong. You do not cause a major disturbance on the nation's biggest highway and then find that only one person is late for work!

Perhaps Weisinger, Guerry, Horwich, Kasner, Fite, and others, could, against all clinical odds, "assume as a working hypothesis that small areas of haemorrhages or of encephalomalacia [softening of the brain]" were responsible for the alleged eye changes in their patients, but three decades later, Burke and his colleagues could no longer do so. Modern imaging techniques leave no such brain pathology unrevealed. There are neither haemorrhages nor areas of softening in the brainstems of whiplash patients. Heavy impact collisions can occasionally cause retinal or vitreous detachment along with transient damage to the macula, or perhaps even the occasional unexplained external eye muscle weakness. But the finding of these well-authenticated signs of injury is a far cry from the reporting of wholesale eye abnormalities in ordinary whiplash patients. The eye is said to be the window to the soul, but the eye doctors are busy turning it into a signpost to a damaged brain.

PART THREE

Fraud and the Medical-Legal Quagmire

15

Post-traumatic Turbulence

> If mental disorders were listed on the New York Exchange,
> post-traumatic stress disorder would be a growth stock worth watching.
> – Lees-Haley and Dunn[1]

> There is probably never a physical injury without some measurable
> psychic trauma. The past 30 years ... have seen the exploitation
> of this truism in workers' compensation and personal injury litigation ...
> resulting in a staggering number of physically fit, mentally competent
> individuals forever being relieved of responsibility for earning a living
> on psychiatric grounds.
> – Martin Blinder[2]

Lawyers no longer learn Latin, but they certainly know the meaning of *post hoc ergo propter hoc:* "This followed that, therefore this was caused by that." Anything that follows an accident becomes attributable to it. *Post-traumatic* is one of the most succulent words in an accident litigation lawyer's vocabulary. Plaintiff experts use it liberally – post-traumatic headache, post-traumatic depression, post-traumatic anxiety, post-traumatic fibromyalgia, post-traumatic neurosis. One Toronto psychiatrist, who makes a specialty of plaintiff whiplash reports, managed on one occasion to put ten different post-traumatic conditions in the same report.

Although any causal relationship with trauma is often dubious, so compelling is "post-traumatic" that it becomes a standing indictment of the accident and of the person who caused it. Assiduous whiplash claimants routinely lay claim to at least two post-traumatic conditions. Their lawyers send them to a rheumatologist to acquire a diagnosis of post-traumatic fibromyalgia and to either a psychologist or a psychiatrist (or both) to acquire a diagnosis of "post-traumatic stress disorder" (PTSD).

A relative newcomer to the medico-legal scene, PTSD became a psychiatric diagnosis with the publication of the *Diagnostic and Statistical Manual of Mental Disorder–III (DSM-III)* in 1980.[3] Actually, the need for this diagnosis was more political than clinical. Veterans returning from Vietnam had been exposed to the horrifying experience of war and had developed "post-Vietnam syndrome," a non-compensable condition. The Veterans' Administration needed a suitable psychiatric diagnostic category by which to compensate its veterans. The American Psychiatric Association produced it.[4] The *DSM-III* states of PTSD:

> [Its] essential feature is the development of characteristic symptoms following a psychologically traumatic event that is outside the range of usual human experience ... The stressors producing this disorder include natural disasters (floods, earthquakes), accidental man-made disasters (car accidents with serious physical injury, airplane crashes, large fires), or deliberate man-made disasters (bombing, torture, death camps). Some stresses frequently produce the disorder (e.g., torture) and others produce it only occasionally (e.g., car accidents) ... The disorder is apparently more severe and longer lasting when the stressor is of human design.[5]

PTSD comprises a miscellany of symptoms. The traumatic event is re-experienced either by intrusive recollections or in dreams and nightmares. The victim is either hyper-aroused with an exaggerated, perhaps "jumpy," psychophysiological response to ordinary happenings, or becomes withdrawn and sluggish with "psychic numbing" or "emotional anaesthesia" so that his emotional responses are reduced, especially in regard to intimacy, tenderness, and sexuality. Depression and anxiety are common, and activities or situations associated with the traumatic event are mostly avoided. The symptoms are said to start soon after the event but may be delayed for months or years. If the symptoms persist for more than six months the disorder is designated as chronic.

From the point of view of generating medico-legal work, PTSD is fantastic. It has become a rising wave of terror, with whiplash often riding on its crest. Within fourteen years of its introduction, the reported incidence of alleged PTSD in victims of MVAs seeking medical treatment had gone from near zero to nearly 50 per cent. The kinds of minor collisions that are said to cause whiplash now often cause PTSD as well.

Less than two decades ago psychiatric complications following accident-induced trauma were uncommon. Ulrik Malt, a distinguished professor of psychiatry at the University of Oslo, studied the psychiatric status of a sample of 107 Norwegians admitted to hospital on account of accidental injury, 46 per cent of whom had been injured in traffic accidents. Using *DSM-III* diagnostic criteria, he performed his study during 1981 to 1982, a year or so after the publication of DSM-III.[6] Comparative statistics show that the health of the Norwegian population corresponds closely to that of white populations of other Western countries, so Malt's findings can legitimately be generalized to other countries of the developed world.[7] The study provides reliable baseline information on the incidence of traffic accident-induced PTSD at a time when the diagnosis of PTSD was still mostly unknown to both lawyers and plaintiffs.

Malt assessed injured subjects in hospital, mailed out packages of questionnaires six to nine months later, and finally re-examined the subjects two years after the accidents using a clinical interview and further questionnaires. Norway's extensive medical record-keeping arrangements enabled Malt to examine his subjects' pre-accident health records. He identified various psychiatric disorders related to the accident. Nine per cent of the subjects had a psychiatric disorder due to actual brain injury.

Apart from such organically induced psychiatric disorders, Malt found the rates of psychiatric disorders following accidents similar to those reported in follow-up studies after physical illness. Only one of the 107 patients fulfilled the *DSM-III* criteria for PTSD, and in this one patient the positive result was only obtained at the interim follow-up examination. Malt's conclusion was that, with a rate of less than one per cent, the incidence of PTSD following accidental injury is low. Since then the rates have steadily edged up to their present epidemic proportions.

In the early 1990s psychiatrist Richard Mayou and his team at Oxford University studied the incidence of PTSD following traffic accidents.[8] There was a twelve-year interval from when Malt had collected his data to the Mayou study, during which lawyers and claimants had time to learn all about the symptoms of PTSD. Mayou studied 200 traffic accident victims consecutively admitted to the Emergency Department of the Radcliffe Hospital in Oxford. The accidents were of varying severity; some victims required hospital admission and others were sent home. The investigators managed to follow 188 of these 200 patients over the next year. They found an 11 per cent incidence of PTSD; more than ten times the rate that Malt had found.

In 1985 psychiatrist Klaus Kuch and his colleagues from the University of Toronto had found that 100 per cent of thirty MVA victims met the *DSM-III* criteria for PTSD.[9] However, there was clearly some selection bias in this group of patients since twelve patients had been referred specifically for psychiatric treatment.

Edward R. Blanchard and his colleagues at the University of Albany Center for Stress and Anxiety Disorders initiated a study of "relatively unselected MVA victims" to determine the psychological morbidity found in such a sample.[10] To enter their study, the subjects had to have been involved in an MVA for which they had sought medical attention within one week of the accident. The authors advertised for suitable subjects through the local media and by flyers sent to healthcare practitioners. They collected 50 MVA victims of whom 46 per cent met the criteria for PTSD, while another 20 per cent showed a sub-syndromal version (the re-experiencing symptom cluster plus either the over-arousal cluster or the avoidance/numbing cluster) of PTSD.

Besides this apparent 45-fold increase in the incidence of PTSD following MVAs over a 15-year period, the accidents that are its alleged cause are actually less severe. All of Malt's patients were injured severely enough to warrant hospital admission; about two-thirds of Mayou's patients required admission. Blanchard's subjects were injured only to the extent that they needed to seek some kind of medical attention within a week of the accident.

The likely explanation of Blanchard's findings is that both the MVA victims and their lawyers perceived the participation in this well-advertised study as a convenient and inexpensive way to establish the presence of PTSD. People commencing a whiplash injury suit were quick to volunteer their services and gave the diagnosis of PTSD a helping hand when answering Blanchard's questionnaires.

Intrusive horrific memories of the psychologically traumatic event are frequently reported in the form of recurrent nightmares; such reports too are on the increase. Malt, from his 1982 to 1983 data, found "there were few reports of [patients] worrying over the injury or its consequences, or of nightmares" amongst his post-accident group of patients. In contrast, Blanchard's team found that 30 per cent of their MVA victims complained of "disturbing dreams." I now find it exceptional to assess an MVA victim who does not complain that his sleep is disturbed by nightmares of the accident.

Along with the increasing reports of nightmares by accident victims, PTSD has become one huge nightmare for the defence bar. The increasing percentages of the incidence of PTSD have large legal implications. In distinction to criminal law, a civil law case is won on the balance of probabilities. Once the medical literature confirms that it has been *scientifically* shown that more than half of MVA victims develop PTSD then, purely on the balance of probabilities, any MVA claimant will be accepted as having PTSD. The medical literature is certainly bullish on PTSD, and it probably will not be long before the 50 per cent mark is regularly surpassed. Any determined MVA claimant (most of whom are whiplash victims), will then be virtually guaranteed compensation for a psychiatric disorder in addition to the compensation for his ongoing whiplash pains and mental impairment from whiplash brain injury.

How has this nonsensical state of affairs come about? For various reasons, even from its inception, the diagnosis of PTSD has been problematic. To start with, there are substantial difficulties with its diagno-

	Whiplash Injury Victim	Car Occupants (excluding whiplash)	Motorcycle Rider
No intrusive memories	3	48	23
Intrusive memories (non-frightening)	62	22	51
Intrusive memories ("horrific")	35	30	27

Fig. 15–1   The smaller the accident the greater the afterthoughts
Percentage of MVA victims from three categories of injury with intrusive thoughts of the accident at post-accident interview. Most of the motorcycle riders and the car occupants required hospital admission. In contrast, none of the whiplash victims required admission

sis.[11] PTSD is not a discrete diagnostic entity, but a hodgepodge of psychiatric disorders – anxiety, panic, phobic, depressive, conversion, somatization, and other disorders – all mixed up together in one disturbing brew of real or alleged psychiatric pathology.[12] And how traumatic must the psychological trauma have been to cause PTSD? The *DSM-III* specifies that car accidents, unless accompanied by serious physical injury, only occasionally cause it.

But how often is "only occasionally"? Any plaintiff lawyer worth his salt will argue that since whiplash is a common cause of permanent disability, whiplash must be a serious injury. And what constitutes "a psychologically traumatic event that is generally outside the range of human experience"? This is a matter of opinion. Being hit with a bag of carrots in a grocery store, and finding a cockroach (not even half a one) in a sandwich are occurrences that have been submitted as alleged causes of PTSD.[13] A medical technician once sued after a doctor gave him a fright by unexpectedly tapping him on the shoulder while he was repairing some medical equipment.[14] The symptoms of PTSD are mostly subjective, and the verification of their presence depends upon the self-report of the patient. Such reports, especially in medico-legal situations, are notoriously unreliable.

The Mayou PTSD study is an example of this problem. These Oxford investigators divided their 200 injured patients into three categories: injured car occupants other than whiplash victims (55 patients); injured motorcyclists (71 patients); and whiplash victims (74 patients). They found "the principal and very strong predictor [for the development of PTSD] was the patient's report of 'horrific' intrusive memories at the post-accident interview." To obtain this information, the patients were asked whether or not they had "intrusive memories" of the accident and if they had, whether these intrusive memories were "non-frightening" or "horrific."[15] Figure 15–1 shows the results in percentages.

The car occupants (excluding the whiplash victims) and the motorcycle riders all required admission to hospital. Both groups scored high on injury severity. In contrast, the whiplash victims had no rateable injuries and were all sent home after the accident. By objective standards, the whiplash victims were far less seriously injured than the patients in the other two groups, yet a higher percentage of the whiplash victims (97%) claimed intrusive memories of the accident compared to the motorcycle accident victims (87%) or the nonwhiplash car-occupant victims (52%). The whiplash-injury victims also reported the highest rate of "horrific" intrusive memories.

How much personal involvement must there be in a traumatic event for it to cause PTSD? A difficult question. In March 1987, the P&O passenger ferry, the *Herald of Free Enterprise,* capsized outside the Zeebrugge Harbour drowning 193 people, including 38 of the 80 crew members. The authorities established a mental health centre which the survivors and the bereaved were invited to attend. Over the next three years, some cross-channel ferry workers, who had had no direct contact with the disaster as survivors, as bereaved relatives, or as helpers, presented themselves to the mental health team with PTSD. It was argued that they were the indirect victims of the "ripple outward" effect of this major disaster.[16]

The British Law Lords (apparently out of the fear of opening the floodgates to an indeterminate number of claimants) ruled that catastrophes communicated by television and other electronic mass media are not an acceptable cause of PTSD, while in the United States, a judge ruled that children who watch scary movies on television can suffer from it.[17] All in all, the medico-legal diagnosis of PTSD is a bit fluffy.

Although emphasis is placed on the psychological trauma of the event in making the diagnosis, factors other than the accident are clearly involved in its aetiology.[18] In 29 people who narrowly escaped death in a bus accident, in friends of adolescent suicide victims, and in a group of fire-fighters exposed to a bush-fire disaster it was found that previous emotional or psychiatric problems or substance abuse played an equal or greater part in the genesis of PTSD symptoms than did the degree of exposure to the traumatic event.[19] Even with the best will in the world, it is no easy matter to disentangle the symptoms of the various pre- and co-existent psychiatric disorders from those of PTSD.

There are many inconsistencies about PTSD. A bad conscience protects against it. While it seems reasonable to suppose that, at least for some people, the responsibility of having caused an accident would augment the psychological horror of the accident experience, it does not seem to. Jerome Platt and Stephen Husband from Hahnemann University in Philadelphia recently examined approximately 150 MVA victims and found only two instances in which the *hitter* sought psychiatric treatment for accident-attributable symptomatology.

Added to all these inconsistencies is the fact that clinicians vary in their clinical assessments. In order to avoid such individual differences, scoring scales such as the Clinician Administered PTSD Scale (CAPS) have been devised to standardize the diagnosis of PTSD. Blanchard and his colleagues, the University of Albany investigators who managed to find an almost 50 per cent incidence of PTSD in minor MVA victims, examined the effects of changing the scoring rules on tests for PTSD. They administered the CAPS to a sample of 100 MVA victims, and then, using the same rules, changed the scoring from a conservative to a liberal interpretation. The diagnosis of PTSD changed from 29 per cent to 44 per cent of the sample.[20] While these tests give the semblance of scientific reliability, they are, it appears, as fallible as mere human assessors, and perhaps even more so since the tests follow a rote and thus are devoid of any moderating human common sense.

The tests for PTSD rely entirely on a patient's honest reporting of his symptoms. Most accidents resulting in PTSD are compensable, and since compensable injuries encourage the embellishment and inaccurate reporting of symptoms, it is necessary to question the reliability of the test under these conditions. At least three excellent studies have demonstrated how easily these tests can be faked.[21]

Human nature being what it is, when test results can be faked, some probably will be; and the evidence is that they are. Some American war veterans receiving treatment and support on account of PTSD due to horrible experiences in Vietnam, for example, were found never to have even been in Vietnam.[22]

Litigation issues so frequently complicate PTSD that it is difficult to ascertain the natural history of the disorder in the absence of legal involvement. The Latin-American refugees that Canada receives, who have been imprisoned and tortured in their own countries, are an illustrative example. Understandably, these refugees often have the characteristic symptoms of PTSD. Federico Allodi, a Toronto transcultural psychiatrist, has many such refugees under his care. He reports that once these refugees have left their strife-torn countries and reached the safety of Canada, their PTSD symptoms usually diminish quickly.[23] Recovery from PTSD induced by a psychologically traumatic event, as with most other physical or mental disorders, is the expected course of the illness. In comparison, PTSD induced by minor MVAs does not seem to remit; indeed, it often appears to worsen with time.

Despite the *DSM's* explicit precautions against the use of its psychiatric diagnoses in the courtroom, lawyers show no hesitation in using it, and tort law reform has done nothing to improve the situation.[24] Landy Sparr, a psychologist who specializes in malingering, in his article "Post-traumatic Stress Disorder: Does It Exist?" comments that psychiatry, having faced the inevitable and acquired this disorder, then discovered that "PTSD had a bevy of nasty lay-legal relatives (e.g., disability and personal injury claims)."[25] Alan Stone, professor of psychiatry and law at Harvard University, is clearly fed up: "No diagnosis in the history of American psychiatry has had a more dramatic and pervasive impact on law and social justice than PTSD ... It has created a cottage industry among both criminal and negligence attorneys and mental health practitioners." He reports that the diagnosis is being used with increasing frequency in routine MVA cases.[26]

In chapter 3, I presented Ms O's account of her alleged whiplash injury sustained in the Toronto subway crash. The lawyers who had launched the $55 million class-action lawsuit against the Toronto Transit Commission (TTC) selected her as one of two typical plaintiffs for cross-examination. They selected Mr G as the other typical plaintiff. Mr G told reporters: "Money would never remove the horror of the crash."[27]

Mr G was a 38-year-old married auto body repairman in August 1995 when the subway crash occurred. He alleged that other passengers fell on him, injuring his left shoulder and low back, and so frightened him that he developed PTSD with nightmares nightly for eighteen months. He attributed his alcohol and wife abuse, as well as his impotence to the crash. Mr G reported that, because of his back injury and psychological problems, he remained inactive and confined to the house for several months. Objective evidence failed to confirm his story.[28]

Surveillance throughout that period showed him as a "strong and active individual." Among other things, Mr G was videotaped mowing his lawn without difficulty; he was followed to an electronic equipment store from which he emerged "carrying three large, heavy boxes of stereo equipment, as well as a bag, all at one time, over 100 feet from the store to his car." He was shown squatting and bending without apparent discomfort.[29]

Although Mr G had claimed previous good health, examination of his medical records showed that he had been injured in two apparently minor car accidents within two years of the TTC crash, for both of which he had received financial compensation. His wife had similarly been involved in two separate car accidents, for which she received cash settlements for injury.[30]

At his cross-examination, Mr G demonstrated so little knowledge of the crash that the TTC took the position that he had not been a passenger on either train. Confronted with this information, Mr G dropped his claim and agreed to pay $2,500 towards the TTC's legal costs.[31] In total, about a third of the 178 class-action plaintiffs also dropped their claims. It is not known just how many of these drop-outs were also frightened off from trying to turn the train crash into a gravy train, but maybe Mr G was a more typical representative plaintiff than his lawyers had originally bargained for.

Psychiatrists are ever-helpful. Mr G's psychiatrist stated in the report about him: "I told [Mr. G] that probably his mental suffering would get a larger settlement [in] the class-action suit [than his physical injury], and he is probably going to discuss this with his attorney."[32] As so often happens, such professional advice landed Mr G in trouble.

Milo Tyndel, a Toronto psychiatrist, introduced the term "nomogenic" to describe lawyer-made diseases, as a twin to "iatrogenic," or doctor-made disease.[33] Long before PTSD became widely epidemic, Tyndel and his neurologist son Felix had commented: "PTSD is the most important and the most frequently seen [of the nomogenic diseases]."[34] Undoubtedly, lawyers make an enormous contribution to the propagation of PTSD, but so do many physicians and psychologists. The term "iatronomogenic" (doctor- and lawyer-created) reflects both more fairly and more accurately the common aetiology of this now extraordinarily common condition. Of course, it is dishonest for plaintiffs to make false claims, but lawyers and health-care practitioners have used the authority of their prestigious professions to create a medico-legal system that actively invites this kind of exploitation.

Canadian psychologist Tana Dineen, in her well-documented book *Manufacturing Victims*, takes her own profession to task:

Psychology presents itself as a concerned and caring profession working for the good of its clients, but in its wake lie damaged people, divided families, distorted justice, destroyed companies, and a weakened nation. Behind the benevolent façade is a voracious self-serving industry that proffers "facts" which are unfounded, provides "therapy" which can be damaging to the recipients, and exerts influence which is having devastating effects on the social fabric. The foundation of modern psychology, its questioning and critical thinking, if not an illusion from its inception, has at the very least been largely abandoned in favour of power and profit, leaving only the guise of integrity, a show of arrogance and a well-attuned attention to the bottom line. What seemed once a responsible profession is now a big business whose success is directly related to how many people become its "users."[35]

These are certainly harsh words, but in view of the number of people who are needlessly disabled by the temptation to prove a diagnosis of PTSD, perhaps her words are well justified. Dineen points out that it is with the manufacture of PTSD that what she calls the Psychological Industry has had some of its greatest financial successes. Emotional incest, satanic ritual abuse, and UFO abduction are now all firmly established in the public's imagination. Of course, most middle-of-the-road kinds of people do not wish to admit suffering from such far-out conditions, but, even for the most rigidly square among us, an MVA has become a perfectly acceptable cause of PTSD.

The astute reader will perceive that PTSD has all the characteristics of a fashionable illness. Doctors and psychologists created a new disorder and described its symptoms and characteristics, and before long a multitude of patients began to suffer from it. Since many of the purported traumatic events are compensable, lawyers refer their clients to psychologists and psychiatrists upon whom they can rely to confirm the diagnosis.

I have mentioned the huge medico-legal briefs that are sent to the various examining expert witnesses. Nestling among their innumerable pages are sometimes found revealing documents inadvertently included in the brief by an overworked legal secretary. One such brief contained a mimeographed letter from the medical director of a large whiplash clinic addressed to the plaintiff lawyer. Attached to the letter was a copy of *DSM-III's* list of symptoms for anxiety disorders. In his letter, the medical director suggested that any whiplash litigant with any of the symptoms contained in this list would benefit by referral to his whiplash clinic. Most people have some anxiety symptoms and it is certainly an unusual whiplash litigant who does not. It is a safe bet that the clinic will find any whiplash litigant referred in this way to have PTSD.

In the wake of major disasters in the developed world come planeloads of mental health workers intent upon the prevention of PTSD. These mental health professionals and the grief counsellors with their certificates from such institutions as the Association for Death Education and Counselling are expensive. "Good Grief," the American federal government bereavement program, paid out $10 million for such counselling but there is no evidence that such counselling works.[36] To study the effects of such programs, psychiatrist Simon Wessely and a research team from Britain's Institute of Psychiatry systematically reviewed the published studies of the effects of such professional intervention. They found them to be ineffective – indeed, they report that, if anything, counselling had both short- and long-term adverse effects. Subjects who had received such counselling had more symptoms and remained in greater distress than did the controls.[37] Disasters, however horrible, unite communities. Faced with a catastrophe everybody starts the unusual process of helping each other. But, as Ivan Illich insightfully observed, "At the first sound of an ambulance siren in a Mexican village everyone stops helping." Outside assistance with physical necessities can be crucially useful but, when it comes to psychological help, stricken communities perhaps do better when comforting their own.

Successful industries are generally encouraged, and PTSD, along with other whiplash complaints, has provided commercially stimulating work for the healthcare and legal professions. PTSD, in particular, has been an extraordinary economic success. There is, however, a price to pay! The tremendous gain in popularity of PTSD over the last few years risks obscuring the fact that we, as humans, have, over millions of years, managed to survive and surmount unspeakable disasters.[38] Our caretakers make us so immature that we are becoming as defenceless as children in facing ordinary everyday calamities. In perceiving a small auto collision as a cause of a persistent and disabling psychiatric disorder we diminish the calibre of our souls. We dissipate our human heritage of courage.

16

The Inverse Paradox and the Period of Meditation

As long as people believe in absurdities
they will continue to commit atrocities.

– Voltaire

My computer typing-tutorial provides aphorisms as practice material for playing *allegro* on the keyboard. While my fingers still insist on playing *lento*, I have learned a lot of aphorisms, one of which is particularly germane to whiplash: "He who cries the loudest is often least hurt." This paradox implying the inverse correlation between the severity of the initial injury and the severity of the subsequent complaints is well recognized, but it confuses the lay public and often physicians as well.[1] If someone appears in constant pain and distress and needs constant treatment and a cane to get around with, then surely he must have suffered an injury. No matter that the accident was small and all the wondrous modern imaging techniques cannot find anything amiss. Failure to understand this paradox results in large awards being granted for little injuries and inadequately small awards for large ones.

When a person is visibly injured in a traffic accident, an ambulance arrives and takes the victims to hospital; there is little choice about who goes. Lots of people have small collisions – gentle little taps in parking lots and small bumps at stoplights. After a quick reassurance that their vehicle is neither dented nor scratched, and perhaps with a glare at the offending driver, most people drive off and get on with their lives. However, a few people, say *x* per cent of the population – either because they need to justify what they perceive as unacceptable symptoms of psycho-social distress, or because they are simply out to make an easy buck (or perhaps both), do not just drive off. They are the small percentage of people who are on the constant lookout to capture any fashionable illness that happens to be *flybuttering* by – a small collision, and a whiplash injury is in the net. They opt to take themselves off to the hospital or to their family doctors, sometimes even visiting their lawyer first. Inevitably their symptoms are here to stay – symptoms that will soon develop into bigger and better ones.

The arithmetic is simple. In any unselected group of severely injured people, most will recover in accordance with the extent of their physical injuries. A fractured shaft of femur takes three months to heal, by which time the patient will return to normal life with few, if any, setbacks. However, as x per cent of this unselected group of injured people are seeking *an illness*, that x per cent will nurture their symptoms with care and their recovery, at least in the estimation of their doctors, will be unexpectedly slow. The percentage of *good recoveries* in this group will be $(100-x)$ per cent. In contrast, 100 per cent of *self-selected* accident victims will foster their symptoms so that probably none, in terms of the expectations of their attendant physicians, will make *a good recovery*.

The value x is not a constant. It varies, among other things, with the morale of the community, the ups and downs of the business cycle, and the level of communal naïveté in regard to illness behaviour.[2] However, for the sake of argument, let us put the value of x as 20. Then 80 per cent of traffic accident victims who are brought to hospital after having sustained a significant injury will, if judged from the standpoint of their injury, make a satisfactory recovery. In contrast, 100 per cent of the people in search of an illness with a minor injury (or even with no injury at all) will not. From the viewpoint of the physicians assessing the recovery, it will appear that the victims with serious injury mostly recover well, while those with a nothing-sort-of-injury seem never to recover at all.

Nortin Hadler, the insightful rheumatologist from Chapel Hill Medical School whose views I cited earlier, suggests: "To be well is not the same as to feel well." Life presents one illness challenge after another and "to be well requires some sense of invulnerability." Perhaps because of past insecurities some people (Hadler suggests a figure of 15 per cent of the population) lack this reassuring sense of being okay. These vulnerable members of the community use the possibility of a disease or injury process to make sense of their feelings of ill-health. The more doctors become concerned about the possibility of an illness or serious injury, the more likely such patients are to believe that they have it.[3]

The paradoxical effect of injury was first observed in "railway spine." Doctors, of course, had an array of physical signs by which to substantiate this diagnosis, but ordinary people could not help noticing that victims of railway crashes who had fractured limbs or dislocated joints seldom suffered from the debilitating effects of railway spine, while the victims without apparent injury often did.

Believers that physical injury was the cause of railway spine needed an explanation for this perplexing paradox. John Erichsen, fellow of the Royal Society and surgeon to Queen Victoria, produced it: "It would appear as if the violence of the shock expended itself in the production of the fracture or dislocation, and that a jar of the more delicate nervous structure is avoided."[4] By way of illustration, Erichsen gave the example of a dropped pocket watch. A watchmaker had told him that dropping a watch usually damages the works, but that such damage rarely occurs if the glass is broken. There is, of course, a fallacy in this analogy. Pocket watches, being small and slippery, often got dropped, but no one would take his watch to the watchmaker unless it no longer worked or the glass was broken. It is easy to see how the watchmaker gained such an erroneous impression. Erichsen was a plaintiff expert witness for railway spine, and perhaps like his twentieth-century whiplash counterparts was not too fussy about the logic of such explanations. The watch analogy conveniently explained away the uncomfortable paradox.

The renowned Swiss psychiatrist Eugene Bleuler, who introduced Freudian theory into hospital psychiatry and the term schizophrenia into psychiatry, was also the first person to describe the dynamics of the inverse paradox. In his 1924 *Textbook of Psychiatry*, Bleuler commented that when a possibility of "morbid gain" exists, whether in the form of financial compensation in peacetime or escape from the horrors of the front in wartime, recovery from even a small injury may be delayed. In contrast, "in non-insured [injuries], in elemental catastrophes, in duel and sports injuries, and in the severer [war] injuries never is any such delay seen."[5]

Foster Kennedy, a former director of neurology at New York's Bellevue Hospital, wrote about this inverse paradox in World War II: "The severity of a neurosis following accident varies inversely as the severity of the accident and its physical consequences. This was so in the last war, and it is true in this war that a man rarely has a severe generalized neurosis and at the same time is suffering from severe physical wounds." He related the inverse paradox to his recollections about shellshock in World War I.[6]

"Shellshock" most unfortunately was coined to describe the various nervous conditions that occurred in war and we officers, young at the time, were impressed by our elders to believe that these conditions were the result of the physical commotion due to gunfire. Then we began often to see for ourselves neuroses in people who had never been near gunfire at all. We also found that a man shot through the spine and paraplegic was emotionally calm, whereas his fellow in the same trench, physically uninjured, was in a state of anxiety or perhaps had acquired a paralysis of physical character.

We did not find that men with serious wounds became neurotic; and this was natural. When a wound comes it protects the individual from the war; when a wound does not occur, there is no protection and a neurosis may occur by suggestion.

A serious injury requires no elaboration. A paraplegic soldier or a worker who has lost a limb can direct all his energies towards recovery. The soldier will not be sent back to the front and the worker is rescued from the distress of financial uncertainty. A broken toenail is another matter. If it is going to provide such protection, then the injured nail requires embellishment. The toenail causes a limp, the limp causes backache, the backache causes insomnia, the insomnia causes fibromyalgia, which then causes disabling pain. Recovery, injured toenail notwithstanding, is resisted tooth and nail.

The less certain the evidence of physical back problems, the more lurid are the accounts of pain. A study from the Rush Medical College, Chicago, demonstrated this paradox. Back patients were given a pain questionnaire containing words that describe pain. They were asked to check the words in the questionnaire that best described their own pain. The patients with no demonstrable organic cause checked the most words, while the patients with an obvious physical cause for the pain checked the fewest. The authors concluded that in low back pain the number of painful sensations is inversely related to the level of demonstrable tissue pathology.[7]

The name of the late Sir Henry Miller sends personal injury litigation plaintiff lawyers into paroxysms of loathing. This distinguished British neurologist caused all the trouble with his 1966 Milroy Lectures on the topic of "Accident Neurosis," delivered before the Royal College of Physicians in London. His address concerned the frequent occurrence of neurotic symptoms following minor head injury – symptoms that he claimed were relieved by settlement.[8] "In whatever way these cases are broken down they demonstrate an inverse relationship of accident neurosis to the severity of the injury. Gross psychoneurosis occurred, for example, in 31 per cent of patients without radiological evidence of skull fracture, in 9 per cent of patients with simple fracture, and in only 2 out of 25 patients who suffered compound fractures of the skull [a fracture in which the broken bone is visible in an open wound]."

In a subsequent study Miller found that "accident neurosis was commoner in male than in female claimants, twice as common after industrial as after traffic accidents, and commoner in members of the lower social classes and occupational groups. It showed no significant age distribution, apart from the fact that it was not encountered in child-hood. Its incidence was inversely proportional to the severity of injury sustained. It was very uncommon after severe head injury and was common after trivial injuries. It bore no relation to any particularly alarming circumstances of the accident."[9]

Other authors have also pointed out that accident neurosis is not seen in children. It is not that children do not exploit illness and injury – they can be highly skilled at doing so when they do not want to go to school – but they have not yet learned to redirect their innate talents for deception to doctors and insurance companies rather than to parents.

It should be noted that Miller's finding that accident neurosis is twice as common after industrial mishaps as after traffic accidents was made before the editors of Britain's two leading medical journals had helped popularize whiplash. This ratio will certainly by now have changed.

As a novice defence expert, I once innocently quoted Miller's name in regard to this inverse ratio. There was a shocked gasp from the lawyers; it was as if I had mentioned Dr Henry Morgentaler at a born-again-Christian family picnic.[10] I assumed Miller must have done or said something awful that I did not know about, so for a while I avoid-ed using his name. In fact, all Miller had done was to provide so lucid a description of accident neurosis that plaintiff lawyers cannot bear to hear his name. They deal with the problem of Miller's findings by wag-ing a continual slur campaign against him. (I will return to his findings in chapter 21.)

Trying to assess the significance of post-traumatic headache is one of the trickier diagnostic tasks in medical practice. The diagnosis is often made more difficult by the inverse relationship between the severity of the head injury and the frequency of complaints of post-accident headache. Most post-head-injury headache studies are made on patients who complain of headache and this bias in the selection of patients has left clinicians with the impression that headache is an inevitable after-effect of head injury.

Much ado is made about post-head-injury headaches. I would be the first to sympathize with anyone who has one, but headache is by no means an invariable accompaniment of head injury. In fact, averaging out the frequency of post-traumatic headache reported in the litera-ture, even when the injury is severe, only about half of head-injury patients have headaches.[11] Despite the headache selection bias, Eric Guttmann from the Nuffield Department of Surgery in Oxford over half a century ago identified an inverse correlation between the sever-ity of head injury and the subsequent prevalence of headaches.[12]

A more recent study from the University of Newcastle-upon-Tyne confirmed this observation. The authors of the study followed up 300 head-injury patients over a two-year period. At each assessment, they found an inverse relationship between the severity of the head injury and complaints of headache, a disparity that increased with time. At the two-year follow-up, 61 per cent of the patients with a post-traumatic amnesia (PTA) of less than one hour complained of headache, while only 39 per cent of the patients with PTA of more than one hour complained of headache.[13]

A controlled study from University of Washington's rehabilitation department compared pain complaints in two groups of patients. In one group the patients had had a mild head injury and in the other a moderate/severe injury. The two groups had no significant differences in regard to age, education, and length of time post-injury. The percentage of patients with pain complaints was much higher in the mild-head injury group than in the moderate/severe group: for headaches the percentages were 89 and 18; for neck and shoulder pain: 51 and 4; for back pain: 45 and 2; and for all other pain complaints including knee, chest, hip, leg, and arm pain: 20 and 2. The authors of the study point out that their findings are particularly contrary to expectation, since an accident that causes severe head injury is likely to be associated with other potentially pain-causing severe injuries as well.[14]

The same inverse paradox occurs with neck injury.[15] In the salad days of whiplash, two neurosurgeons from Michigan followed up two groups of patients; those with "whip lash" and those with neck fractures.[16] The whiplash patients appeared to have sustained only minor injury, but there was no doubt about the severity of neck fractures; they resulted from diving, severe vehicle accidents, or falls – and one was from a kick by a cow. Six of the neck-fracture patients died in the early stages of injury, including the one kicked by the cow. The authors traced 30 of the surviving fracture-group patients. When asked about neck complaints, 38 per cent of the survivors had minor post-fracture complaints, while 62 per cent replied that they had no complaints.

The whiplash patients reported a much less satisfactory recovery. Seventy-four per cent of them reported they still suffered from the effects of their injury. The authors speculate about the reason for this difference: "The two series were compatible in time of follow-up ... which leaves one wondering why the 'whip lash' patients should fare so poorly. Possibly, the answer may be in the personality of the individual patient as expressed by the type of letters they sent in reply to the questionnaire. Most letters from the 'whip lashed' patients were angry and found fault with treatment, doctors, judges, and lawyers. No letters from the fracture group were derogatory; in fact, most of the patients expressed unsolicited remarks of deep appreciation for the care in the emergency room from the resident and nursing staff as well as the physician in charge of the case."

The inverse paradox is central to understanding the problem of whiplash. In the early 1970s, John D. States and his colleague orthopaedic surgeons from Rochester pointed out in an article "The Enigma of Whiplash" that prolonged symptoms and disability nearly always follow minor accidents with very little vehicle damage. They noted how "perplexing and frustrating is the absence of physical, radiologic[al], or other objective evidence of injury."[17]

Not surprisingly, the perplexing inverse nature of whiplash symptoms soon puts doctors at loggerheads. A medical contretemps in the *Medical Journal of Australia* illustrates what I mean. Some Australian physicians attributed complaints of chronic whiplash pain to bad behaviour, while others – championed by David Champion – attributed them to "central sensitization of nociception."[18]

In case you don't know what Champion was talking about (in which case you have lots of company) "nociception" means "pain sensation," and the "theory of central sensitization" suggests that the pain victim becomes particularly sensitive to pain in the same way that some people become particularly sensitive to bee stings. The fight waxed strong. Mark Awerbuch, a rheumatologist from Adelaide, labelled the proponents of the two sides as the behaviourists and the nociceptionists, each about as friendly to each other as are cities competing to host the Olympics.[19]

William B. Maguire, a Brisbane surgeon from the behaviourist camp, pointed out that the theory of central sensitization does not explain why chronic pain often follows trivial rear-end collisions but does not occur in quadriplegics whose necks have been literally torn apart. The inverse paradox cannot be explained on a pathophysiological basis.

Maguire did have one good thing to say on behalf of central nociceptive hypersensitivity: "The acceptance of the theory would have the positive merit of protecting those patients with this syndrome from the operative fusion of a disc showing an abnormality on discogram [contrast x-ray of disc] or magnetic resonance imaging – the operation with a 100 per cent failure rate!"[20]

Robert L. Leopold and Harold Dillon from the Departments of Neurology and Psychiatry at the University of Pennsylvania also found an inverse relationship between the severity of whiplash symptoms and the severity of neck injury. They produced a psychoanalytical explanation for it – Freud's concept of anal eroticism![21]

The authors, writing in the 1960s, describe what they regarded as the prevailing attitudes to whiplash symptoms, including the widely held belief that the desire for gain motivates exaggeration of symptoms on both a conscious and unconscious level. They alluded to the tendency to attribute ongoing symptoms to pre-existing factors: "Some mention is made of personality patterns as determinants of emotional reaction to these injuries, with allusion to personal peculiarities, personal stamina, pre-existing tension, tension-proneness and the like ... Great stress [is placed] on [the] aggravation by the whiplash injury of pre-existing psychiatric illness. A widely prevalent attitude says in effect that the victim was disturbed before the accident; the injury just made his disturbance more apparent!"

To clarify these issues, the authors studied 47 whiplash patients referred by their attorneys for a neurological examination. They divided these patients into four groups according to the severity of the neck injury and the severity of acceleration of the head (though they do not say how they managed to assess the severity of this acceleration):

Group 1: Patients in whom the motion of the neck had been mild;
Group 2: More severely injured patients, in whom there had been only moderate acceleration of the head;
Group 3: Much more severe neck injuries with immediate and severe symptoms;
Group 4: The severest cervical injuries; all had prolonged periods of unconsciousness.

The authors failed to note the actual length of this "prolonged period of unconsciousness." They also reported a history of unconsciousness in 29 per cent of the patients in Group 1 and in 78 per cent of the patients in Group 3. Such a high reported rate of unconsciousness accompanying whiplash is so far out of line with other people's findings that I can only assume that Leopold and Dillon got the "unconsciousness" of head injury mixed up with the unconsciousness of psychoanalysis.

Leopold and Dillon went on to refute the idea that whiplash plaintiffs have pre-existing emotional difficulties: "It should be pointed out that careful medical and psychological histories were obtained from all patients and that, of the 47 patients here reported, only one gave a significant history of clear-cut pre-existing psychological difficulty." I in turn should point out that such a conclusion is valueless. As a reader of this book you too must well know by now that it is characteristic of patients with a fashionable illness to give a history of everything having been hunky-dory before the occurrence of the fateful event to which they attribute their illness. No pre-accident whiplash medical history is reliable unless substantiated by a patient's previous medical records. The authors give no indication of having examined these records.

However, it is the relationship between the severity of the injury and the severity of the subsequent emotional disturbance that is the central issue of this study. Leopold and Dillon found that patients in Group 1 (the least seriously injured patients) had the most numerous and severe emotional problems, while patients in Group 4 (the most seriously injured patients) had the fewest.

The authors then provided their explanation for this inverse ratio: "One could speculate that the patients who have really prolonged unconsciousness have suffered organic brain change and are thus less sensitive to endogenous stimuli." They went on to dismiss this organic explanation and delineate the factors for an emotional explanation: "A tedious investigation follows the accident, which adds to the anxiety of the bewildered and uncomfortable victim ... Meanwhile, he has had ample opportunity to develop considerable hostility toward the driver of the offending car. His anxiety is increased by fear that he will not be able to convince the doctor who will testify for him in court of his suffering. On returning to the doctor, he will try harder and harder to justify his complaints. He may go from doctor to doctor trying to find someone who will believe him, thus building anxiety upon anxiety."

The psychoanalysts then provided what they described as a typical case history: a 37-year-old man who was a back-seat passenger in a stationary car forcibly struck from the rear by another vehicle.

The impact of the collision caused his head and neck to be snapped sharply backward and then to rebound against the back of the front seat ... There was no loss of consciousness, but this man immediately experienced pain and dizziness which persisted to the time of the examination (Group 2) when he complained of headache, stiffness of the neck, marked irritability, and eye fatigue. Somatic examination was unremarkable ...

This patient is quite typical of the patients in the study. The somatic and neurologic abnormalities were not striking, and do not account for the multiplicity or the severity of his symptoms, nor was he rendered unconscious. Yet the predominant psychologic changes were his irritability, his tension, and especially his bewilderment. This was so pronounced that one month after the accident he did not know what had hit him, or why. It is the frequency and severity of such instances of bewilderment that we feel is so striking, and so different from phenomena observed in other injuries.

My own opinion is that Leopold and Dillon, determined to inflate the seriousness of whiplash, managed to induce in the patient an acute iatrogenic regression. Most of us are easily made anxious about our health, and it seems likely that in this particular instance the two doctors had worried the patient into losing his mind. The doctors themselves had a more psychoanalytic explanation for the patient's catastrophic emotional reaction to whiplash. They pointed out that whiplash usually occurs in a stationary or slowly moving vehicle; a situation in which "the occupants of the car feel quite secure." The assault then occurs violently from the rear. "Fear of such assault from the rear is well known from the association of patients in psychoanalysis, and this dread appears to be operative here. The need to deny the possibility of such an attack during childhood, with its anal connotation, seems to apply also to the problem of rear-end collisions."

By the generous employment of psychoanalytic jargon and appropriate legalese, the authors forestall the common criticisms levelled against whiplash litigants. They make it clear that all the disproportionate fuss that whiplash plaintiffs make has nothing whatsoever to do with such irrelevancies as the small force of the impact, compensation, psycho-social circumstances, or the psychological make-up of the claimant; it is due to the accident *per se*. It is a case of anal rape that leaves these victims feeling ravaged. The perpetrator pays in spades.

No one can accuse my profession of lacking in ingenuity when it comes to finding injury-related explanations for neurotic symptomatology. However, Leopold and Dillon have a problem with internal consistency. Freudian teaching holds that it is the uptight male who is prone to morbid apprehension about such penetration, the female having, at an early age, (consciously or unconsciously) already resigned herself to her fate. This being so, how is it then that far fewer men than women have an untoward reaction to rear-end collisions? Unfortunately, the authors provide no information as to the gender of their 47 whiplash patients, though if their whiplash claimants were like everyone else's they would have had more women than men.

If, dear reader, you were to suppose that medicine has now progressed to a greater level of psychological sophistication, you would be wrong. Orthopaedic surgeon Martin Gargan, and his colleagues at the prestigious Bristol Royal Infirmary in England, within three years of the close of the twentieth century, quoted Leopold and Dillon's article in support of their position that whiplash *per se* is the cause of psychological disturbance.[22]

The inverse paradox and meditation go together. While a "period of meditation" may indicate a short respite from life's exigencies into a state of beatific calm, in accident litigation it means something quite different. To personal injury litigation plaintiff lawyers in particular it is a concept that most certainly brings no peace of mind. The concept of meditation has been attributed both to Charcot, the mastermind of hysteria, and to Babinski, his pupil of plantar reflex fame.[23] Both of these august physicians applied this term to the period of time following a compensable accident during which the victim considers how best to put the accident to good use. During the period of meditation, symptoms escalate.

Foster Kennedy, who re-introduced "the period of meditation" to twentieth-century medicine, described in occurrence:

After an injury there usually occurs what Charcot called "the period of meditation" – of about three days' time, when relations, friends and lawyers pour their tales of other injuries into the sick man's ears ... One will not find a neurosis developing in a person with a dislocation of the cervical spine; one will not find it in a compound fracture of the knee joint or at least I do not think so; but a person who has a twisted back, or has had a knock on the head described as "a concussion," that kind of individual, that kind of injury is the very soil on which a large superstructure of symptoms becomes erected.[24]

Charcot used the period of meditation to refer to the period of delay between the accident and the onset of hysterical (unconsciously motivated) symptoms, but it equally applies in frank malingering.[25]

While "about three days" may well be its average duration, the period of meditation can be much shorter or much longer, depending on the degree to which the soil has been previously prepared. In communities where the whiplash lottery is a going concern and bumper stickers with "Hit me, I need the money" are everywhere, the period of meditation barely lasts an instant. The whiplash victim heads straight to the ER and from there to the lawyer's office.

Two contrasting studies unintentionally illustrate the difference in mediation periods very nicely. The first, by Gargan and his colleagues at the Bristol Royal Infirmary (the authors who cited Leopold and Dillon), was performed in rural England and demonstrates a delayed period of meditation. The authors wanted to study the psychological and physical evolution of whiplash symptoms. They gathered 50 consecutive "patients" who attended the hospital emergency department following a rear-end collision.[26] Each of the participants in the study had been sitting in a stationary vehicle which was impacted from the rear. Noting that sometimes the onset of whiplash symptoms is delayed, the investigators opted to include all the vehicle occupants (i.e., friends and relatives who had accompanied the patient to hospital) whether or not they had any symptoms at their first attendance.

These investigators recorded the symptoms and administered the General Health Questionnaire with 28 questions (the GHQ28) within one week of the accident (mean 5.5 days), and again at three months and two years. (The GHQ28 is used as a measure of psychological distress.) This prospective study was atypical in that the investigators lost none of their subjects during the follow-up period, an indication perhaps that their subjects were unusually eager participants in the study.

The results of the study are fascinating: Within one week of injury, 82 per cent of the subjects had normal psychological test scores, but by the three-month assessment 81 per cent of them had developed abnormal scores, as well as intrusive or disabling symptoms. The scores remained abnormal in 69 per cent of subjects at the two-year follow up. The authors report that in retrospect, the clinical outcome after two years could be predicted with 82 per cent accuracy by using the three-month assessment scores. They found no correlation at all between the initial scores and the final outcome. Clearly these whiplash subjects had developed their significant symptoms, which were to become semi-permanent, somewhere between the first assessment (5 days or so after the accident) and the 3-month assessment.[27]

The second study, by Bogdan Radanov and the group of Swiss whiplash experts, demonstrates a more abrupt onset of "meditation." In many articles these experts had maintained that it is injury and not psycho-social circumstances that is primarily responsible for the chronicity of whiplash symptoms. In this study they set out to demonstrate that they were right. They asked physicians to refer new whiplash victims to them, and so obtained 92 suitable volunteers for their study, of whom 78 remained until the end.[28] By definition, these patients had no evidence of direct head injury or skeletal injury of the neck. All were covered by insurance schemes that allowed them to remain off work with pay until recovery. As in the English study, the mean time interval between the accident and the investigators' initial assessment was approximately one week.

The assessment included a semi-structured interview and three self-assessment inventories: the Well-being Scale (WBS) for the sense of well-being; the Freiberg Personality Inventory (FPI) for personality traits; and the Cognitive Failure Questionnaire (CFQ), a measure of cognitive impairment. On a scale of 0 to 10, the investigators rated each patient for the reported intensity of the initial headache and neck pain.

After obtaining their data, the investigators used the results of the six-month assessment to divide the 78 patients into two groups – a group of 21 patients with persistent symptoms, and another of 57 fully recovered patients. They then examined the material obtained at the initial assessment for the patients in both groups. After a sophisticated analysis of the data, they found that three initial findings significantly predicted the six-month outcome. These were: "Injury-related cognitive impairment on the CFQ; the initial neck pain intensity; and age."

Having had success with their study, the Swiss whiplash experts four years later published an expanded version of it.[29] They added more subjects, used more tests, and lengthened the final assessment to two years. Their results were the same as before, although on the second time round they found that not only did the intensity of the initial neck pain significantly correlate with a two-year poor outcome, but so also did the initial intensity of the headache.

Thus these two sets of investigators, using an almost identical methodology, obtained conflicting results. The English investigators found that there was no correlation between the data from the initial assessments and final outcome, whereas the Swiss investigators found that the initial data strongly correlated to outcome. Why were their findings so different, and what did the investigators say about their findings?

The English team interpreted their results this way: "If patients with severe symptoms [at the two-year assessment] were those with a low threshold for anxiety or a predisposition to psychosomatic reaction, it would be reasonable to expect that the accident would precipitate these [reactions] early. This was not so since the psychological disorder [as measured by the GHQ28 scores] developed in these patients between one week and three months and was associated with reported pain and neck stiffness." In good whiplash tradition, the authors dismiss litigation and other psycho-social factors as a possible aetiology for the patients' evolving symptoms and suggest: "The symptoms of whiplash injury have both physical and psychological components, and ... the psychological response develops after the physical damage."

In other words, they say that there was nothing wrong with these patients when the accident occurred, litigation circumstances had no influence upon the course of the psychological symptoms, and symptoms developed in response to the delayed pain and dysfunction of the neck injury. The whiplash victims need treatment (more work for the boys!) and the hitter pays all.

The Swiss authors say of their findings: "By contrast with previous studies, our results suggest that psycho-social factors have little power to explain the course of recovery from common whiplash." Again, work for the boys and the hitter pays all!

Taking account of the period of meditation provides a more realistic interpretation of the findings of these two studies. The Swiss study was performed in a whiplash-sophisticated community in which individuals were well aware of the financial and other advantages of a whiplash claim. Any subjects who wished to take advantage of their injury did so very soon after their injury, so that their initial complaints correlated well with the final outcome.

The English study, on the other hand, took place in a rural setting in which people were still unfamiliar with the potential benefits of whiplash. A number of study subjects were initially not even patients, having just been other occupants of a rear-ended car who accompanied *an injured victim* to the emergency department. Some of the accompanying subjects were children: the youngest female in the group was twelve years of age and the youngest male was ten. In normal circumstances children do not complain of ongoing whiplash symptoms. It is improbable, therefore, that these fellow travellers (especially the children) would have become patients but for the fact that the authors enrolled them in their whiplash study.

Once in the study, some of the subjects were eventually made anxious by the doctor fuss. They were, no doubt, also pressured by friends and lawyers to sue for compensation. At some time between the initial assessment within a week of the accident and the three-month assessment the penny dropped and about a third of the group "meditated." Any patient can raise his scores on the GHQ28 by providing slightly more pessimistic answers to its 28 questions. Any patient can report pain symptoms, and any patient can have a stiff neck on examination if he holds his neck stiffly. In no way were the authors' physical and psychological tests reliable. The English meditated, but for very understandable reasons took much longer to do so. The period of meditation varies with the time and the place.

The Gargan study usefully illustrates how illnesses such as whiplash are spread. It took obstetricians over half a century to accept Semmelweis's clear evidence that it was they themselves who, with germs from their unwashed hands, were killing one parturient mother after another.[30] Similarly, present-day doctors seem reluctant to acknowledge that it is they, with their whiplash studies and focused interest, who are spreading the contagion. When it comes to manipulating the system, the English are as quick to learn as everyone else is. No doubt, the English by now meditate with as much alacrity as do the Swiss.

Semi-structured interviews and self-assessment questionnaires give the impression of scientific authenticity, but patients, being human, are likely to answer the questions in accordance with the impression that they wish to convey to investigators. A patient can easily demonstrate brain damage on tests of cognitive function by indicating an impaired capacity to reason. Radanov and his Swiss colleagues naïvely accepted the data at face value, failing to take even the most elementary precautions of checking them against their subjects' previous medical records.

Journal editors like statistics. Not, of course, that there is anything wrong with statistics *per se* for they are often an essential part of the scientific process. But then "there are lies, damned lies, and statistics!" A Swiss Rolex watch may keep perfect time 200 meters below the surface of the ocean, but its reliability is a snare and a delusion if the watch was set wrong in the first place. The Swiss psychiatrists did just so. They used the precision method of statistics but then they fed in erroneous material. Garbage in; garbage out! The conclusions are wrong, but all dressed up in statistical garb they caught the eye of a *Lancet* editor who used Radanov's findings to support the contention that whiplash symptoms have a physical basis, and so helped bring whiplash to the United Kingdom.

17

Lawyers, Junk Science, and Chicanery

Lawyers can't go to the beach anymore. Cats keep trying to bury them.
— Jess M. Braillier

If all the lawyers were hanged tomorrow, and their bones sold
to a mahjongg factory, we'd be freer and safer, and our taxes
would be reduced by almost half.
— H.L. Mencken

Without inordinate disrespect towards an august profession, I am perhaps entitled to relate lawyer jokes because there are probably even more jokes about psychiatrists, and, while lawyers are customarily portrayed as sharks, psychiatrists are depicted as stumblebums, and I would rather be seen as a shark. Such lawyer jokes reflect a longstanding disgruntlement with the legal profession. Nevertheless, as most of us, when we are in trouble, hire a lawyer as our verbal Rottweiler, it is perhaps unseemly to complain if we happen to get bitten.

Not that I have an aversion to all lawyers; an esteemed aunt and a much-loved niece are both of the profession. I learned early from my aunt that the law and justice have little to do with each other. She once enlisted the family to collect aluminum milk bottle tops, which she needed to defend a client who had stolen a bottle of milk. The dairy owner claimed to have identified her client as the culprit by the code number on the aluminum top of the stolen bottle. In court, my upright Quaker aunt tipped out a sackful of the bottle tops collected from dozens of places around England and so confused the dairy owner with bottle top code numbers that she soon discredited his testimony. Her client, whom she later acknowledged to her perplexed nephew as being undoubtedly guilty, was acquitted.

My professional involvement with personal injury litigation has consistently confirmed my earlier impressions of the law. My aunt's use of confusing information to discombobulate the dairy owner provides a perfect paradigm for the way courts function today. Ingenious lawyers devise creative ploys to confuse and demoralize hostile witnesses. The outcome of a case has much more to do with the ability of plaintiff and defence lawyers to discredit their opposing expert witnesses than with the rights or wrongs of the case. A comment in *U.S.A Today* sums up the situation: "In most civil liability cases before the bar, you can count on more chicanery, lying, and misrepresentation than a household with a cheating husband, a spendthrift wife, and a teenage delinquent."[1] Of all the chicanery, lying, and misrepresentation that occur in personal injury litigation, the habitual misuse of science is perhaps the most egregious.

In our science-dependent society, science carries enormous prestige, although relatively few people have any inkling of how science actually works. It is a perfect situation for exploitation, in which any preposterous assertion can be easily made to sound scientifically plausible. Expert witnesses, however dubious their expertise, can be very expert in bogus science. *Medical experts* are prepared, for a price, to use junk science to prove practically anything that the retaining lawyer wants proven. Nobody needs a PhD to recognize that this abuse of science is endemic in our courts.[2] Elizabeth Whelan, president of the American Council on Science and Health, describes junk science as "a distortion of scientific fact and exaggeration of risks."[3] When faced with personal injury litigation, lawyers are junkies for junk science.

Peter Huber popularized the term. He is a fellow of the Manhattan Institute for Public Research and a partner in a Washington law firm. He writes of the courtroom corruption of science:

When they learn of these legal frolics, most members of the mainstream scientific community are astounded, incredulous, and exasperated in about equal measure ... Eccentric theories that no respectable government agency would ever fund are rewarded munificently by the courts. Batteries of meaningless, high-tech tests that would amount to medical malpractice or insurance fraud if administered in a clinic for treatment are administered in court with complete impunity by fringe experts hired for litigation. The pursuit of truth, the whole truth and nothing but the truth has given way to reams of meaningless data, fearful speculation, and fantastic conjecture. Courts resound with elaborate, systematized jargon-filled, serious-sounding deceptions that fully deserve the contemptuous label used by trial lawyers themselves: *junk science.*[4]

In his book *Galileo's Revenge: Junk Science in the Courtroom,* Huber provides an account of how the medical profession once mass-produced spurious scientific material to prove that bruises and other trauma sustained at work can cause cancer.[5] On the basis of scant evidence, Richard Wiseman, an eminent seventeenth-century English surgeon, introduced this idea to medicine. He treated two patients with cancer, both of whom reported that it followed upon a bruise.[6] It only takes one person of stature to make an assertion about health and a huge following is likely to believe it. However, by the mid-nineteenth century this erroneous medical belief had more or less been put to rest, and physicians accepted that, while chronic irritation and chemicals (such as tobacco smoke) might cause cancer, simple trauma did not.

In 1884 German Chancellor Bismarck introduced the world's first workers' compensation program. Then, as now, cancer was a health catastrophe. If cancer could be attributed to a work-related injury it would be compensable; workers, their lawyers, and their doctors would all benefit. The worker would receive compensation, the lawyer could litigate, and the doctors' fees would be generously covered by insurance.

The medical profession set to work on the aetiology of cancer. Old medical textbooks were pressed into service and trauma was reinstalled as the guilty party. Doctors amassed the appropriate *scientific evidence*. In the sixteen years between the introduction of workers' compensation and the end of the century, 2000 new books and papers on *carcinogenic trauma* were published in Germany alone.[7]

By the early 1920s all but eight American states had also introduced workers' compensation programs. The traumatic cancer epidemic invaded the New World. In 1939, Richard J. Behan, a surgeon from Pittsburgh, Pennsylvania, was so irritated by such cancer claims that, like me – but with greater eloquence – he wrote a book to vent his indignation. His excellent 400-page book documented false claims of cancer-causing trauma that had been accepted by the court. Behan raised the question of motivation behind these claims: "Opinions were expressed for which there was no basic support in theoretical or actual knowledge. In some instances hypotheses were elaborated which for pure imagery rivalled the concepts of fiction. It is possible that in some instances the expressed belief was earnest and incorporated the ideals of honest conviction, yet in many other cases it is not fanciful to suppose that the formulated thought was moulded by the dictates of self-interest."[8]

The self-interest persisted, and since such a good idea could not be wasted only on workers, it crossed over to ordinary tort cases as well. Anything that could be "bumped, banged, or collided with" became a potential cause of cancer: street cars and orange juice cans, metal bobbins, slippery floors in grocery stores, hot-water heaters, umbrella handles, car dashboards and a box of cheese represent a small sampling of these claimed carcinogenic agents.[9]

Even rear-end collisions were implicated. In 1963 Jack Murdock claimed that a rear-end collision threw him violently against his fastened seatbelt. A doctor testified: "Trauma induced by pressure from a seatbelt might have led to an inflammatory condition of the testicles," which might then "conceivably" have triggered cancer in the left testicle. A Georgia court of appeals agreed.[10] Quite apart from whether or not trauma causes cancer, even the mechanical evidence in this case is shady. In a rear-end collision, the vehicle occupant is forced backwards into the seat, and so Mr Murdock would not have been thrown violently against the seat belt – with the forward acceleration produced by a rear-end collision, it would not have locked anyway. However, in personal injury litigation, seldom do courts allow such simple facts to keep the defendant from being found financially liable for the plaintiff's problems.

Although cancer frequently cannot be cured by medical science, at least a great deal is now known about its causes. There is no acceptable evidence that a single traumatic event *ever* caused cancer. American physician Reynold Crane in 1959 commented cynically on the escalating cancer claims attributed to single trauma: "Neither single trauma nor insurance alone has ever to my knowledge been proved to produce trauma, but the carcinogenic properties of the combination increase in potency each year and in direct proportion to the broadening of insurance coverage."

Lawyers have always had to make a living, but now the difficulties of doing so have become more pressing. A population explosion of lawyers in the 1980s increased their numbers by 48 per cent.[12] Currently, America has three times as many working lawyers per capita as anywhere else in the world. With so many lawyers needing employment, everything that can be disputed is disputed. The American legal business has grown so big that it rivals the auto industry.[13]

While most lawyers live too grandly to have to eat junk food, many of them live off *junk science*. Lawyers tend to go where the pickings are the juiciest – the manufacturing industries. By the judicious misuse of science, lawyers have proven that a vast array of industrial products cause harm. Beginning in the 1980s, they initiated hundreds of thousands of product liability suits against manufacturers for alleged injury or disease attributable to their products: pharmaceutical, household, and automotive products along with numerous medical devices. The fallacious science used in such cases is often so ludicrous that even a bright tenth-grader can point out its fallacies.[14]

Once a suggestion is made that a product might cause harm, all its users can join forces to sue and harass the manufacturer. By means of a class action suit a lawyer can service hundreds or even thousands of plaintiffs at the same time. In the States, and now in Britain and Canada, under the contingency "no win, no fee" fee system, the lawyer is entitled to receive 30 to 40 per cent of the client's award – and this after all his costs associated with the case have been deducted. When collected from a thousand or so clients, this cut of the takings turns lawyers into *tort billionaires*.

In chapter 5, I provided two examples of product liability cases: billion-dollar claims against the American and Canadian governments for alleged harm from UFFI; and the thousands of claims against Digital, IBM, Apple, AT&T, and other computer manufacturers for alleged wrist injury induced by keyboard use. I discussed the kinds of scientific evidence (or lack of it) upon which these claims were based.

Certainly some plaintiffs have legitimate claims, but in countless class action suits the claims are clearly specious. Plaintiff lawyers, using means as varied as TV commercials or union shop stewards, round up would-be plaintiffs, and many just go along for the ride. The sheer size of the numbers – sometimes up to a quarter of a million plaintiffs – makes it impossible for a manufacturer to dispute each case. Even without any hard evidence that their products have caused harm, manufacturers are often forced to settle or even be pushed into bankruptcy. The story of silicone breast implants illustrates how lawyers used junk science lawyers to manufacture another "useful illness."[15]

Lawyers have a penchant for small breasts. It is not that the legal profession has a fetish for anorectic women, but small breasts, or rather the silicone implants used to make them bigger, are a legal cornucopia. Women now claim to be victims both of men's desire for large breasts, and of the harm that these implants, by way of satisfying men's concupiscence, have caused them.[16] I am indebted to Marsha Angell's recent book *Science on Trial* for much of my material. Angell is an editor of the *New England Journal of Medicine,* the world's most influential and prestigious medical journal and Angell herself is particularly well versed in the assessment of scientific material.

In the early years of this century, injections of paraffin wax were used to enlarge women's breasts. The wax sometimes melted and gravitated down the body, forming bumps under the skin, giving a sort of multi-breasted Diana of Ephesus effect. Then, just before World War II, using sand and oxygen, chemists created silicone gel, a substance which, as far as the body is concerned, is remarkably inert. After the war, Japanese prostitutes, in a bid to satisfy the American occupation force's desire for large Western-style breasts, used injections of this gel to bring their breasts up to par. Las Vegas showgirls and aspiring actresses followed suit.[17] Not surprisingly, the consequences of having silicone gel injected haphazardly into breast tissue were sometimes awful; many women were left with painful, scarred, hard, and unsightly breasts.

By the early 1960s, cushion-like silicone implants with a firm exterior and a soft filling which were inserted through a small surgical incision, replaced the injections. While undoubtedly an improvement on the previous technique, these cushions sometimes caused local tissue irritation and, especially when treated roughly, could rupture or leak. The implants were also used for breast reconstruction after cancer surgery, and in both cases most women appeared satisfied with the results. The manufacturers claimed the implants were safe, though in fact they had done little research to confirm it. Between 1979 and 1992, each year about 100,000 to 150,000 American women received breast implants.[18]

In 1976 the Food and Drug Administration (FDA) had been given responsibility for body implants, but it showed little interest in them until 1988, when women who had had them reported developing connective tissue disease. The FDA gave the breast implant manufacturers thirty months to produce data on their safety. Two years later, buoyed by a groundswell of public concern, Connie Chung clearly conveyed the message on her CBS TV show "that implants were dangerous devices foisted off on unsuspecting women."[19] Like shouting, "Fire!" in a crowded auditorium, Connie Chung's program had results.

In December 1991 a federal jury in San Francisco found implants to have caused a mixed connective tissue disease and awarded Marianna Hopkins $7.34 million.[20] The following year the FDA announced a virtual ban on breast implants, which inevitably conveyed the impression that they were, indeed, causing serious trouble. With no evidence that they actually did so, doctors and scientists concocted theories to explain how breast implants caused an immune response leading to various connective tissue disorders. Perfect ammunition to fire off in court.[21]

Women activists were divided about the ban. Some resented being denied the chance to decide for themselves, while others were outraged that a male-dominated society had thrust these implants upon them. They were, they maintained, allowed no more choice in the matter than were African women with clitoridectomy.[22]

In the next two years over 1000 lawyers filed more than 16,000 lawsuits on behalf of women with breast implants.[23] Pamela Johnson, a 46-year-old Houston administrative assistant, claimed that an implant had ruptured and given her an autoimmune disorder. Although she had no actual evidence of such a disorder, she felt as if she had "a bad case of flu all the time."[24] The courts awarded her $25 million.[25]

In 1994 Judge Sam Pointer, in a class-action suit, awarded breast-implant plaintiffs $4.25 billion.[26] All that the women with breast implants needed to tap into this fund were subjective symptoms: a complaint of joint and muscle aches, disturbed sleep, fatigue, and burning pain in the chest could fetch up to $700,000. A quarter of a million women claimed such symptoms.[27] This happy windfall for many women turned into a painful blow for lawyers. They had felt entitled to 40 per cent of the $4.25 billion award, but Judge Pointer reduced the percentage to 25 per cent, diminishing their share to only $1 billion.[28]

A dubious court decision is soon reinforced by similar decisions, its dubiousness being reduced with each repetition. What was initially regarded as an audacious attempt by a smart lawyer soon becomes a well-established legal precedent.[29] Silicone was now a proven cause of disease and the courts gave short shrift to any medical evidence to the contrary.

In the silicone gold rush that followed, plaintiff attorneys extended their reach to other silicone devices. Dan Bolton, a San Francisco lawyer who had already had phenomenal success with breast implants, filed on behalf of 300,000 men with silicone penile implants inserted for the treatment of impotence. Another attorney asked for $50,000 on behalf of each member of a similar class-action suit – surely the world's best example of putting sexual impotence to good use.[30]

Teenage girls were also a lucrative resource. Norplant is probably the most reliable contraceptive on the market, particularly for sexually active teenage girls. The contraceptive comes in six very small silicone-coated rods implanted under the skin of the arm, its protection remaining effective for five years. As with breast and penile implants, lawyers actively recruited clients to sue the manufacturers, filing nearly fifty class action suits on behalf of Norplant users.[31]

Apart from an occasional local tissue reaction, there was no hard evidence that silicone caused the plaintiffs harm. The American Cancer Society, the American Society for Clinical Oncology, the American Medical Association, the British Council on Medical Devices, the board of directors of the American College of Rheumatology, and the commissioner of the FDA, as well as other august scientific organizations, have all concluded that there is currently no evidence that silicone breast implants induce connective tissue disease, yet lack of hard scientific evidence has not at all deterred the courts from making astronomical awards.[32]

In hindsight, the silicone implant manufacturers were caught with their pants down when it came to defending themselves against these trumped-up allegations. They had not collected data on the safety of their products – an oversight for which they paid dearly.[33] Studies were belatedly initiated to determine the safety of silicone implants, but such studies take many years to complete. Sherine Gabriel and her colleagues from the Mayo Clinic produced the first reliable study two years after breast implants had been removed from the market.[34] Using women from Olmsted County (in which the Mayo Clinic is located), the study compared 749 women who had received breast implants with 1,498 of their neighbours matched for age who had not. The implant group had no higher incidence of connective tissue disease (or related symptoms and abnormal blood tests) than did the other women.[35]

Two other huge studies on the safety of these implants have now been published. One of them looked at 400,000 American women in the health professions, about 11,000 of whom had received breast implants.[36] The results showed a slight increase in reports of connective tissue disease among women with breast implants, although unfortunately no attempt was made to use medical records to verify these claimed diagnoses. The study was performed following the publicity and legal activity surrounding implants, something that could easily have biased the results. The other study was of 90,000 nurses, of whom 1,183 had received breast implants. In this case, no differences were found in the health indices of the two groups.[37]

All other studies have also failed to demonstrate any connection between silicone implants and rheumatological illness.[38] Of course, these studies cannot prove that silicone does not cause illness; they can only demonstrate that any illness that it may cause is so rare as to be scientifically undemonstrable. That the courts found so many women to have been made ill by silicone is yet another example of the defeat of science by the law.

How did the law come up with such abysmally wrong findings? First of all, in the United States the scales of justice are weighted strongly in favour of the plaintiff. Letting the plaintiff win encourages more litigation, and it is litigation that keeps lawyers in business. The contingency system of payment, the right of lawyers to advertise, and the absence of financial penalties for losing a case all encourage personal injury litigation.

While the scales of justice are unbalanced throughout the States, they are totally askew in Texas. In Texas, judges are elected and plaintiff lawyers may make unlimited contributions to a judge's campaign funds. Texan judges are beholden to plaintiff lawyers and award astronomical sums to their clients.[39] Unfortunately, there is an infectious *universality* about the law. As soon as one jurisdiction sets a precedent others follow suit. Just as flu viruses incubated in the crowded conditions of pigs, chickens, and people in Asia sweep around the world, so these devastating court rulings incubated in Texas swept through the courts of the developed world.

Good science is a standing threat to such profitable rulings, and lawyers do what they can to discredit any reliable expert witnesses, a process that was only too evident in breast implant litigation.[40] Angell was the editor responsible for the publication of Gabriel's Mayo Clinic breast implant study in the *New England Journal of Medicine*. She was instructed by a Texan subpoena to produce the documents revealing how much the implant manufacturers had paid her to publish Gabriel's study.[40] Prestigious medical journals may have their faults but they are not corrupt in this way.

Gabriel and her co-workers were even more insultingly treated. The *New York Times* described their ordeal.[42] The Texas lawyers subpoenaed over 800 manuscripts, hundreds of databases, dozens of filing cabinets, and the entire records of all Olmsted County women, whether or not they were in the study. These sorts of requirements are a ludicrous waste of a researcher's time and energy; they certainly compromised Gabriel's ability to do her work. Such harassment has a chilling effect on investigators. Few people are prepared to be on the receiving end of such legalized gang-warfare; serious scientists stay away.[43] If the women of Olmsted County are not concerned that their medical records have fallen into the hands of such consummate entrepreneurs, they should be!

In a complicated world we need experts; in the medical field they are easy to find. The Medical Legal Consulting Service of Rockville, Maryland, for example, assures lawyers: "If the first doctor we refer doesn't agree with your legal theory, we will provide you with the name of a second."[44] Self-proclaimed experts have been a longstanding irritant. As far back as the 1850s a judge complained that "opinions of persons professing to be experts may be obtained to any amount ... wasting the time and wearying the patience of both court and jury, and perplexing, instead of elucidating, the questions involved.[45]

In 1942 the American Law Institute, in introducing its *Model Code of Evidence*, stated of expert testimony: "The abuses which have developed since experts have come to be witnesses for litigants are everywhere deplored. Not only by the bench and bar but also by members of the other learned professions ... Expert witnesses are all too frequently merely expert advocates. The most shocking exhibitions occur in criminal prosecutions and personal injury matters, but the evils are not thus confined."[46]

In 1994 Erwin Griswold, dean of Harvard Law School and later attorney general of America, wrote: "I have been greatly depressed, though, to see the number of 'phoney' experts who are allowed to appear in court and advance most unlikely views."[47] In science, truth is necessarily always *provisional* – an uncertainty about which lawyers manage to be scathing. *Their* experts always know for sure.

American-type experts now infiltrate the British courts. Lord Woolf, Master of the Rolls, comments: "You can get experts in every imaginable field. Some cases have dozens of experts." In 1998 Lord Woolf announced that the British government would slash the £100 million that it provides for their payment.[48] All this adds up to the fact that, for a price, plaintiff lawyers can obtain medical expert witnesses to attest to anything they want.

Do-gooders often do bad! In the 1960s and 1970s, academic lawyers, like everyone else in those nostalgic decades, wanted to be social participants. They took up social engineering. Accidents are expensive, and the purpose of liability, they enthusiastically argued, should be to control the costs of accidents; the person who should be made to pay is the person who might have prevented it most cheaply in the first place. In the execrable jargon of economics, this was the accident's "cheapest cost avoider."[49]

The search was on for the *culprits* who might have made the accident avoidable: the car manufacturer who could have installed better brakes, the municipality who could have repaved the road, the owner of the car who should not have lent it, and the restaurant owner who served too many drinks. Everyone was responsible except the person who had the accident. He was the unfortunate victim deserving of compensation.

These good intentions had sparse hope of success in the first place but, as the *me generation* of the 1980s and 1990s replaced the social activists of the 1960s and 1970s good intentions turned into greedy behaviour. The search for remote causes became a search for money. In her book *A Nation Under Lawyers,* Mary Anne Glendon writes: "While some lawyers were touting litigation as a quick fix for social ills, others were teaching there is someone with deep pockets, the government or a large corporation, who can be sued and made to pay."[50]

Implementing social policy by imposing punitive awards, a third of which goes to the plaintiff's lawyer, is akin to allowing policemen to keep a third of the fines they impose. Few of us would be able to drive down the street without getting a ticket. Inspired by such incentives, no pockets, however remote from the cause of harm, are now safe from the long fingers of the law.

The case of a Kentucky supper club that got hot should send cold shivers down the backs of all small manufacturers. In 1977 an aluminum wire short was deemed to be the cause of a fire that burned the supper club down, killing 165 people. The club had minimal insurance and all its records were destroyed in the fire, making it impossible to determine the manufacturer of the allegedly faulty wire. Undeterred, lawyers launched a class action suit against all the manufacturers of aluminum wire in the country – over 1000 of them – on the grounds that they were all liable for having manufactured a faulty product. The suit generated $50 million in damages, of which $6 million went to the law firm involved. The lawyer who had undertaken the suit then moved onto silicone breast implants, which proved even more lucrative.[51]

Nobody wants to be driven into bankruptcy by a liability suit. The effort to avoid such a catastrophe has caused competent obstetricians to stop delivering babies, manufacturers to withdraw socially desired products from the market, and cities to close recreational facilities desired by the community.[52] Silicone and other plastics can serve as an example, as they are used far more extensively outside the realm of medical care than within it. Fearing that such a trivial part of their business will land them in a multibillion-dollar product liability suit, chemical manufacturing corporations are now reluctant to sell their products to makers of medical devices. What will happen if they stop selling altogether? In a year or so, you or one of your family may need a new heart valve or one of the many other neat gadgets that are used to keep us alive or make our lives more comfortable. We may just have to need; the chances of obtaining such medical devices are getting slimmer.[53]

As an instrument of social engineering, product liability litigation does little to increase either public safety or civil justice. Only about 15 per cent of the insurance dollar is returned to injured claimants to cover economic losses, and the individuals who allow harmful products to remain on the market or sanction the suppression of information about them are seldom the ones hurt by litigated penalties.[54]

The effects of lawyers' activities on a country's economy are controversial.[55] Lawyers can be useful, but, it seems, only in small numbers. Stephen Magee, a professor of finance and economics at the University of Texas, is a leading expert on the economics of the legal profession. Using a mass of data, Magee has calculated that up to a ratio of 23 lawyers per 1000 white-collar workers lawyers add generously to the economy. At higher ratios the story is different; they detract from it badly.

The United States has 38 lawyers for every 1000 white-collar workers (some 40 per cent or 300,000 lawyers too many) each costing the American economy $1 million a year.[56] A pessimistic economist has calculated that if the last two decades' trend in increased legal activity continues, then "within a mere 100 years, [the United States] will have a gross national product of minus $1.25 quadrillion in today's prices."[57] Many Americans would love to reform the calamity of their legal system, but it is difficult to curtail the abuses of the Mafia let alone the abuses perpetrated by the very people whose job it is to prevent them.[58]

In seeking to reform scientific testimony, it would be easy to jump from the frying pan into the fire. Judges and lawyers are largely untrained in science, and courts are hopeless at assessing the validity of scientific testimony.[59] The Frye rule, which became a precedent in 1923, was a useful tool to aid judges in their deliberations. James Alfonso Frye had been convicted of murder, but claimed innocence on the grounds that he had passed a systolic blood pressure deception test (a precursor of the modern polygraph lie detector). The court rejected the evidence of the deception test on the basis that such a test had not gained general acceptance in the particular scientific field in which it belonged.[60]

The Frye rule, which has been directly quoted in nearly 1000 court cases, came to mean that the reasoning used by an expert to reach his or her conclusions need not be addressed; all that was required was that the expert's conclusions be in keeping with accepted scientific practice.[61] When the opinion of the medical expert was in doubt, the courts focused on the expert's credentials and the certainty with which he expressed his opinion, while the validity of the scientific argument leading to his conclusions was ignored.[62]

A recipe for disaster! Assessment of a witness's credentials is often a waste of time. Charlatans have always had the knack of presenting themselves and their ideas convincingly, a proficiency that is a necessary part of their identity. Competent scientists, on the other hand, are likely to be, and perhaps even should be, somewhat diffident about their expertise and their opinions – they are open-minded enough to know their fallibility. Courts are in the business of distinguishing between the upright citizen and the delinquent, but if required to distinguish between responsible scientists and disreputable experts, they seem incapable of doing so.

A change was needed. In 1975 the American Congress made a rule requiring judges to ensure that expert testimony was credible. The rule turned out to be so vague and the task so daunting, however, that judges faced with this disconcerting obligation for the most part stuck firmly to the security blanket of the Frye rule. Scientific evidence in the courts remained as monumental a mess as ever.[63] Then suddenly, in 1992, all the legal passions that saturated these contentious issues crystallized around the case of Daubert *v.* Merrell Dow Pharmaceuticals, Inc.[64] Daubert was one of two women who had taken the pharmaceutical company's anti-nausea drug, Bendectin, and whose children were born with stunted limbs; the parents sued.[65]

The company asserted that over a 25-year period, 33 million people had taken the drug without apparent harm; 30 published studies had shown no statistically significant link between the drug and birth defects. The plaintiff's experts argued that their own work, which they had not published, showed that such a link might exist. The lower courts ruled the parents' scientific evidence inadmissible, holding that the only good science – the only science acceptable in court – is science that is "generally accepted" and published in peer-reviewed journals.[66]

While the court's ruling was perhaps a useful refinement of the Frye rule, it left many observers, albeit for different reasons, indignant. As a reader of this book you will know that medical journals, even reputable, peer-reviewed ones, sometime publish nonsense. Publication, even in a reputable journal, does not ensure scientific reliability. Furthermore, the issue unleashed a torrent of other concerns. Some prominent scientists, including Gerald Holton and Stephen Jay Gould, pointed out that conventional science can be wrong and that much mainstream science started as heresy. They filed a brief urging the Supreme Court to overturn Frye.[67] Again, the Supreme Court had to tidy up the mess.

In 1994 the Court held that a judge must rule on scientific testimony not on the basis of peer review but on his own evaluation of the science-in-question. A judge must ensure that "the reasoning or methodology underlying the testimony is scientifically valid," and must determine that the conclusions presented in the testimony are "relevant and reliable." Scientific evidence was too important to be left to scientists.[68] As few judges have much understanding of science, the new ruling, as the Chinese proverb would say, leaves the chickens talking to the ducks!

Like an adolescent's bedroom, some messes are too awful to be tidied up, and the Supreme Court's ruling has scientists and many legal experts even more upset. William Harvey, an Indiana University specialist in litigation involving scientific evidence, writes of junk science: "We're sinking under the stuff and now it is going to be worse." The Court's ruling "is a ghastly decision."[69]

Unravelling complex scientific issues will tie up the courts with thousands of hours of high-priced second-rate scientific debate. Plaintiff litigation lawyers already trot out novel theories to explain how a company's product or a small accident freakishly injured their client. Science "starting-as-heresy" is likely to prove particularly golden as many an exuberant quack takes the stance in court that he is a misunderstood scientific innovator. Like the Norwegian whiplash expert who claimed he was breaking new ground with his vaginal examinations for whiplash, charlatans like to compare themselves to Galileo. "Most ideas are wrong," and for every Galileo there are probably are hundreds of scientific crackpots. Juries and judges already have a predilection for junk science and the new Supreme Court ruling encourages them to wallow in it.

George Levy, a chemist and scientist from Syracuse University, puts it best: "No matter how many respected scientists the defence brings in, the plaintiffs need only one fringe scientist to sow enough doubt in the jurors' minds to allow them to find for the plaintiff." In a recent illustrative case, a jury awarded $1 million to a woman who claimed a CT scan had wiped out her psychic powers.[70]

I am among the first in line to agree that modern medicine does not do as much for health as doctors would have us all believe, but had doctors stuck to their poisonous potions, the cautery, and their unhygienic ways, they most certainly would not have been *any* good for our health. The legal profession remains tradition-bound. Lawyers have, of course, raised up their fees faster than other professions, and become even more prolix, but they still conduct trials in much the same way that they did when they tried witches in the fifteenth century.

As a way of determining truth, trials did not work well then, and when adjudicating on scientific evidence, trials do not work well now.[71] Trials now have all the sluggishness of the participatory process without its benefits, except, of course, for the lawyers who clock up their expensive hours. Evidence about how frequently courts come up with wrong answers is now embarrassingly apparent. A slew of cases in Britain, the United States, Canada, and Australia, in which DNA testing has been applied retrospectively to people convicted of murder, reveal how often the courts convicted the wrong person![72]

In this hothouse of injury-litigation, whiplash quietly and inconspicuously flourished. While it would be difficult to round up would-be whiplash litigants to make one massive and profitable class action suit against all New York taxi drivers, whiplash provides steady work for thousands of small-time lawyers. In *The Fortune Cookie,* a 1966 Billy Wilder movie, an unabashedly dishonest lawyer's medico-legal activities earned him the nickname of Whiplash Willie. Whiplash Willies abound in real life also. Ambulance chasers hand out specialist lawyers' business cards. Billboards proclaim: "ACCIDENTS HAPPEN: IT IS NEVER TOO EARLY TO CONSULT A LAWYER." Partnerships of lawyers beaming out from television screens entice accident victims to visit them, and soft-spoken radio advertisements offer legal solace for whiplashed necks.

While lawyers' use of mass media to promote their business is new, the problems they inflict upon the community are not. The Roman Empire is credited for having taught the art of law to the world, but the world would perhaps have been better without this legacy from the past. Jérôme Carcopino, in his *Daily Life in Ancient Rome,* provides an account of how Roman law was actually practised. "From the reign of one emperor to another," he writes, "litigation was a rising tide which nothing could stem."[73] People took their grievances to court and "the hearings exhausted everybody." The advocates used the opportunity to practise their eloquence and hired "a low rout of claqueurs" to applaud and generally interrupt the proceedings. While the claqueuring has gone, it has been replaced by the mind-softening drone of pseudo-science.

Robert Burton's *Anatomy of Melancholy* is the most famous book on depression ever written.[74] Burton assigned to seventeenth-century lawyers (though to physicians as well) a central role in the production of melancholy. He suggested that the presence of many lawyers and many physicians is "a manifest sign of a distempered, melancholy state." Burton also saw the divisive effects of litigation as no new problem: "Plato long since maintained [that] where such kind of men [lawyers] swarm, they will make more work for themselves, and the body politic diseased, which was otherwise sound."

Burton's account of the "insensible plague" of lawyers in his own day is scathing: "Never so many of them are now multiplied as so many locusts ... and for the most part a supercilious, bad, covetous litigious generation of men. A purse-milking nation, a clamorous company, gowned vultures, thieves and seminaries of discord: worse than any pollers by the highway side, that take upon themselves to make peace, but are indeed the very disturbers of the peace, a company of irreligious harpies, scraping catchpoles."

What could well have been written about our contemporary law courts, Burton wrote of lawyers' aptitude for creating dissension: "If there is not a jar [a quarrel], they can make a jar out of the law itself. They find some quirk or other to set them at odds and continue causes so long, I know not how many years before the case is heard, and when 'tis judged and determined by reason of some tricks and errors ... they have enriched themselves and beggared their clients."

It is perhaps the most convincing justification for the study of psychology that human behaviour remains remarkably constant. The behaviour of lawyers has changed little over the millennia, although when Burton wrote his famous treatise, lawyers' activities were on a very small scale compared to the huge legal machinations of today's world. There are legitimate taxonomic reasons for excluding "nomogenic [lawyer made] disorder" as a separate entity in a modern classification of psychiatric disorders. As a practising psychiatrist who has comforted numerous patients through protracted and bankrupting divorce and other legal proceedings, however, I have no doubt that the work-generating activities of the legal profession remain a significant cause of human distress. Civil justice has become an expensive mechanism for holding someone else responsible for the inevitable problems of life so that a lawyer can acquire a goodly portion of the proceeds.

Like the citizens of many developed countries, Canadians cherish their government-financed health service. With medical costs now out of hand, this service is uncomfortably underfunded. Some see private enterprise as the solution to this endemic shortage of healthcare resources, but many Canadians understandably fear that such a solution would lead to the development of a two-tiered healthcare system. What Canadians fail to realize is that they already have a two-tiered health service: a disorganized service that struggles haphazardly to reduce the ills and suffering of Canadians; and an extraordinarily costly and wasteful service tightly orchestrated by lawyers committed to the creation of compensable chronicity in as many Canadians as possible.

Marsha Angell calls her book on the breast implant bonanza *Science on Trial*, but there is nothing wrong with science. "Science," as Thomas Huxley pronounced, "is simply common sense at its best; that is, rigidly accurate in observation and merciless to fallacy in logic."[75] Such rigorous application of common sense is what scientific medicine and justice should be about, but in medical and legal practice, the observation is blurred and the logic askew. Science remains the best way, and perhaps the only way, to determine what causes what. The problem lies not with science but with the doctors and lawyers who exploit the authority of science for their own ends. Rule by law is one thing, but rule by lawyers another.

Courts may be good for TV drama but they offer an inhospitable environment for a constructive discussion of the intricacies of symptom formation following upon minor accidents. Lawyers groan, look bored, and interrupt. Science is complicated and often dull. The slow process of sifting the complex evidence required by science is doomed to failure in court, while the drama of pseudo-science thrives in the court environment. Junk Science and the courtroom are natural partners in deception. Whiplash is one of their oversized progeny.

18

Pain and Suffering: Calculating the Incalculable

Two hundred thousand dollars isn't really enough, Your Honour.
After all, my client deserves something, too.
– A considerate lawyer

A lawyer is a man who helps you get what is coming to him.
– Lawrence J. Peter

Drivers cause damage to themselves, their cars, other people, and other people's property, and it is in everyone's interests that the cost of such damage be covered by insurance. There are two categories of auto insurance systems, tort liability and no-fault; the systems are often combined. "Tort" just means "wrong." If someone does wrong by causing an accident, the injured party goes to court, and presents his case in an effort to be awarded damages. Even though most cases settle out of court, this kind of system can involve endless arguments as to who caused the accident and therefore whose insurance company ought to pay. No-fault insurance, at least for smaller accidents, does away with these arguments; the insured's own company pays, irrespective of which driver was at fault.

No-fault removes the need for expensive arguments about liability, but its disadvantage, at least as far as the claimant is concerned, is that the claimant's own company cannot be made to compensate as generously as can the other driver's insurance company. No-fault usually only applies in less serious accidents because in more serious cases of injury, the other driver is held at fault and his insurance company remains liable for damages. For this to happen, the injury needs to be severe enough to reach *threshold*. Thresholds are usually *monetary* or *verbal*.

To reach a monetary threshold, medical expenses and other expenses must exceed a certain dollar value – it is just a matter of arithmetic. A verbal threshold is often less certain – a requirement that certain specified criteria, such as a permanent disability, or a determined level of severity must be present. These are all grounds for uncertainty. Many words may be needed to determine if a threshold has been reached, hence the epithet *verbal*.

Differing insurance schemes affect whiplash- and auto injury-claiming behaviour, and legislatures try to moderate the deleterious effects of each system. The diversity of insurance schemes complicates the straightforward comparison of whiplash insurance claims between jurisdictions, but when allowance is made for these differences, interesting facts emerge.

In the United States, the number of serious auto accidents is declining. Countrywide between 1980 and 1993, auto accident fatalities fell from 51,091 to 40,115, and property claims per 100 insured vehicles fell from 4.94 to 4.00, a decrease of 19 per cent. Credit for this remarkable improvement must go to the efforts of federal and state regulators to reduce automobile accidents and increase passenger safely. Laws mandating the wearing of seatbelts, the installation of airbags, a more robust construction of the car body, enhanced vehicle safety standards, better road design, and campaigns against drunk driving have all helped.

Despite these impressive improvements in road safety, however, Americans now make more claims for bodily injury, referred to as BI. Between 1980 and 1993, the number of BI claims per 100 insured vehicles rose 33 per cent, from 17.9 to 29.3, and the likelihood of a BI claim being filed in an accident that involved a property damage claim rose 64 per cent in the same time period.[1]

The *whippies*, as the insurance industry calls whiplash claimants, account for this huge increase in BI claims. For the purpose of insurance statistics, whiplash is recorded as "sprains and strains," and since these sprains and strains nearly all involve the neck and the back, it is reasonable to equate them with whiplash. From 1987 to 1992, claims for sprains and strains increased in proportion to other injuries. In 1987, 75 per cent of BI claims were for sprains and strains, and 45 per cent for "all other injuries." (These percentages add up to over 100 per cent because some people claimed sprains and strains along with other injuries.) By 1992 sprains and strains had risen to 83 per cent and all other injuries had fallen to 40 per cent.[2] This trend is no isolated oddity, for similar changes have happened elsewhere. In Japan annual collision deaths peaked at 4900 in 1993 and fell to little over 4200 by 1997, while over the same period the number of whiplash claims rose from 228,000 to 252,000.[3]

The fact that whiplash claims went up just when other bodily injury and property claims were going down made whiplash sceptics even more sceptical. Plaintiff lawyers, using a little legal elasticity, produced two explanations to confound their critics: the wearing of seatbelts and the altered collision behaviour of cars.

In chapter 2, I discussed the evidence (or rather the lack of it) for seatbelts being a cause of whiplash. What about altered collision behaviour of cars? Theoretically there are two kinds of collisions: elas-

tic and plastic. Plastic in this sense has nothing to do with the ubiquitous synthetic materials that sully our environment; it simply means
something that can be moulded. The collision of billiard balls is elastic; the balls bounce apart. The collision of two soft clay balls is plastic;
the soft balls just mould into each other. Plaintiff lawyers argue that
these two kinds of collisions are of relevance to whiplash since, in varying proportions, a motor vehicle collision is either elastic or plastic;
the transfer of the kinetic energy of impact to the head of the vehicle
occupant is greater in elastic collisions. The more rigidly a vehicle is
constructed, they claim, the more elastic it becomes, and the more
likely are its occupants to sustain whiplash.[4]

Plaintiff lawyers argue that since modern cars are more robustly constructed than older cars, they are more elastic and hence their occupants are more likely to sustain a whiplash injury. The brochure for
The Permanency of Whiplash, a travelling seminar for lawyers run by
Integrity Seminars Inc., advertises that its seminars include analyses of
"plastic *vs* elastic deformation, law of conservation of linear momen-
tum, magnification of acceleration, and the effect of seatbelts and
head restraints." The brochure promises: "You will learn how soft tissue and closed head injuries occur, why over 50 per cent suffer a permanent impairment, and how to prove damages. The common myth
that 'minor vehicle accident damage means inconsequential injury' is
completely refuted. Twenty-one checkpoints to determine a mild head
injury are examined."[5]

All their analyses go toward ensuring that whiplash is considered a
bona fide injury. By attending at these seminars lawyers earn
Continuing Legal Education (CLE) credits, which they require to reassure their licensing bodies that they are sufficiently sharp to be an
asset to their profession – that they remain up to date in fleecing the
public!

The elasticity of collision of modern cars sounds convincing and,
since courts deal in junk science, the argument goes over well. There
is, however, no actual evidence that modern cars predispose to
whiplash, and a perusal of the insurance statistics shows that the
lawyers' argument is probably bogus. If strongly constructed modern
vehicles really did predispose to whiplash, then the increase in bodily
injury claims (the majority of which are for whiplash-type injuries)
should at least be somewhat consistent across the United States. They
are not. I have taken my data from publications of the Insurance
Research Council.

In 1993 Metropolitan Los Angeles had 98.8 BI claims per 100 property damage claims, while Franklin County, Florida, had only 8.8 such
claims. This wide variability in the rates of BI claims compared to auto

damage claims extends throughout the States and appears independent of the insurance system in use and of the probable *elasticity* of
vehicles involved. In 1993, North Dakota had 5.6 BI claims per 100
property damage claims, while Massachusetts had 34.8; both are *no-
fault* states. Wyoming had 17.6 such claims compared to California's
60.7; both are *tort* states.[6]

I doubt if Californian cars are really more elastic than Wyoming
cars, but whiplash plaintiff lawyers are persistent. They may well argue
that trendy Californian cars are indeed more elastic than the old
clunkers driven by the staid inhabitants of North Dakota. Again this
potential argument is unsupported by statistics. Similar cities within
states also have very differing rates. For the years 1989 to 1991, San
Diego had a BI claim rate of 39.8 per 100 property damage claims
compared to Los Angeles's 98.8. Pittsburgh's was 18 compared to
Philadelphia's 78.5.[7] There is no reason to suspect that cars are any
more or less bouncy in either one of these pairs of cities.

Strains and sprains have usually been regarded as minor injuries,
and it might be innocently supposed that since a larger proportion of
claims are now for minor injuries the claims would be cheaper. They
are not. The cost of BI claims has increased. Between 1987 and 1993,
the average cost of a BI claim per car insured in the United States rose
from $138 to $212, an annual growth rate of 7.4 per cent, while the
average cost of a property damage claim per car insured rose from $54
to $63, an annual growth rate of only 2.7 per cent. Again, these injury
costs varied markedly from one place to another: $75 per car insured
in North Dakota to $504 in New Jersey, a state in which whiplash
enthusiasts are particularly active.[8]

Many variables affect BI costs, so a straightforward comparison of
these costs in different locations is meaningless. For instance, while
there are fewer accidents in rural than urban areas, rural accidents
often occur at faster speeds in which more serious injuries are sustained. In one setting, only 4 per cent of people involved in city accidents required admission to hospital while 18 per cent of those in
rural accidents did so.[9] Also healthcare costs, like other costs, vary in
different parts of the country. The *injury cost index* (the ratio of BI
claim costs to property damage claim costs) neutralizes these variables.
If the accident is severe, the injured person may require much more
attention, but so also will his damaged vehicle. If the accident happens
in Manhattan, the medical bills may be large but so will the vehicle
repairs. The *injury cost index* therefore provides more meaningful
information on BI claiming behaviour in different parts of the nation.

Across America, this index rose from 2.57 in 1987 to 3.36 in 1993;
i.e., in 1993 the cost of repairing humans was over three times greater

than the cost of repairing their crashed vehicles. The index varies widely. For tort states, Nebraska had the lowest at 1.99 and Delaware the highest at 5.24. For the no-fault states, Kansas was bottom at 1.81 and Hawaii top at 5.73.[10] At first glance, it is difficult to understand these huge cost differences in repairing humans and repairing their cars from one place to another, but then cars, unlike humans, do not put in claims for *pain and suffering*. To understand the significance of pain and suffering, at least in the insurance sense, it is necessary to know yet more about insurance.

A bodily injury payment (excluding fatalities, which involve funeral expenses) consists of separate parts: replacement of the person's economic losses; and an award for pain and suffering. The economic losses comprise the medical costs, lost wages, and miscellaneous expenses. Medical costs are the lion's share of the economic losses – an enlarging share that went from two-thirds of the economic losses in 1977 to three-quarters in 1992. The claimant is, of course, out of pocket for the economic loss. The pain and suffering award is different. The claimant (and his lawyer) get to keep the money; not only is the award pure financial gain but it is also a public acknowledgment of the claimant's real or alleged ordeal.

There is no earthly way to determine the monetary value of pain and suffering, so judges, to save themselves the pain and suffering of trying to calculate the incalculable, use a simple formula to arrive at this value – a formula based on the economic losses. The pain and suffering award works out to nearly double that of the economic losses; i.e., for every $100 added to the economic losses, the claimant gets to keep an additional $187 for pain and suffering. The longer the claimant stays off work and the more investigations and treatment he receives, the greater his pain and suffering award; and, of course, the greater the lawyer's share.[11] Naturally enough, claimants and lawyers hike up their economic losses. In 1977 the average economic loss was $1,162, the final settlement being $4,532; by 1992 it was $2,666 with the final settlement of $8,460.[12] If any two things are guaranteed to make whiplash worse, it is medical interventions and staying off work.

Although some 10 to 15 per cent or so whiplash claimants (the illness capturers) make a big deal of their injury and rapidly develop disabling *pain behaviour*, most claimants do not bother even to appear injured – in, fact, just the opposite – they do not interrupt their daily routines or take time off work; they do, however, lodge an insurance claim. In 1977, 40 per cent of bodily injury claimants lost no days off work; by 1992 this figure had risen to 59 per cent. It is too expensive for insurance companies to question these claims; they just pay up. As

Macnab observed forty years ago, the claimant receives the price of an expensive holiday in the sun.

The big-time whiplash claimant must raise his economic losses. Besides being off work he needs investigations and treatment. Healthcare practitioners have powerful financial incentives to provide these and, of course, the necessary sickness certificates. The medical management of compensable injury is, and has for a long time been, a substantial source of medical income. In the early 1960s Hirschfeld and Behan, in their classic studies of chronic pain, found that the medical bills of the physician and his adjuvants about equalled the amount received by the client (see chapter 11).

Thirty-five years later, the costs of pain and suffering and the medical costs have remained about equal, though perhaps the healthcare practitioners have benefited the most. The auto injuries they now treat are usually far less serious than previously, so less professional effort and expertise is required for their care.

Nowadays it is not only doctors who get this money; other healthcare practitioners have muscled in on the act. Between 1987 and 1992, the treatment provided by a variety of medical practitioners other than physicians increased dramatically. Now, under bodily injury liability, only 40 per cent of the money paid to healthcare practitioners goes to physicians. Chiropractors account for 25 per cent of the medical costs – physical therapists for 14 per cent, osteopaths for 3–4 per cent, dentists and psychotherapists 1–2 per cent each, and 12–13 per cent went to "other medical professionals" (this includes costs for such things as CT scans and MRIs).[13]

Physicians still hold the largest corner of the market because they see more whiplash claimants than other healthcare practitioners, but when non-physician practitioners obtain a toehold in treatment, they generate more claimant visits and are more costly than physicians. Chiropractors and physical therapists (when involved in the treatment of a patient) had the highest average number of visits and generated the largest medical bills per claimant treated.[14] Similar changes have occurred outside the United States. In Quebec, for example, $1.5 million was paid to physiotherapists (physical therapists) as compared to $230,000 to physicians.[15]

This change in healthcare practitioner usage is not surprising. The symptoms of whiplash can last forever, but physicians, cannot do much more than say, "Alas and alack!" every few weeks and prescribe some more pills. Chiropractors and physical therapists can keep whiplash patients attending several times a week for months on end.

Post-traumatic stress disorder, cognitive impairment due to alleged brain injury, and TMJ disorder have become frequent subsidiary diag-

Health Practitioner	Average Number of Visits	Average Cost of Treatment in US$
Chiropractors	25	1,999.00
Physical therapists	19	1,676.00
Psychotherapists	11	1,610.00
Other unspecified healthcare practitioners	9	3,974.00
MD/osteopath other than the ER visit	8	1,266.00
Dentists	7	1,607.00
Unspecified medical professional	6	1,318.00
MD/osteopath ER visit	1	635.00

Fig. 19–1 Getting a foot in the door for treatment.
The average number of visits to a healthcare practitioner once the claimant comes under the practitioner's care. Also the average cost of services that the practitioner then provides.

noses of whiplash neck injury. The first two diagnoses often entail ongoing psychological treatment, and TMJ disorder keeps a dentist busy with splints and worse. When any of these professionals are involved in the BI claimant's care, the costs are likely to be high. For 1992 the number of visits and the costs involved for each type of practitioner are shown in Figure 19–1.[16]

Under the *tort* system of auto insurance, it is to BI claimants' financial advantage to build up their medical expenses, but *no-fault* insurance pays no money for pain and suffering so, from the point of view of the claimant's financial advantage, all money spent on medical care is wasted. To avoid this waste, a no-fault case must be turned into a tort, which can only be done by reaching *threshold*. To bring about the conversion from no-fault to tort a threshold (monetary or verbal) has to be reached.

Clinical ingenuity may be required to finesse a whiplash sprain to the level of threshold. New York, for instance, has a threshold that restricts claims to serious injury – a category that does not easily include a sprain of the neck. Radiologists solved the problem. In New York State, MRI of the spine, an investigation that is excellent at revealing degenerated intervertebral discs, is used to investigate 24 per cent of BI whiplash claimants.[17] The fact that it is almost normal to have some degenerated discs is conveniently overlooked. The *abnormal* discs are attributed to injury from the accident. Disc problems have an unwarranted reputation for being serious, so the whiplash claimant and his lawyer are away to the races. In Ontario it was neuropsychologists' demonstration of whiplash brain injury that enabled the whiplashed to reach verbal threshold by the busload.

With a monetary threshold, the sum of medical and other expenses must surpass a set limit. Inflation quickly erodes low monetary thresholds, so that reaching threshold becomes a cinch. Connecticut, until 1994 when it abolished its no-fault insurance, had a threshold of $400. A raging bull elephant is about as likely to be stopped by a picket fence as BI claims by such a piddling sum. From 1983 to 1993, Connecticut's BI claims rose 149 per cent – from 10 BI claims per 100 property-damage claims to 24.9.[18] At the other extreme, a high monetary threshold serves as a professional challenge to the local medical and legal communities. In 1989, to discourage tort cases, Hawaii raised its monetary threshold to $7,000. This sum again provided little barrier; Hawaiians have now raised it to $10,000. Whiplashed Hawaiians may soon have to take up residence with their chiropractors, but the chances are that this new threshold will provide little discouragement to litigation.[19]

In an Insurance Research Council survey, American households were asked what services their attorneys performed for them. Eighteen per cent of households reported that their attorney advised them which doctors and which clinics to use for the treatment of their various injuries.[20] Such advice comes into it own in the management of whiplash. In the United States, lawyer involvement in BI claims rose from 47 per cent in 1977 to 57 per cent in 1992. The rate of lawyer involvement varies with location; it is higher in cities than in rural areas.[21] In New York, lawyers represented 95 per cent of BI claimants compared to 23 per cent of claimants in Wyoming. The lawsuits mostly involve the posturing of the opposing lawyers; in the end only one per cent of cases actually go to court; and of those that do, 40 per cent settle before a verdict is reached.[22]

High rates of legal involvement raise claim costs. In the United States, for instance, while there is no evidence that injuries are any more serious in one state than another, medical costs are much higher in states where there is high lawyer representation. In 1992, in states in which attorneys represented less than 40 per cent of BI claims, the cost of BI claims averaged $84 per car insured. In states with 40 per cent to 50 per cent attorney-representation, this cost was $114, and in those states with over 50 per cent lawyer representation the cost was $144 per car insured.[23]

The average economic loss for whiplash claimants with lawyer representation was $4,098, and without lawyer representation was $1,237; medical examinations and investigations accounted for about 75 per cent of this increase.[24] I must point out yet again that the vast majori-

Legal Representation	Average Economic Loss	Average Gross BI Payment	Average Net Payments to Claimants
Attorney involved	$4,098	$7,918	$1,207
No attorney involved	$1,237	$2,480	$1,243
The difference	$2,861	$5,438	$(36)

Fig. 19–2 A no-win situation.
Average payouts to whiplash claimants: with and without legal representation. A lawyer usually reduces the money received by the claimant since his fees are often greater than the extra winnings he generates.

ty of these added investigations and treatments not only are unnecessary but also do harm.

On the face of it, for anyone intent on playing the whiplash lottery, the decision to hire a lawyer seems to make financial good sense since, by doing so, he should about treble the *winnings*. Perhaps the real pain and suffering turns out to be that the claimant does not get to keep the extra money; the lawyer walks off with it. On average, the whiplash plaintiff wins more dollars without a lawyer's help. These disillusioning statistics are shown in Figure 19–2.

The arithmetic is simple. American lawyers are paid on a contingency basis, taking 30 per cent or so of the total payments made to the claimant. Sometimes there are court costs and other legal expenses that the claimant has to pay in full. The claimant is already out of pocket for the economic losses, and by the time the lawyer has taken his 30 per cent cut on both the recovered economic losses and money for pain and suffering, not much remains. The award needs to be large if the whiplash victim is to get any sizable pickings. In the end, the whiplash victim is often more the victim of the lawyer and all the various healthcare practitioners than of the person who actually rear-ended him.

That whiplash litigants are left aggrieved by the results of their long-sought-after court award is nothing new. Two American surgeons writing in 1966 about the unfortunate effects of litigation upon the course of whiplash, quote follow-up letters from their whiplash patients: [25]

From a housewife not recovered after ten years – no damage to car: "All we ever received from the accident was $1,500 if you call that fair. I never seen such a farce in all my life. No it didn't begin to pay for bills ... If my husband was no so understanding we would have been divorce by now. I still take pain pills."

From a housewife several years after the accident: "I received 2,500 for my accident it just barely covered my doctors fee and lawyers fees, I had very little left, I feel this is wrong because of the misery one goes through with and is still going through."

"Win your lawsuit, lose your money." The old Spanish proverb has not lost its punch.

Doctors, lawyers, chiropractors, physical therapists, dentists, and psychologists have all come to rely upon their whiplashed clients to bring home the bacon. Ecclesiastical endeavour is missing from this impressive professional array, though even so *the higher calling* is not entirely forgotten. Douglas L. Baker of Integrity Seminars, the company that puts on the Permanency of Whiplash seminars, writes to his legal colleagues about his programs:

This presentation is so powerful I make the following unqualified guarantee. If, by the break, you have not received information beneficial to your personal injury practice, return the course materials and I will give you a full refund. I am convinced this information will enable you to settle cases more effectively, and for much greater dollar amounts than other whiplash cases in the same geographic region.

Settlements and awards should depend upon the nature and extent of injuries suffered. More often than not, it is the competency of the attorney that determines the amount of compensation to the auto injured. This course of study will greatly improve your proficiency. But setting aside the monetary benefits to be derived, when we are able to properly evaluate and represent auto-injured people, we are able to respond to the higher calling of our profession as lawyers.

A "higher calling" their profession may be, but when anyone threatens their incomes lawyers soon revert to more mundane levels of existence.

In chapter 3, I reported the 28 per cent fall in whiplash claims that followed the 1995 change from tort to no-fault auto insurance in Saskatchewan. The Saskatchewan Government Insurance (SGI) commissioned the University of Saskatchewan, Toronto's Institute for Work and Health, and Stockholm's Karolinska Institute to study the effects of this changeover on claims. The study by these high-powered academic institutions was published in the *New England Journal of Medicine*. Besides showing a significant fall in the incidence of whiplash, the study showed that consultation with either a lawyer or a chiropractor (with or without a physician involved) significantly decreased the rate of claim closure and, by inference, the recovery from whiplash. The authors concluded: "The elimination of compensation for pain and suffering is associated with a decreased incidence and improved prognosis of whiplash injury." In the last sentence of their report the authors suggest: "Legislators may wish to consider the advantages of removing payments for pain and suffering from the compensation system."[26]

Well! David Cassidy, the senior author of the study, was unprepared for the assault. Lawyers accused him and his colleagues of fixing the data to satisfy the requirements of SGI, who had funded the study. The *National Law Journal*, one of the American legal profession's biggest newspapers, reported: "[In contrast] to their usual boredom with things north of the border ... lawyers are now paying the sort of attention baseball fans might if the Expos won the World Series." The president of the Association of Trial Lawyers announced: "[Unless the study] is exposed for what it is – nothing – it will fuel efforts by people who have agendas to bring about tort reform."[27] Lawyers established a Web site to castigate both the study and its authors. Merskey and Teasell, members of the group of whiplash experts from the University of Western Ontario and perennial advocates for the dangers of whiplash, joined the attack.[28]

Universities are sensitive to accusations of academic fraud. Faced with this criticism, the University of Saskatchewan impounded the research data and held an enquiry. Nothing was found amiss; the study was impeccable. However, it is one thing to be found innocent and another to live through a deluge of personal and professional accusations. The researchers report that the investigations were unpleasant and time-consuming.[29] The higher calling soon became a back-alley brawl. However, by changing over to no-fault insurance, Saskatchewan, a province of a million people, has in five years saved half a billion dollars that would otherwise have gone to its medico-legal systems.[30] Lawyers do not like being deprived of this much money.

What about the insurance industry? Is it also the victim of whiplash? The answer is a resounding "No!" Certainly, individual insurance companies vigorously combat exorbitant whiplash claims, but the behaviour of the industry at large is the opposite. The insurance industry makes its profits through insurance premiums; the bigger the whiplash payouts the higher the premiums have to be.[31]

Nobody likes paying these escalating premiums. We would scream loudly if it were shown that the industry was making an unjustifiable profit, but who can complain when the profit is only 10 per cent or so of its annual turnover? Other industries have larger profit margins. Without whiplash claims, the need for large auto insurance premiums would plummet and the industry's turnover would drastically shrink – a non-compensable disaster!

Despite the advantages of whiplash to claimants, lawyers, healthcare practitioners, and the insurance industry, we all become whiplash losers. In a 1995 national survey, 34 per cent of Americans reported that the purchase of automobile insurance at an affordable price was a major concern, and another 27 per cent said it was a moderate concern.[32] In Ontario the government has just introduced fines of up to $50,000 for driving without insurance coverage, fines intended to discourage the million Ontario drivers who now either cannot afford these sizable premiums, or who optimistically hope to get by without paying.[33] The whiplash lottery may be fun, but not, I expect, at the cost of no longer being able to afford to keep the family car on the road.

19

Jumpers and Add-ons;
Slippers and Yankers

The quacks are the world's biggest liars, except for their patients.
– Benjamin Franklin
None of us could live with a habitual truth teller,
but, thank goodness, none of us has to.
– Mark Twain
There's one way to find out if a man is honest – ask him.
If he says, "Yes," you know he's a crook.
– Groucho Marx

To be a contented psychiatrist, although not necessarily a good one, it helps to be a voyeur of people's lives. Although a psychiatrist is privileged to hear all manner of interesting things, most patients still prefer to put their best foot forward; even in a psychiatrist's office, as with priests in the confessional, there are lots of things that a person prefers not to mention. Divorce mediation is a different matter. The contending partners reveal horrendous behaviours about each other as justification for their marital break-up. It was in one such situation, about twenty years ago, that I first learned about fraudulent claims for whiplash.

The husband was a lawyer and the wife a nurse. Three years previously the couple had been rear-ended while waiting at a stoplight. Neither was the slightest bit hurt and only minimal damage was done to the car. After the usual collision formalities the husband and wife sat in their car to decide which of them should make the claim. As the husband's earnings were greater, he would be the better compensated, but his job was going well and the wife was discontented with shift work. It was the wife who developed whiplash. Her family doctor put her on sick leave and prescribed tranquilizers and analgesics. She had no reason to take them, but she was a compliant, traditional woman who did what her doctor suggested.

Up until the accident the marriage had apparently gone well. After the accident the wife stayed off work and soon began to add vodka to her regime of tranquilizers and painkillers. Two years later her health and her behaviour had both deteriorated. Her enraged husband protested that there had been nothing wrong with her in the first place and that her behaviour was inexcusable. The discord escalated until separation was inevitable and they came to me for divorce counselling. Their minds were set and there was little to be done except to admit the wife to a drug and alcohol program. I never heard the outcome of her whiplash litigation, but some years later I met her in a shopping mall with two handsome children. She looked well and reported that she was happily remarried.

The Hippocratic oath has, except perhaps for its now anti-woman stance on abortion, served both doctors and patients well. However, "Hear no evil, see no evil, speak no evil" is a closer approximation to the way the practice of medicine is actually conducted. Clinicians do not like to see or report bad things about their patients.

One has only to glance through the newspapers to see how frequently parents abuse their children. Every week there are reports of children being rescued by a children's aid society from a parent's murderous rage. Most doctors, I expect, see themselves as students of human nature, but in these cases they had failed to see, and certainly to report, this aspect of family life. The sufferings of their smallest patients went unrecorded. It was a radiologist not involved in direct patient care who in 1946 described "the battered child syndrome."[1] In reporting on x-rays ordered for the investigation of children's injuries, John Caffey from Columbia University, New York, noticed that the radiographs sometimes showed not only a recent fracture but also previous fractures in various stages of healing, and sometimes evidence of a previous head injury as well. These battered children had received multiple injuries during their short lives. Clinicians had seen these injured children but somehow managed to deny the distressing realization that the injuries were caused by the parents and not by accidents.

Much the same sort of denial happens with malingering. The patient/doctor relationship is regarded as one of trust in which the doctor and patient should unquestioningly each believe the other. If the patient states he is ill and in pain, then he is ill and in pain. Even when the complaints are implausible, physicians seldom consider the possibility of malingering; they search instead for a disease explanation.[2] Alan J. Cunnien, a psychiatrist with the Mayo Clinic, makes the point well: "Clinicians are trained to believe patients and often maintain an undiscerning naïveté about the potential for deception in their subsequent professional practices. When eventually confronted with the reality of simulated illness or fraudulent information, mental health professionals may unfairly personalize such behaviour and assume that deceptive patients 'pervert the very basis of the doctor-patient relationship, which is founded on trust.'[3]"4

There is, however, overwhelming evidence that the deliberate feigning of whiplash and other injuries is widespread. I will start with some examples from public transportation: *jumpers and add-ons.*

By 1988 the Southeastern Pennsylvania Transportation Authority (SEPTA), faced with a payment of $53 million in settlement of the 15,000 personal injury claims filed against it each year, had had enough. SEPTA initiated a Fraudulent Claims Program. The program's briefing package notes that information about claims was computerized and carefully scrutinized.[5] They found that the number of claimants sometimes exceeded the number of passengers on the vehicle at the time of the accident. Several claims were submitted after the crash of a SEPTA vehicle that was returning empty to the garage. Some injuries were fabricated or previous injuries attributed to a SEPTA accident. "Claims involving excessive treatment coupled with excessive disability period are all too pervasive." In some instances, claimants actually had staged crashes with SEPTA vehicles.

SEPTA asked the FBI to investigate suspicious claims and press charges against claimants and physicians or lawyers when any claims were found fraudulent. In a typical incident, a SEPTA trolley jumped its track and crashed into a car, killing the driver. Seven passengers filed claims for injuries sustained in the crash, but only one passenger was on the trolley at the time of the crash. The six allegedly injured passengers were indicted by a grand jury for fraud.[6] A 73-year-old doctor known "to many, many, many, many people as a very good man and a caring physician who had served as a role model to young physicians" was sentenced to fifteen months in jail and fined $100,000 for providing false testimony in regard to the alleged injuries.[7] Similar convictions followed. Once it became known that SEPTA was after the cheaters, injury claims against the transportation authority fell by 60 per cent and law suits by 50 per cent, resulting in multimillion-dollar savings for the financially strapped mass-transit agency.[8]

Following the publicity, Philadelphia became known as the Fraud Capital of the World, even though Newark's insurance fraud problems were just as bad or even worse.[9] One small New Jersey bus company with fifty to sixty buses was plagued by injury claims. Although few of its 100 or so collisions a year were anything other than small fender benders, they were followed by a spate of expensive whiplash claims. The company was powerless to confront the claimants because their injuries were always medically authenticated, either by ordinary family doctors and specialists, or by physicians specializing in personal injury cases. The company asked the New Jersey Insurance Fraud Division to investigate.

In "Operation Bus Roulette," the fraud division staged ten bus accidents throughout the state of New Jersey. The same bus could be used on each occasion as none of the rear-end collisions was serious enough to cause even a dent or scratch the paint. Staff from the fraud division rode on the bus and each accident was videotaped. Connie Chung of CBS with her *Eye to Eye* team, participated in one of the staged crashes, and reporter Roberta Baskin, outfitted with a black wig, rode on the to-be-rear-ended bus.

The *Eye to Eye Undercover Report* was aired in August 1992.[10] It showed seventeen members of the public, who happened to have been walking by when the crash occurred, quietly entering the bus before the police arrived. Subsequently, all seventeen of these passengers submitted injury claims, mostly for whiplash. Baskin followed some of the *jumpers* to a lawyer. Although she never complained of an injury, the lawyer suggested that she should report pain in the neck since this is what the "others mostly do."

A film clip was taken of Baskin in conversation with the lawyer. He suggested that she visit the chiropractor regularly for two months, after which time she would probably be awarded $10,000. She, the lawyer, and the healthcare practitioners would then split the money. Baskin's initial doctor's examination was also secretly videotaped. The examination took less than five minutes, for which the doctor charged the insurance company $150.00. Another film clip showed Baskin receiving her regular treatment – sitting on a hot water bottle for five minutes. On one occasion, when Baskin was late for her appointment, the doctor quickly examined her in the parking lot – an examination for which he then charged the insurance company.

The sum of the fraudulent claims for each crash ranged from $30,000 to $400,000. Armed with the videotapes of bystanders entering their bus and with the false medical reports, the bus company was able to challenge the plaintiffs' symptoms and especially the medical reports that had previously seemed so incontrovertible.

Operation Bus Roulette caught at least 107 people ripping off insurance companies, including ten doctors and four lawyers. The claims were filed either by the *jumpers,* who climbed onto the crashed buses, or by *add-ons,* people who did not bother to get on a bus but merely submitted a claim stating they had been on the bus when the crash occurred.[11] Two Newark police officers were caught putting add-ons onto the list of passengers of a crashed bus (see Fig. 19–1).[12]

Insurance crime is about the easiest of all crimes to perpetrate. The police regard it as a victimless crime and assign insurance fraud a low

Accident Occurrence	Number of Jumpers	Number of Add-ons	Total False Victims
Sept. 1992	7	2	9
Oct. 1992	3	2	5
Dec. 1992	12	4	16
Feb. 1993	9	1	10
March 1993	17	2	19
May 1993	3	0	3

Fig. 19–1   Riding the whiplash bandwagon.
The number of *jumpers* and *add-ons* caught in six intentionally staged bus crashes in New Jersey State.

rank on their list of priorities. Claims, be they honest or fraudulent, both serve to swell the size of the insurance industry's business, so the industry has not been overly concerned about such fraud. Except for the odd SEPTA- and New Jersey-type insurance fraud sting, most people who perpetrate insurance fraud have had a free ride. This situation is changing. In an attempt to control the rise of premiums, various North American jurisdictions have enacted legislation forcing insurance companies to establish special investigation units (SIUs). It is the work of these SIUs that is uncovering the high prevalence of health insurance fraud.

It is not easy to be in the right place at the right moment to hop on a crashed bus, and anyone in need of an injury or wanting to make money from one needs to take a more proactive approach. There is no end to the ingenuity by which this is done. Recycling old injuries is one of the easiest. One man, having sustained a compression fracture of a vertebra in the early 1980s, discovered that these compression fractures retain their original x-ray appearance almost indefinitely. During the 1990s he *sustained* the identical injury in at least seventeen new accidents. Perhaps he had done the same in the 1980s but as the insurance industry did not keep any overall records there is no way of knowing.[13] Removing the cast from a recent fracture and presenting at a hospital emergency department along with a story of a car crash effectively turns a non-compensable injury into one that is compensable.

In other attempts at fraud, insalubrious objects like broken glass are added to hamburgers or other restaurant food. Doctors, probably innocently, confirm the harm that these additions to the meal have caused. Videotape surveillance of grocery stores not only catches the person who quietly pockets a tin of sardines but also it provides a record of the *yankers* and the *slippers*. The yankers deliberately pull products down onto their heads and then claim injury from the cascading merchandise, while the slippers find loose tiles and lettuce leaves on which to slip. Some habitual slippers carry a plastic water bottle to prime the floor; one fraud ring even had their own home-cooked slip-sure faked vomit concocted from boiled potatoes and mayonnaise.[14]

Whiplash is the prince of all faked injuries. Nothing succeeds like whiplash because no objective evidence of injury is needed. In the minds of judges, juries, and some doctors such soft tissue injuries can be permanent. Claimants, lawyers, and healthcare practitioners all want more of it. They go out and get it.

The simplest way to harvest potential whiplash claimants is to inter-cept police and ambulance emergency calls, locate the accident sites, and send *runners* or *cappers* to befriend them. The cappers shepherd any would-be whiplash claimants to specific doctors and lawyers who pay a kickback for the service rendered. The cappers also recruit will-ing insurance fraud perpetrators who are willing to participate in staged or simulated collisions and then attend a *medical mill.*

Simulated accidents are contrived by placing previously wrecked cars up against a hydro pole or upside down in a ditch. There are many ways of staging accidents. A currently popular method is to hold a seat-sale in a vehicle that is to be crashed. Rental cars or old cars are frequently used. The organizers keep the money from the seat-sales and the car occupants take their necks to stipulated lawyers and healthcare practitioners. Innocent occupants of the crashed-into cars have been severely injured or even killed.

A medical mill consists of a group of healthcare practitioners who work in conjunction with a lawyer; the two professions *ping-pong* the whiplash victims back and forth. Such mills are numerous; the degree of their fraudulent activity depends upon the amount of risk the healthcare practitioners are prepared to take. Since many of the patients have only spurious injuries, some mills offer little or no actu-al treatment. They provide certification of injury and treatment.

Much of my information about American insurance fraud comes from *Spotlight on Insurance Crime,* a publication of the National Insurance Crime Bureau (NICB). The NICB now enters insurance claims into its ClaimSmart computer program, which searches for sus-picious claim patterns – claims, for instance, in which fifty claimants of many separate accidents all have the same address, claims where the names of lawyers and health practitioners are repeatedly linked, or multiple claims that are submitted by a particular claimant to different insurance companies.

I have selected some examples of whiplash scams, reported in *Spotlight,* which were broken by the NICB in 1996 and 1997. In

"Operation Backbone," a female undercover agent posing as an MVA victim in New York State visited lawyers and healthcare practitioners. The lawyers referred her to various chiropractors who billed the insurance company for treatments she did not receive. Twelve chiropractors, four lawyers, an orthopaedic surgeon, and various administrators were arrested.[15]

"Operation Paper Accidents" targeted fraud rings involving medical clinics and law offices in California. The operation received its name because in some instances the participants did not even bother to stage accidents; they simply submitted false claims for fictitious collisions. The conspirators shared the insurance settlement money. Undercover officers, posing as victims and cappers, recorded the conversations of lawyers, doctors and office personnel. Arrest warrants on fraud charges were issued for seventeen people including five doctors and chiropractors, one lawyer, and several office administrators.[16]

"Operation Side-swipe" was a four-year investigation in the Houston area. A driver of a car filled with college students hungry for cash would stage collisions with empty vehicles. The wrecked vehicles were filled with college students wanting to make extra cash. The organizers would claim the insurance money. When exposed, the ringleader received a 99-year jail sentence, a lawyer 30 years, and two doctors 20 and 10 years respectively.[17]

In Brooklyn, New York, nine people operating medical clinics were charged with defrauding seventeen insurance companies of $2 million by staging vehicle collisions and filing false or inflated claims.[18] In Philadelphia an attorney was sentenced to three years in prison and ordered to pay nearly $70,000 in restitution for his role in an 18-month, $7-million insurance scam involving fabricated and inflated personal-injury claims and medical bills.[19]

With the help of ClaimSmart, investigators are bagging fraud perpetrators in record numbers. In 1995, the latest year for which statistics are available, 1097 claimants, 114 medical practitioners, and 53 legal providers were charged with fraud following NICB-assisted investigations.

Canada likes to see itself as the honest neighbour above the forty-ninth parallel, and Toronto, the capital city of Ontario, was for many years known as "Toronto the good." In whiplash matters, however, the goodness and honesty are hard to find. In fact, Toronto is an ideal home for whiplash and, since it is my home also, I am especially familiar with its whiplash machinations.

Whiplash fraud flourishes in many North American jurisdictions but circumstances have made Ontario a particularly hospitable place for this kind of fraud. In the 1970s and 1980s, Ontario citizens had an ongoing grievance against insurance companies for being slow to pay claims. The provincial government decided to teach the insurance industry a lesson. At the same time, the government let itself be persuaded by the rehabilitation industry that more and immediate rehabilitation was required to reduce the high rates of chronicity and disability associated with vehicle accidents. In 1990 the government enacted a new auto insurance law that forced insurance companies to pay all claims within fourteen days without quibble and to make $1 million available for treatment and rehabilitation of any MVA victim who required it.[20]

Ontario neuropsychologists immediately showed that whiplash victims were brain-damaged, and the whiplashed found they needed specialized and ongoing treatment. Ontario's whiplash rehabilitation industry blossomed. Between 1990 and 1994, the average cost of Ontario accident benefits increased 119 per cent from $12,000 to $26,800.[21] However, in order to cover the costs of these benefits, auto insurance premiums jumped up. Ontario citizens were even more disgruntled with high auto insurance premiums than they had been with slow payment. The government had to enact another insurance law.

Perhaps unwittingly this time, the Ontario government gave another helping hand to whiplash. Following the example of some other North American jurisdictions, it sought to economize on police time by establishing Collision Reporting Centres. Except for cases of bodily injury or suspected criminal activity (such as drunk driving) the police were no longer required to attend traffic accidents; drivers had to report their accidents to a Reporting Centre.

This new law is a charter for the would-be whiplashed. No longer is there any officially confirmed record of an accident. No one verifies the extent of the vehicle damage or even who was in the crashed vehicle. A driver who crashes his car (accidentally or on purpose) into a hydro pole on his way home from work, can simply add his wife and children, a few aunts and uncles, and an odd family friend to the list of the car occupants. Neither he nor any of his extended family, he claims, appear to have been hurt in the accident so it was appropriate just to report it to a Reporting Centre. Everyone knows that whiplash sometimes only begins to hurt a few hours after the accident and once the report is lodged the necks of all the family and friends begin to ache. Soon everyone is in intractable pain.

The Ontario College of Physicians and Surgeons also aided whiplash. Most North American medical regulatory bodies have stringent rules that forbid a doctor from referring a patient to a clinic for treatment in which he or a relative has a financial interest. The Ontario College has no such rule; instead the doctor is obliged to inform his patient and the college of this financial connection before the service is rendered. For a patient and doctor interested in a little whiplash exploitation, no arrangement could be more propitious. The claimant needs treatment to build up his case and the doctor is delighted to treat the patient in the clinic in which he has a financial interest. Both the patient and the doctor are comfortably assured that each will look after the other's interests. The patient will ensure that he is available for treatment and the doctor will ensure that the patient's injury is suitably authenticated.

A hundred Ontario physicians are now under investigation for such collusion.[22] A lawyer writes of this problem: "Evidence suggests that some physicians are making fraudulent self-referrals 'outside the bounds of medical necessity'; others, who are referring patients to particular clinics, 'are receiving excessive fees for providing patient information' ... [It] is likely that millions of dollars are being paid fraudulently to alleged accident 'victims' and to clinics which excessively treat patients who are not injured or whose injuries are exaggerated. [In some clinics, patient well-being is ignored, and health services are] continued until insurance resources are exhausted, simply to benefit the owners of the clinics."[23]

These auspicious political circumstances have guaranteed the flourishing of whiplash fraud in Ontario.[24] Here is a selection of its activities in and around Toronto. Two employees pleaded guilty to fraud while working in a Toronto lawyer's office. An undercover officer told one of these employees that he had bumped his knee in an auto accident and, although the knee had recovered, he wanted advice. The employee supplied the officer with lists of other injuries for which to claim, chores he could not do, and doctors to visit to verify his injuries. One employee admitted to having aided about 100 fraudulent claimants while working at the law firm.

The firm's lawyers denied any knowledge of these fraudulent activities. They pointed out that the Law Society of Upper Canada had twice reviewed their firm and had voiced no concern.[25] Whether the Law Society performs a poor job of these reviews or whether it just considers this kind of activity to be in keeping with normal legal practice is open to speculation.[26]

In another case, an undercover police officer visited a chiropractor. He recounted that he had a minor knee injury sustained in a collision. The knee had quickly healed but he wanted advice on submitting an insurance claim. The chiropractor submitted insurance documents indicating that his patient suffered from neck and back pain, headaches, insomnia, generalized weakness and stiffness that required twelve to fifteen weeks of treatment. At the request of the police, the

College of Chiropractors visited the chiropractor's office and pulled the files of twenty-four motor vehicle accident cases. In most of these cases the chiropractor had made exactly the same diagnosis, provided the same treatment, and recommended several months off work or free from household chores.[27]

In the summer of 2000 the Toronto police in "Project Slip" charged thirty-five people, including five doctors, in a multimillion-dollar insurance scam. Their investigations revealed several incidents of staged car accidents and tumbles on city buses and streetcars. The awards ranged from $10,000 to $25,000 per incident. Ontario Hospital Insurance Plan (OHIP) paid the doctors and chiropractors for their services; the victims and the recruiters shared the awards.[28]

Claiming injury from rear-end collisions can be hazardous. One Hamilton man, an expert at stopping unexpectedly at yellow lights, had been rear-ended a total of thirty-two times, and each time had sued the hapless driver behind him. His last victim was a member of the Hamilton underworld who, in revenge, firebombed his house. It is claimed that when running from the burning house the claimant had been seen in public for the first time in years without a neck collar.[29]

A Toronto man driving a rental car deliberately ran an Ottawa stop sign and broadsided a car in the intersection. The driver of the broadsided car sustained a fractured pelvis, sixteen broken ribs, and a punctured lung, and her teenage son was injured in the jaw and the back. The three passengers in the rental car each collected more than $50,000 in auto insurance. The driver made no claim, but is alleged to have received money from *seat-sales* to his passengers. The driver was found to have been involved in four or five previous incidents and subsequently was involved in at least as many again.[30]

Jim Adams, the police detective who investigated this string of accidents, reports that following this accident the police launched Canada's biggest auto insurance fraud investigation ever.[31] Their searches uncovered a large Toronto auto insurance fraud ring responsible for 257 suspicious claims worth $10 million. More than sixty staged accidents were involved. Fifty-four people were charged and the names of the implicated physicians and chiropractors were given to their respective colleges.[32]

Some of the claimants had paid up to $1000 for a seat in the accident vehicle and $1000 for bogus employment records to inflate their insurance claims.[33] One Toronto man was found to have made $20,000 a month in seat-sales for staged crashes. One new Canadian, on the pretext of helping his fellow countrymen on their arrival in Canada, offered to obtain driver's licenses for them but put his own picture on the license. By crashing vehicles and submitting claims under twenty-five different names, he was making $28,000 a week in accident benefits.[34] Of course, such behaviour is an exploitation of our insurance system but, with Canadian lawyers and healthcare practitioners so ready to offer their services to confirm a neck injury, claiming for whiplash must seem to any newcomer to Canada as North American as apple pie.[35]

Dramatic as these staged crashes are, they are only the tip of the iceberg of fraudulent whiplash claims. A study by the Insurance Research Council estimates that while about 36 per cent of all auto insurance bodily injury (BI) claims in the United States involve some element of fraud, only a scant 3 per cent of them actually involve premeditated criminal acts such as faked or staged accidents. According to the council, *opportunistic acts* by doctors, lawyers, and claimants are responsible for about 33 per cent of all claims.[36] My own opinion is that the council is somewhat naïve in putting this estimate so low. The council, however, does comment that bodily injury is unlikely to occur in collisions at less than 10 mph or in which the damage to the vehicle is less than $1,000. The council found that when injury claims for such low-impact collisions are singled out for special investigation, 90 per cent of these claims are dropped.[37]

Staging a faked accident requires a decision to commit a criminal offence with all the attendant risks of exposure. Most of us are probably either too upright or too scared to fake an accident or even to claim we have been in a crash when we have not. For a person actually involved in an accident, the opportunistic exploitation of the accident incurs no such risks. It may not even include any conscience-pricking mendacity. It is not difficult to find a little stiffness here and a little pain there, or perhaps even some anxiety, that can, without too much stretching of the truth, be attributed to the accident.

It would indeed be surprising if the attribution of symptoms to a *bona fide* accident were *not* common behaviour. In my experience, the medical records of claimants who are later shown not to have been in the crashed vehicle are essentially no different from the records of claimants who have been in genuine collisions. In both cases, various healthcare practitioners, with a variety of injury-related diagnoses, certify that the claimant's symptoms have been caused by the accident. It is reasonable to suppose that the whiplash-claiming behaviour of the couple I saw for divorce counselling is so common as to come within the realm of normal behaviour.

Insurance fraud is expensive; it is second only to tax evasion as the most costly white-collar crime in the United States. Conning & Company, a research and asset management company that monitors insurance trends, estimates that $120 billion is lost annually in the States through insurance fraud, of which $95 billion comes from health-care claims.[38] Like the billions of stars in a galaxy or molecules in a drop of water, the billions of dollars lost to health care insurance fraud soon become meaningless figures. Let me put these figures into more human proportions.

The 50-km-long under-the-sea link between Britain and France, the Eurotunnel, is Europe's largest construction project within living memory and certainly one of the greatest engineering feats of the twentieth century. It cost $15 billion to build.[39] A small calculation shows that the amount of money lost through fraudulent healthcare claims in the United States would build at least six Eurotunnels every year. Much of the healthcare fraud money that could build these six Eurotunnels makes its way into the pockets of healthcare practitioners.

In the past, doctors, along with the lay public, believed that liars were easy to detect. Freud, the master mind-reader, emphasized just how difficult he believed successful lying to be: "He who has eyes to see and ears to hear may convince himself that no mortal can keep a secret. If his lips are silent, he chatters with his fingertips: betrayal oozes out of him at every pore."[40] Jones and Llewellyn, in their book *Malingering or the Simulation of Disease*, also express this belief: "It is around the eyes that we may discern most clearly the natural language of slyness, cunning, craft or other sparks of deceit. The conscious malingerer is uneasy, fearful of detection, his unrest betraying itself by the restless wavering of the eyes, their sidelong furtive glance through veiled or drooping lids."[41]

The problem is that these colourful descriptions of the fraudster do not hold water. Freud certainly had remarkable, albeit somewhat androcentric, insights into the inner workings of the human mind, but he seems to have been hopeless at seeing through people's every-day behaviour.[42] His colleagues saw him as a poor *Menschenkenner* (knower of people).[43] He may have caught out his guilt-ridden patients trying to cover up their sexual secrets, but with his expectation of seeing every liar chattering with his fingertips and oozing guilt from every pore, he would have made a very inadequate customs officer.[44]

After William Hamilton, Edward O. Wilson, and other sociobiologists had published studies on the evolution of patterns of deceptive behaviour in animals, evolutionary psychologists began to question traditional beliefs about our own lying.[45] These psychologists hold that humans are innately good both at lying and at getting away with it, and that through our long mammalian ancestry we have at least come by our dishonesty honestly.

Nature is the absolute mistress of deceit; indeed deceit is almost her stock in trade. Tasty moths mimic the appearance of foul-tasting ones. Fireflies, instead of flashing at a rate to attract a mate, flash at a rate to attract someone else's; snap, an easy breakfast. There is no end to Nature's deceptions and Mother Nature has certainly not deprived humans of any such useful survival strategies.

When our species evolved in the savannas of Africa, according to evolutionary psychologists, we were faced with a trying predicament: we like meat – big game – but as we are small and puny with no sharp claws or fearsome teeth, the only way to catch dinner was to cooperate. In the case of procreation, on the other hand, we remained (or at least our genes did and still do) in competition. Being friends and competitors at the same time is not easy; the answer to the dilemma, in the view of these psychologists, is deceit. We became highly skilled at appearing to do one thing while actually doing another.

Our big brain has caused biologists a problem. Darwin, in his 1871 *Descent of Man,* suggested males needed it for the acquisition of hunting skills; Elaine Morgan in her 1972 *Descent of Woman,* suggested women needed it for the acquisition of food-gathering and nurturing skills.[46] But evolutionary psychologists suggest that our big brain developed for less seemly reasons. We needed it for deceit. When Fido devours yet another slipper under the bed we know at once of his misdeed; his hangdog look of canine culpability is unequivocal.

To escape detection, in this theory, the telltale signs of guilt require eradication, a skill for which a bigger brain was needed. Life gives no points to suckers; a still bigger brain was needed to detect deception.[47] Soon human brains were leapfrogging over each other to keep ahead in a rat race of mendacity, and in a flash of geological time, we had acquired our unconscionably enormous brain. (Of course, it is well possible that this explanation for our big brain may be purely a figment of the imagination of deviously minded ethnologists inspired by the deceptive ploys of their academic colleagues.)

Richard Wiseman, a psychologist at the University of Hertfordshire in England, is an excellent amateur magician who spends his life in skilled deception. In 1994 he designed the world's largest experiment in lie detection. It involved the cooperation of Sir Robin Day, Britain's best-known television host. Wiseman interviewed Day twice about his favourite film. Before the interviews, Wiseman had arranged that Day tell the truth in one interview and tell nothing but lies in the other. The BBC aired both interviews on radio and television, and the *Daily Telegraph* published the transcripts.[48]

Viewers, listeners, and readers were asked to identify the interview in which Day was telling the truth. Forty-one thousand people participated. The TV viewers did little better than chance, only 52 per cent identifying the truthful interview correctly. The *Telegraph* readers did somewhat better with a 64 per cent success rate, while 73 per cent of the radio listeners identified the truthful interview. Clearly humans are not particularly good at lie detection. That the TV watchers faired so poorly was odd, because they received the most information with which to inform their decision; they could see Day's eye movements, facial expression, gestures, and posture. This more complete exposure seems to have been a disadvantage for, expecting liars to have "chattering fingertips" and "wavering eyes," they were misled. Skilful deceivers know very well how people think, and good liars fake honesty by controlling these visual giveaways.

We are perhaps now sophisticated enough in our understanding of lying to know that sociopaths are consummate liars. Devoid of what the rest of us call conscience, they feel free to weave a skilful web of untruths for such projects as fleecing vulnerable people of their life savings. Herein lies another problem, however, as many of us, including, it would seem, large numbers of healthcare practitioners, believe that it is only sociopaths who lie effectively. It is not true. Many people who would never dream of taking a penny off an old lady tell lies and do so adroitly.

I certainly do not wish to imply that everyone with competence in deception chooses to deceive. There are sturdy advantages to honesty: lies soon poison business and personal relationships, and being prepared to stand behind actions and thoughts perhaps gives the truthful a greater sense of personhood. Nevertheless, deception is part of the package of primate cognitive skills. In dealing with governments and large corporations, many of us clearly have no qualms about putting our biological heritage to profitable use.[49] We pay huge taxes and high insurance premiums, we rationalize; it can seem financially prudent to recoup our losses when the opportunity arises.

In the United States, approximately 17 per cent of adults say it is acceptable to cooperate with lawyers, doctors, or chiropractors to file false or exaggerated workers' compensation claims.[50] The Insurance Bureau of Canada comments: "Canadians don't consider insurance fraud a serious breach of the law, or they pass it off as something 'everyone' is doing, so it's okay."[51] The (Canadian) National Task Force on Insurance Fraud reports a revealing story of an obsessional Vancouver burglar who kept detailed records of all his thefts. After he was eventually caught, the insurance claims of his victims were checked against his carefully stored records. Only one of forty claimants had not in some way inflated their claim.[52]

"Lord, Lord, how this world is given to lying," is no doubt true, though now we are perhaps less intent than our forebears on trying to deny our deceit. Chuck V. Ford takes a deep look at our lying behaviour, both the good and the bad things about it, in his recent book *Lies! Lies!! Lies!!!: The Psychology of Deceit.* Perhaps lies are beginning to take their rightful place in society – rightful insomuch as, like it or not, we tell lots of them.[53]

People seldom see what they are not looking for. Richard Rogers, professor of psychiatry at the University of North Texas, is a world authority on malingering. "I am continually dismayed," he writes, "at the number of clinicians [who], despite decades of practice, have never observed a single case of dissimulation. The problem is circular. If we never investigate dissimulation, then we may never find it. I believe that our working assumption in clinical practice should be that an appreciable minority of evaluatees engage, at some time, in a dissimulative response style. If we accept this working assumption, then we also accept the responsibility to screen all referrals and actively consider the possibility of malingering and other forms of deception."[54]

It would be out of keeping with what is known about both whiplash and human behaviour if many or even the majority of whiplash plaintiffs did not lie about their symptoms, or at the very least, exaggerate them. They have received a heaven-sent ticket to the whiplash lottery; it would perhaps exhibit unseemly prodigality to dispense with such good fortune. Physicians who insist that malingering is rare have nothing but their naïveté to support their belief.[55] The hard evidence is all to the contrary. There is no doubt that malingering and fraudulent whiplash claims are common, but perhaps a reasonable doubt remains as to how common.

Anyone interested in winning a whiplash suit needs a gullible physician, but for the serious business of getting better, most patients want a doctor whom they can trust. Litigants often keep one set of doctors for their litigation problems and another for their illnesses about which they have genuine concern.

Hirschfeld and Behan relate a telling incident on this subject. "A well-educated secretary was interviewed by two sets of physicians, some called by her attorney, and some by the company. Following the court testimony, in which the favourably reported examinations won the patient an award, she crossed the courtroom and asked the psychiatrist who had testified against her for treatment. She openly expressed contempt for the doctors who had accepted her story!"[56] When push comes to shove, competent healthcare practitioners are perhaps more useful that gullible ones!

20

Hysteria and the "M" Diagnosis

The mind is a place of its own, and of itself can make
a hell of heaven or a heaven of hell.
– John Milton, *Paradise Lost*

Awareness is a region with ill-defined and porous borders.
The truth, or certain aspects of it, may float in and out of awareness
or hover on the periphery, present yet not distinct.
– Robert Wright, *The Moral Animal* [1]

Milton may have been correct about the mind, but sometimes a few days on Prozac can also change the hell of despair, if not to a life of heaven, at least into one of earthly satisfaction. A distraught young husband whose emotional state is tied to the roller coaster moods of his wife's menstrual cycle complains that it is difficult to know what is mental and what is physical. Philosophers, with amazing mental gymnastics, have tried over the centuries, usually rather unconvincingly, to define the relationship, or even the non-relationship between mind and body. Nowadays, at least scientifically, it is accepted that mind and body, like the two sides of the same coin, are so interconnected that they cannot be separated.[2] Whiplash experts, never slow to latch onto the vanguard of scientific thought, are in the forefront. "If the mind and body are one and the same thing," they say, "then it makes no difference if a person's neck was injured or not in the accident; if he believes it was and is in pain, then it is the same. The defendant caused the neck pain, so he is financially liable."

While it may be scientifically indefensible to separate mind and body, there seems little hope of teasing out the intricacies of personal injury litigation unless we assume that, at least at some levels of human activity, a difference remains. Preponderant evidence indicates that it is the *mind* rather than the *body* that is responsible for generating persistent whiplash symptoms. It does so either because the symptoms serve as a convenient expression of psycho-social distress or because the victims choose to report symptoms because it seems beneficial to do so.

Psychiatrists, faced with the lack of any demonstrable physical injury and with evidence that the symptoms (unconsciously or not) serve a purpose, must make a psychiatric diagnosis – and this diagnosis easily becomes contentious. The American Psychiatric Association's *Diagnostic and Statistical Manual of Mental Disorders (DSM)* provides criteria for the diagnosis of each psychiatric condition.[3] These diagnostic criteria are useful when they are used properly, since everyone involved in a case has at least a chance of knowing what disorder is being talked about, and its classifications are used in many countries besides the United States.

Its usefulness notwithstanding, the *DSM* inevitably imbues its diagnoses with an aura of scientific authenticity despite the reality that many of its diagnoses only delineate patterns of socially devalued behaviour, patterns sometimes shaped by unacknowledged expectations of healthcare practitioners.[4] The *DSM-IV* provides three possible diagnostic categories for psychologically induced persistent whiplash symptoms: the *somatoform disorders* (these include pain disorder); the *factitious disorders*; and *malingering*.[5]

- The common feature of the somatoform disorders is the presence of physical symptoms that suggest a general medical condition that are not fully explained by a general medical condition, by the direct effects of a substance, or by another mental disorder. [The symptoms are not intentionally produced or feigned as in factitious disorder or malingering].
- The essential feature of factitious disorders is the intentional production of physical or psychological signs or symptoms. The presentation may include fabrication of subjective complaints, self-inflicted conditions, exaggeration or exacerbation of pre-existing general medical conditions, or any combination or variation of these. External incentives for the behaviour are absent ...[The symptoms of the factitious disorders are] intentionally produced or feigned in order to assume the sick role ... The judgment that a particular symptom is intentionally produced is made both by direct evidence and by excluding other causes of the symptom.
- The essential feature of malingering is the intentional production and presentation of false or grossly exaggerated physical or psychological symptoms, motivated by external incentives such as avoiding military duty, avoiding work, obtaining financial compensation, evading prosecution, or obtaining drugs.

For the diagnosis of malingering, the *DSM* provides four additional criteria of which the presence of two makes "malingering a strongly suspected" diagnosis. These are:

- Medico-legal context of presentation (e.g., the person's being referred by the attorney to the clinician for examination);
- Marked discrepancy between the person's claimed stress or disability and the objective findings;
- Lack of cooperation during the diagnostic evaluation and in complying with the treatment regimen;
- The presence of Antisocial Personality Disorder.

While theoretically these three diagnostic categories may seem neat and tidy, in practice they are a hen's breakfast. The *DSM* cautions that its diagnoses are not valid in certain legal judgments and in the determination of compensation, which are, of course, exactly the times when they are most needed. The *DSM*'s caution is necessary since much psychiatric diagnosis assumes that the patient reveals the true nature of his symptoms; but in a medico-legal setting this revelation may be very distorted. Disclaimer or no disclaimer, many forensic psychiatrists use the *DSM*'s nomenclature anyway. A few psychiatrists take this sanctioned opportunity to create their own psychiatric diagnoses instead – often with fanciful and exotic results.

Whatever lawyers like to think, claiming to have the symptoms of a particular psychiatric disorder and actually having that disorder are two different things. Medical schools sometimes use actors as surrogate patients on whom their students can practise diagnostic skills. A competent actor can soon learn to feign any number of psychiatric disorders, and so, for that matter, can anyone else.

Intentionality is the ingredient that differentiates malingering, factitious disorders, and the somatoform disorders. In malingering, the illness behaviour is intentional. In the factitious disorders, the simulation of illness is intentional, but the motivation to adopt the illness behaviour is unconscious and therefore unintentional. In somatoform disorders, the motivation to simulate illness and the simulation itself are both unconscious and hence unintentional. For the most part patients fall confusingly somewhere in between these diagnostic descriptions. The decision to place a patient into a particular category then depends upon the whim of the examiner.

You may be thinking that this arbitrariness is of trivial importance; if so you are wrong. Courts regard malingering as a non-illness and a malingerer as a *persona non grata* – certainly not deserving of any compensation. They regard a somatoform disorder (since it is an involuntarily generated disorder) as a *bona fide* illness for which the patient is entitled to full compensation. When it comes to factitious disorder, however, courts are stymied; there is cliffhanging uncertainly as to whether the plaintiff will or will not be awarded compensation. If you are involved in this kind of stuff, as a plaintiff or as a lawyer or healthcare practitioner whose fortunes rest on the court's findings, these diagnostic issues become highly charged politically as well as financially.

Many authors have pointed out how much these three diagnoses have in common.[6] Let us look at them more closely. Malingering, the intentional feigning of illness to achieve some obvious goal, may be as old as humankind, for once our ancestors began to feel sympathy for their sick kith and kin, malingering entered as an option in the wide gamut of manipulative strategies. It is sympathy to other people's distress that allows malingering to work. Amnon, son of King David, "lay down and made himself sick" so he could force himself upon Tamar when she brought him food for his ailments.[7]

The term was originally used for anyone who, under the pretense of sickness, evades duty.[8] The first Earl of Northumberland in the year 1403 "lay craftily sick" to avoid taking part in the battle of Shrewsbury.[9] Lieutenant George Bass, an early explorer of Australia, used illness as a pretext to leave the navy and commence his profitable business venture: "I shall most certainly be sick and make the best of my way home in a whaler that no time shall be lost ... I have quitted the *Reliance* invalided. Behold me embark in trade."[10] Hector Gavin, a wily Edinburgh physician, wrote his 1843 book *On Feigned and Factitious Diseases* from his experience in the devastating French wars which gave young men cogent reasons to avoid conscription by any means they could.[11]

The *DSM-IV* suggests the presence of an antisocial personality disorder as one of the four findings that make malingering a strongly suspected diagnosis, and most authors consider malingering to be intimately associated with this personality disorder. Amnon feigned illness so that he could rape Tamar. Tamar was not only his sister, but having raped her he treated her despicably into the bargain. Even after three millennia and in a different cultural context, it is perhaps not unreasonable to make a diagnosis of antisocial personality disorder (psychopathy).

However, Amnon is more the exception than the rule. There is no reason to think that all the young Frenchmen who feigned illness to avoid conscription had antisocial personality disorder; perhaps just the opposite – they had no taste for killing and cruelty. Nor is there any reason to think that Lieutenant Bass, a courageous and successful man, had anything wrong with his personality. He was a competent man intent upon making the best use of his opportunities. I belabour the point because, in my experience, most people who feign illness to obtain compensation after minor auto collisions do not have an antisocial personality disorder; they are perfectly nice normal human beings trying to do their best for themselves and their families. The exaggerated perception that malingerers are "psychopaths" results in misdiagnosis; malingering is overlooked as the appropriate diagnosis.

Since malingering is not classified as a medical condition, some more *sticky* psychiatrists and judges insist that it must be detected rather than diagnosed. It can, for instance, be detected by videotaping the plaintiff doing something that he reports himself unable to do – perhaps digging all afternoon in his garden when he reports that his pain forces him to rest all day long in bed. Videotape surveillance is often revealing. I recently reviewed a videotape of a young woman who, following a trivial bang on the head in the office, alleged such severe brain injury that she had lost the sense of depth perception. She claimed she could no longer cook for her family, since on trying to do so she blistered her arms on the burners. The tape showed her playing baseball for the local team, making home runs and some fantastic catches.

The somatoform disorders are a group of somewhat disreputable conditions, and, like people of ill repute, they frequently change name. Originally, these disorders were simply known as *hysteria*. For the most part, the condition continues to masquerade as a physical disorder when its true identity often remains undetected.

Hysteria's pedigree goes back a long way. Plato believed that it was caused by the *hysteros,* or womb, which, being frustrated by sterility, wandered around the female body causing mischief (an anatomical supposition that necessarily confined hysteria to women).[12] Charles Lasègue, a French physician after whom two psychiatric syndromes are named, observed, "Hysteria has never been defined and never will be."[13] An English physician called it "the mocking-bird of nosology."[14]

All the young women confined to Bath chairs on the supposition that they were victims of spinal disease have long since disappeared from the fashionable seaside resorts of Regency England (see chapter 4). Hysteria may vanish but it always returns, and, as far as the cervical spine is concerned, its present incarnation is as whiplash.[15]

Despite the longstanding preference of both healthcare practitioners and patients to accord hysterical symptoms a physical basis, its largely psychological component has long been recognized. At the end of the nineteenth century, Charcot demonstrated that hysteria's symptoms are at least partly psychogenic. Using hypnosis, he got his hysterical patients to turn their symptoms on and off like a tap.[16] While Hermann Oppenheim, a leading neurologist, and his colleagues in

Germany were using hidden brain injury ("traumatic neurosis") as the explanation for railway spine, Charcot disagreed. To prove his point, he told his hypnotic subjects that when he slapped them on the back they would be paralysed. Slap, they were paralysed. Instant railway spine produced by a perfectly harmless and unfrightening slap. No shock was needed – psychological or otherwise.[17]

The question still remained as to whether these hypnotically induced symptoms were voluntary. In some subjects the symptoms seemed to come and go through an unconscious mechanism of suggestion, but other subjects could produce their symptoms at will. They would often do so on purpose to please the great master, who then allowed them to participate in the celebrated public displays of hysteria held weekly at the Salpetrière. Charcot was a realist; of malingering he said: "It is found in every phase of hysteria and one is surprised at times to admire the ruse, the sagacity and the unyielding tenacity that especially women, who are under the influence of a strong neurosis, display in order to deceive ... especially when the victim of deceit happens to be a physician!"[18]

The snake of sex has always been a popular explanation for many varieties of ills. Freud attributed hysterical symptoms to hidden childhood memories of seduction fantasies. When powerful adult sexual impulses threaten the re-emergence of these anxiety-provoking memories, he claimed the impulses are quickly and safely converted into physical symptoms, a *mental mechanism* that provides several advantages (gains) to the hysterical patient. The *primary gain* is the relief from anxiety obtained by the conversion of the distressing memories into physical symptoms.[19] An updated concept of primary gain might be the inner sense of relief obtained by a person who, hampered by a guilty sense of superiority towards others, adopts an illness that makes him less able to compete. *Secondary gains* are all the advantages that accrue from having that illness: escaping from a difficult situation, getting attention and sympathy, manipulating family and friends, and acquiring disability payments or compensation.

Freud's definition of secondary gain notwithstanding, when it comes to accident compensation there is seldom anything *secondary* about secondary gains; they are often a very primary purpose of an illness. Secondary gains are not esoteric; all that is required to detect them is an adequate history and an elementary understanding of human behaviour. Is the patient generating his useful symptoms intentionally? Many Freudian-minded psychiatrists still hold that both primary and secondary gains are produced unconsciously (unintentionally), though more sceptical psychiatrists wonder how the patient can remain oblivious to his unconsciously motivated behaviour when he so transparently puts his symptoms to such profitable use.

In the unspeakable horror of World War I trench warfare, soldiers developed *shellshock,* a concept derived, as we have mentioned, from the spinal shock concept of railway spine; the force of exploding shells caused brain damage.[20] To some doctors shellshock looked like hysteria; but were its symptoms intentional or not? Perhaps the shell-shocked soldier, having had enough of blood and mud, sensibly decided to develop symptoms that would permit his escape from the frontlines.

Except, perhaps, for a few stiff-necked generals, most people were happy to collude with the exculpatory diagnosis of shellshock, for without such medical absolution soldiers in large numbers would have been shot for treason, creating, among other things, an unnecessarily unfavourable impression on the civilians back home. It was much more politic to send the soldiers home as wounded war heroes. Unfortunately, the result of this otherwise constructive solution to the plight of these desperate men was to entrench in the minds of both doctors and the public alike the involuntary nature of hysterical symptoms.[21]

While consolidating hysteria's position as an unconsciously generated condition, the war plainly demonstrated that hysteria is not just a female complaint. It was embarrassingly apparent that males, if subjected to unpleasant enough circumstances from which they had no legitimate escape, also developed hysteria. A new name for hysteria was needed, one that was both gender-neutral and divorced from the implication of a childhood sexual aetiology. Somatoform disorders are now, more or less, hysteria's modern equivalent.

Psychogenic symptoms and sickness exploitation are so deeply interwoven into the patterns of our everyday behaviour that it is difficult to separate hysteria from normal behaviour. The more thoughtful members of the medical profession readily admit this difficulty. Eliot Slater, a distinguished British authority on hysteria from the Maudsley Hospital, wrote: "It is generally agreed that no one has yet framed a satisfactory definition of hysteria ... The only thing that hysterical patients have in common is that they are all patients."[22]

Where does sickness end and where does the ordinary human propensity to deceive begin? It is not easy to tell. Jones and Llewellyn, the physicians who wrote about the giveaway signs of malingering, point out, "Nothing resembles malingering more than hysteria; nothing resembles hysteria more than malingering."[23]

Foster Kennedy, director of neurology at the Bellevue Hospital, shortly after the end of World War II wrote of these intertwined conditions: "It is hard to say where hysteria stops and malingering begins ... The two are often mixed. The soldier who is a neurotic begins with an unconsciously assumed hysteria, and he may be quickly cured in the security and comfort of a hospital and very understandably does not want to go back to the lines. He starts to malinger. It is clear that after three days of meditation [see chapter 16] an injured man may malinger, but if he is allowed to malinger long enough he gets to believe his own malingering and then he is a hysteric."[24]

The distinction between hysteria (somatoform disorders) and malingering "depends on nothing more infallible than one man's assessment of what is going on in another man's mind."[25] Hysteria and malingering following minor accidents are, in essence, both motivated by a desire for compensation or some other secondary gain, the distinction between them being dependent upon the fallibility of doctor's assessment of the claimant's mind.[26]

"Factitious disorder" is the art of making oneself sick. Playing sick is a time-honoured way of getting sympathy and nurturance, a convenient excuse for avoiding something we do not want to do. In factitious disorder the patient takes playing sick to extremes. Last year, for example, I examined a nurse who was missing an arm and leg, both of which had required amputation after she surreptitiously injected her knee and elbow joints with faeces.

Mark Feldman and Charles Ford, the aforementioned psychiatrists from University of Albany, are authors of a well-informed and readable book on factitious disorders, *Patient or Pretender*.[27] Ford is also the author of *Lies! Lies!! Lies!!!*, the two books having a common theme since factitious disorder is, of course, another form of lying. Feldman and Ford identify the various degrees of factitious disorder:

- *Total fabrication*: the patient groans about severe back pain but is not really having any pain at all;
- *Exaggeration*: the patient claims to be having devastating, incapacitating migraines but really only has the occasional mild tension headache;
- *Simulation of diseases*: the patient spits up "blood" that was actually concealed in a rubber pouch inside the mouth;
- *Self-induced disease*: The patient has fever and pain after having induced an infection by injecting herself with bacteria or dirt.

Factitious disorder is common among healthcare practitioners, for not only does illness play a large part in their lives but also they are well versed in the signs and symptoms of serious diseases. By all sorts of ruses they can mislead their fellow practitioners. A thermometer is put in a hot drink, or egg white added to urine to mimic the proteinuria of kidney disease. Some, using a large hypodermic needle, deliberately bleed themselves to become anaemic, while others, taking enormous risks with their lives, induce anaemia by suppressing the bone marrow with anticancer drugs. They swallow or inject various substances as a way of becoming ill. The real cause of their symptoms often remains undiscovered.

There is much speculation as to what drives a person to be so self-destructive.[28] Feldman and Ford provide an insightful explanation:

During the perpetration of their factitious illnesses (which sometimes last for years), these people live within private hells of their own creation, unable to experience the fullness of life because all their experiences must revolve around sickness. And what makes their plight so sad is that they honestly believe that they must go to such outrageous, desperate extremes to obtain support and attention in their daily lives. Yes, some factitial patients are full of rage, and defeating caregivers is a way to express their rage. They may be especially delighted when the physician finally becomes aware of how badly he or she has been deceived. Others feel they've lost control of their lives, and "outsmarting" doctors allows them to feel "in control." But in any case, playing sick in lieu of communicating one's real needs or emotions is unhealthy, destructive, sometimes dangerous, always pathetic, and almost certainly more common than we know.[29]

It is so easy to fool doctors with symptoms that it's like stealing candies from children; there is not much sport to it.

The late Richard Asher, although a distinguished British neurologist in his own right, was best known for being the father of Jane, the Beatles' girlfriend. Asher described the Munchausen syndrome as a variant of factitious disorder, "a common syndrome which most doctors have seen, but about which little has been written."[30] He named his syndrome after Baron Karl Friedrich Hieronymus von Munchausen (1720–1791), a one-time war hero in the German cavalry who enchanted listeners with tall stories of his military adventures.[31] Although Munchausen did not show any inclination towards the sick role, his tall stories were so similar to the *pseudologica fantastica* (fantastic fabrications) of Asher's factitious patients that Asher appended the baron's name to his newly described syndrome.

Munchausen patients use self-induced symptoms to gain admission to hospital. They are the *hospital hobos* who in their peregrinations around the country go from one hospital to the next. Despite the concerted efforts of hospitals to keep them out, Munchausen patients, with their plausibility, expertly manage to penetrate the barriers. These *professional patients* "are relentlessly self-destructive, encouraging and submitting to countless unnecessary surgeries and dangerous diagnostic procedures during their lifetimes."[32] Factitious illness keeps up with the times. Perfectly healthy people join Internet support groups created to provide mutual support for various disabling conditions. Sometimes these factitious sufferers are exposed because their symptoms and misfortunes escalate to such implausible levels that nothing in life could really be so awful.[33] Sometimes parents or childminders induce or report illnesses in a child by way of getting the doctors's attention for themselves – a condition known as *Munchausen's by proxy.*

At the end of the nineteenth century, Siegbert Ganser, a German psychiatrist, described *hysterical pseudopsychosis* in prisoners. Ganser syndrome has become another well-recognized variant of factitious disorder. Ganser patients appeared to mimic madness, usually as a means of avoiding unpleasant events or obtaining sick privileges. Without familiarity with psychotic illness, florid madness is difficult to simulate. Ganser patients do what *hysterics* do when simulating physical illness. They present the signs and symptoms of disease as they imagine them to be.

Ganser patients give crazy answers to simple questions. "How many legs does a cow have?" "Three." Such answers give the Ganser syndrome its other names – the "syndrome of approximate answers," or the *three-legged cow disease.* Of course, dissimulators familiar with psychotic illness, either through close acquaintance with a psychotic person or from a prior psychotic illness of their own, present a much more credible performance, one that may be indistinguishable from the genuine article.[34] Psychiatric textbooks generally classify Ganser syndrome as a hysterical illness, but that is perhaps because most psychiatrists prefer to see all motivation as *unconscious.*

Psychiatrists have traditionally regarded the malingering use of mental illness as rare. In the words of a distinguished British professor of psychiatry, "It is universally agreed that purposive feigning of mental illness is first uncommon and second, extremely difficult to carry out in a sustained and convincing way."[35] Doctors, as I have shown, and even psychiatrists, it seems, often prefer to perceive illness as a mechanistic process unadulterated by any intentional hanky-panky.

Actually, one needs only recall a number of murder trials in which the two expert psychiatrists did not agree as to the sanity of the defendant, to realize how difficult the determination of sanity can be. Benjamin Braginsky, a Yale social psychologist, and his co-workers provided a more formal demonstration of how easily psychiatrically trained professionals can be manipulated. In their study *The Methods of Madness* they examined the interaction of mental hospital patients and the staff who care for them. By means of simple but clever questionnaires they demonstrated how adroitly such patients presented themselves to be *sane* and ready for discharge or *insane* and requiring further confinement to hospital. By "impression management" the patients blatantly manipulated the psychiatrists and other hospital staff and the staff fell for it. "While it is not surprising that patients are seen as 'out of touch with reality,' we were amazed to find a similar 'perceptual deficit' in the psychologists and psychiatrists who care for them."[36]

A mental hospital offers many tangible benefits for someone lacking financial and emotional resources: the accommodation, food, and recreational facilities are good. Sexual favours are readily available from other patients (the staff often regarding such activities as "bush therapy"), and the staff members are mostly friendly and supportive. Mental hospitals can provide a useful refuge from the law and from abusive relationships. It is not surprising that some people who lack any definable psychiatric illness opt to live in them. They make a *career* of being a mental hospital patient.

A study in a large Toronto mental hospital showed how successfully many of these "professional patients" conducted their careers. The psychiatrists' duty roster was regularly posted in a local tavern, so that any would-be patient could choose to arrive at the hospital when a particularly diffident psychiatrist was on duty, and late at night when his resistance was likely to be at its lowest. A public threat of suicide or injury to another person, a brick through a shop window along with a few peculiar remarks, and a mention of being a mental hospital patient ensure a free cab ride to the hospital in a police cruiser. Confronted by any dalliance by the hospital over his admission, the patient ups the ante. "I might have to take all my pills; my friends will know you would not let me in." If out of indignation a rejected patient carries out his threat and accidentally kills himself since the pills were more lethal than he believed, the denying doctor will be held responsible for his death.[37] The patient is admitted! In the event of an unwanted discharge, the patient re-enacts the admission strategy with, of course, escalating hostility from the police, the public, and media for discharging such an unfortunate man. The professional patient stays inside! The study found that professional patients accounted for one-sixth of all in-patient hospital days.[38]

In addition to having difficulty distinguishing between real and feigned mental illness, psychiatric staff also fail to recognize normality when they see it. Rosenhan, in his celebrated study *On Being Sane in*

Insane Places, nicely demonstrated this incapacity. Rosenhan organized eight very sane volunteers to get themselves admitted to twelve sample mental hospitals in locations throughout the United States.[39] Each volunteer was instructed to contact the hospital, report hearing voices, and say, "My life is hollow and empty." Apart from falsifying identifying information, the volunteers were to provide honest accounts of the events of their lives. Once admitted to the ward the volunteers were to behave normally and report that they were then feeling better.

The length of stay of these pseudo-patients varied from 7 to 52 days (average 19 days), and in no case was the subterfuge detected by the staff. All of them were discharged with a diagnosis of "schizophrenia in remission" with the exception of one who was diagnosed as an (active) schizophrenic. The psychiatrists tended to pathologize the personal histories of these normal adults, and the nursing staff also perceived them in terms of illness, charting such observations as "the patient indulges in writing behaviour." A total of 2100 pills was administered to the volunteers during their hospital stay.[40] On hearing of the study's findings, the staff of a different psychiatric teaching hospital maintained that such an error would not occur in their hospital. The staff were informed that during the following three months one or more pseudo-patients would attempt to gain admission and the staff were asked to assess on a ten point scale the likelihood of any new admission being fraudulent. No pseudo-patients were actually sent to the hospital but during the specified three months 193 genuine patients were admitted for treatment. Forty-one of these patients were confidently alleged by at least by one member of the staff to be a pseudo-patient, nineteen by a psychiatrist. Rosenhan's conclusion was unequivocal: "It is clear that we cannot distinguish the sane from the insane in psychiatric hospitals."

Doctors, like other people, see what they expect to see. Once labelled *psychiatric,* all patient's behaviour is perceived as abnormal. Like beauty, psychiatric illness is often in the eye of the beholder.[41] The actual prevalence of factitious disorder in the community at large is difficult to determine since only the unsuccessful cases are recognized and reported. From the large number of cases and studies in the medical literature, Feldman and Ford estimate that factitious illness is both under-recognized and more prevalent than ever.

While it is often difficult to distinguish between factitious disorder and malingering, it is equally difficult to distinguish between factitious disorder and the somatoform disorders, if only because somatoform patients sometimes deliberately exaggerate their illness. A Danish study examined 282 frequent hospital users who had had at least ten general admissions over an eight-year period. The investigators identified 56 of these patients who had had more than six admissions for medically unexplained physical complaints or symptoms, and designated these patients as the "persistent somatizers."

Eighteen per cent of these 56 patients were found on at least one or more of their admissions to have had a factitious disorder consisting of a self-inflicted illness denied by the patient. The simulation of illness included adding blood to urine or vomit and injecting joints to induce arthritis and simulated fever. The investigators compared the demographical characteristics of the factitious disorder patients with those of the other persistent somatizers. The only difference they found was that the factitious disorder patients tended to have a larger number of medically unexplained admissions.[42]

If 18 per cent of these Danish somatoform patients were found to have cheated by deliberately fabricating symptoms, it seems reasonable to assume that some others in this group of somatoform patients also cheated but did so too cleverly to be found out. It would be a brave or mendacious physician who could claim with certainty to be able to differentiate between somatoform and factitious disorders.

Apart from military or penal institutions and family life (a hothouse of manipulative behaviours), these three look-alike conditions were probably rare until the industrial revolution. This catastrophic economic upheaval devastated people's lives, and laws were appropriately enacted to soften the plight of the seriously injured – laws that permitted financial recovery for injury from railway companies and industrial employers. Few things are ever exempt from the law of unintended consequences. It was these humane laws that initiated the ongoing epidemic of feigning illness (unconsciously or intentionally).[43]

Are these three look-alike conditions really all just different presentations of the same condition? Some psychiatrists think so. Jeffrey M. Jonas and Harrison G. Pope from the Mailman Research Center and Harvard Medical School, perceive malingering, factitious disorder, and somatoform disorders to have so much in common that they should be united as a single entity, the "Dissimulating Disorders." Jonas and Pope pointed out: "[These] psychiatric disorders [are] characterized by symptoms or signs that are not *real* in that they do not appear due to a "*genuine* medical or psychiatric illness."[44] Jonas and Pope note the similar demographic features of the three conditions, which usually start in adolescence or early adult life and are often chronic, with multiple and varied medical conditions often being simulated over a lifetime. All three have a high rate of dysfunctionality in the family of origin and respond poorly to treatment.

The only demographic variance between the three conditions is in their gender ratios. More women have somatoform disorders and factitious illness (excluding the Munchausen and Ganser variants) and more men malinger. The authors suggest that this is yet another form of gender discrimination, the described differences having more to do with diagnostic bias than with any real gender differences. "We tend to diagnose [somatoform] disorders primarily in women – as we believe these women are the preferred victims of unconscious conflicts and lack voluntary control. On the other hand, men are more often assigned a diagnosis of malingering – implying that men tend to be conscious of their motivations and in command of their actions." Medicine is male chauvinistic and psychiatry particularly so. Jonas and Pope are probably right!

Attempting to fit all whiplash plaintiffs properly into one of the three look-alike diagnostic categories would be a Herculean task if it were attempted. Few experts even bother to do it. Most expert witnesses, both for the plaintiff and the defence, opt for the diagnosis of a somatoform disorder. This convenient diagnostic choice conveys to the court that the plaintiff's symptoms are authentic (he really experiences them). Since the symptoms followed upon the accident, the court is reassured that the plaintiff has a genuine medical disorder and grants a generous compensation. This systematic favouring of an illness diagnosis rather than one of "malingering" inevitably perpetuates the whiplash epidemic.

Based on *DSM* diagnostic criteria, "malingering should be strongly suspected" in every plaintiff with persistent whiplash. After all, virtually without exception every whiplash plaintiff presents in a "medico-legal context" and every such plaintiff has a "marked discrepancy between [his] claimed stress or disability and the objective findings" (see diagnostic criteria above). Nevertheless, doctors seldom consider the "M" diagnosis, let alone actually make it. Why not?

There are many reasons. It goes without saying that the plaintiff's expert medical witnesses will not support such a diagnosis, and neither will his personal physicians. The plaintiff sees his lawyer as his champion and he expects his doctors to behave with even greater solicitude. Everyone knows lawyers are devious but doctors, after all, are members of a caring profession; and they should care![45] A doctor who supported the "M" diagnosis would quickly be left without his patient.

Even if defence internists and surgeons suspect such a diagnosis, they seldom make it. A psychiatric diagnosis is seen as outside the realm of their professional competence. The plaintiff's lawyer could give a non-psychiatrist a hard time in court for going beyond his professional competence. Defence psychologists and psychiatrists are in a position to make the "M" diagnosis but they also seldom do. Why not?

Every specialty has its stock in trade. For surgeons it is the scalpel; for psychiatrists it is the unconscious. Many psychiatrists see their skill in terms of understanding unconsciously motivated behaviour. They eschew straightforward explanations of behaviour. Henry Miller, the English neurologist (the one who upset lawyers with the assertion that settlement cures) provides an illuminative example of psychiatrists' blinkered reluctance to see malingering. I have shortened his original account.

A 30-year-old labourer from a distant city was struck by a piece of iron-ore that fell on his head causing a scalp laceration. He remembered the event clearly and was never unconscious. The laceration was sutured in hospital, where the labourer was not retained and he returned to work next day. Two hours later he complained of dizziness and left his job to report to the hospital. During the next three weeks he began to stammer. He had never had previous difficulty with speech. He became depressed and three months after the accident was referred to a psychiatrist.

The patient's depression was resistant to a battery of psychotropic drugs and after five months of fruitless treatment he was given electric shock therapy (ECT), after which he did not speak at all. When Dr Miller examined him, the patient had not been heard to speak for two years, despite expert surveillance by a private detective, extensive investigation in a psychiatric unit of a teaching hospital, and examination by other psychiatrists. Diagnoses of post-traumatic cerebral thrombosis, hysteria, and schizophrenia had been made. His mutism completely resisted an injection of thiopentone [the "truth serum"]. The last psychiatrist had recommended referral to one of the societies for mutes.

While Dr Miller examined the patient, the wife did the talking. All communication with him, much of which was about his continuing headaches, was done by written notes. Physical examination was completely negative. Dr Miller was convinced that the patient was malingering and so arranged to have a colleague follow the patient unobserved as he left the office. The patient took the train back to the Midlands and Dr Miller's colleague followed him.

The patient exchanged his first few remarks with his wife as the train drew out of Newcastle station, and by the time the train reached Durham the whole compartment was engaged in uninhibited and cheerful conversation on matters of the day.

None of the previous eleven psychiatrists who had reported on this man's condition had even raised the possibility of malingering.

There are other reasons for failing to make the "M" diagnosis. Psychologists know no medicine, and most North American psychiatrists are not much better, having long ago divorced themselves from ordinary medical practice. Physical diagnoses easily intimidate them. They are professionally on shaky ground and so are reluctant to stick out their necks and dismiss these nonsensical physical diagnoses.

And the "M" diagnosis rocks the medico-legal boat, a boat that expert witnesses depend upon for their livelihoods. If it were to become widely accepted that whiplash patients malinger, then both the plaintiff and the defence bars would suffer. I, as a sometime defence expert, may expatiate on the excesses of the plaintiff experts, yet the unrestrained exorbitance of their claims provides me with a professional income, an intellectual diversion, and even a vent for moral indignation. The defence may question the extent of a plaintiff's alleged physical and psychological injuries, but it is not likely to argue that they do not even exist. It is in the interests of neither bar to have whiplash completely stripped of its legitimacy.

"Every time you are right someone loves you a little less," is a saying that certainly applies to physicians' being right about a plaintiff's complaints not being genuine. The doctor may not only be right but he may also be "dead right." In *Malingering: A Dangerous Diagnosis*, Neville Parker, a psychiatrist from Melbourne, Australia, gives an account of a worker with chronic backache who, after being told there was nothing physically wrong with his back, killed two orthopaedic surgeons who had made this diagnosis and severely injured a third. The dead doctors had been right; the worker also killed himself and an autopsy showed that there was, indeed, nothing physically wrong with his back.[46] Actually, the killing of doctors is rare. Parker reports that only six such cases were recorded over a 25-year period in the whole of Australia. When doctors fail to produce the needed diagnosis, however, it is not uncommon for them to be threatened and sometimes seriously assaulted.[47]

The "M" diagnosis also makes judges crotchety. In a recent case of a women suing for injuries allegedly suffered in three motor vehicle accidents, the Supreme Court of British Columbia made it clear in a 1994 decision that forensic psychologists, however much evidence they have gathered on a plaintiff's unreliability, are not to comment on the plaintiff's credibility.[48] I would be the first to agree that expert witnesses, both plaintiff and defence, have often shown themselves to be no better at judging a plaintiff's credibility than anyone else, but this decision unbalances the fact-finding process.

Courts have always allowed plaintiff experts to provide their dubious opinions on the questionable results obtained by their unreliable investigations. When these opinions come from highly qualified physicians, they provide a crucial input to the court's deliberations. Psychologists now have well-designed and well-validated tests to evalu-

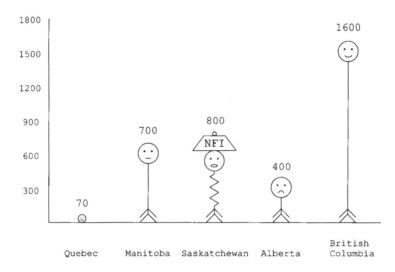

Fig. 20–1   Go West, young man?
Published annual whiplash claims per 100,000 of population for various Canadian provinces for 1997. For anyone wanting to exploit whiplash, the pickings seem larger toward the West.

The Ontario information is missing from this graph since its auto insurance is in such a mess that nobody knows what its figures are. However, various indicators suggest that Ontario has the longest neck of all. Perhaps a young man in search of easy money should not go West but come to Ontario instead.

Saskatchewan's whiplash claims recently fell after the province imposed *no-fault* insurance.

ate a plaintiff's credibility, tests that are certainly better validated than most of the tests used by orthopaedic surgeons to confirm a diagnosis of whiplash or low backache disability.

By disallowing defence psychologists to provide the results of their tests on the plaintiff's credibility, the Supreme Court of British Columbia has virtually guaranteed that physical injury will be the only acceptable explanation for the plaintiff's ongoing complaints. Figure 20–1 shows just how successful British Columbia judges have been in augmenting the vulnerability of West Coast necks. If you are aiming to make your fortune from the whiplash lottery, Indiana newspaperman John Soule's advice, "Go West, young man," remains as pertinent, at least in Canada, as ever!

Not surprisingly, plaintiff personal injury lawyers regard malingering as a despicable diagnosis and, despite any legal nicety about not intimidating witnesses, do all they can to harass any expert psychiatrist or psychologist who is bold enough to make it. They commonly lodge complaints to an expert's licensing body, or have his financial records subpoenaed on the grounds that he must have received large payments for making such an erroneous diagnosis.

Canadian orthopaedic surgeon John McCulloch joined Gordon Waddell, the Scottish back expert, to do seminal work on the non-organic nature of industrial low back pain.[49] On returning to Toronto, McCulloch applied their research findings to patients with low back pain attributed to motor vehicle accidents. Finding all the signs of non-organic back pain, he was prepared to diagnose either symptom magnification or malingering.[50] Toronto lawyers gave him a very bad time until, tired of their continual harassment, McCulloch moved his practice south of the border. This was certainly Canada's loss and America's gain.

The licensing bodies of the various professions are charged with the task of protecting the public from the improper professional behaviour of their members but these bodies inevitable tend to be protective of their profession's interests as well. The management of a head injury or psychological stress resulting from an accident provides only a small portion of the activities of the medical profession. Medical licensing bodies have little concern with protecting such a minor portion of their bailiwick. A short letter of complaint from an aggrieved lawyer may land an expert medical witness with hours of report-writing to answer to queries from his licensing body, but, providing he has behaved appropriately, such legal harassment is just a time-consuming nuisance.

For PhD psychologists, such complaints may be another matter. In Ontario, as elsewhere in North America, a significant number of psychologists make their livelihood by testing and rehabilitating the victims of either alleged minimal head injury or alleged post-traumatic stress disorder attributed to minor vehicle accidents. Such activities provide a substantial proportion of psychological practice. The Ontario College of Psychologists is, therefore, likely to be protective of this area of psychological practice. A psychologist who makes a diagnosis of malingering calls into question much of this remunerative activity.

Frank Kenny, the neuropsychologist whose tests caught out the Surfer, was threatening the market with his diagnostic tests for malingering. Claimants like the Surfer are literally worth millions of dollars to the rehabilitation and psychological industries. In another notable case, Kenny assessed an automobile accident claimant on behalf of a large insurance company and, after a thorough neuropsychological examination of the claimant, concluded that the claimant was consciously feigning impairment for personal gain. Kenny made a diagnosis of malingering/factitious disorder and suggested that the insurance company was neither liable for an injury nor required to provide further funding for head injury treatment. The plaintiff's lawyer complained to the Ontario College of Psychologists, and the College filed charges against Kenny.

The complaint led to many years of legal wrangling. No one disagreed with Kenny's finding. The plaintiff was clearly fabricating symptoms intentionally. However, the College found Kenny guilty on the spurious technicality of having used the words "liable" and "funding" which the College claimed went beyond the professional competence of a neuropsychologist. The College applied a minimal penalty but Kenny refused to accept it. The case, several hundreds of thousands of dollars later, went to the Divisional Court of Ontario. Mr Justice Rosenberg, in speaking for the unanimous opinion of the three-member Divisional Court panel, stated: "Counsel before us acknowledges that there is no allegation that Dr Kenny's diagnosis was wrong. In our view, the proper forum to attack Dr Kenny's report was in the cross-examination in the court proceedings. The Complaints Committee and the College should not have allowed themselves to be used by the solicitor who lodged the complaint to circumvent the appropriate route for civil litigation. As a result of allowing these proceedings to go on, Dr Kenny has suffered irreparable harm."[51]

The College was instructed to pay all Kenny's costs from the beginning. Kenny was totally vindicated, but in many ways his was a Pyrrhic victory. The litigation had dragged on for four years, during which time Kenny's practice had disintegrated. Kenny won his fight but at enormous personal cost.[52] The College, although landed with huge costs, had certainly sent a clear message to all its members that a diagnosis of malingering would not be tolerated. Few psychologists have either the financial means or the courage to conduct such a fight. Ontario psychologists can safely continue their lucrative trade of rehabilitating allegedly brain-injured plaintiffs without actual brain injury, and of treating PTSD claimants with unremitting symptoms consequent upon the most minor of accidents.

As every demagogue well knows, big lies work better than little ones. "My neck has been hurting ever since the accident" may well be dismissed as an understandable exaggeration aimed at augmenting damages, but juries and judges find it hard to doubt that someone confined to a wheelchair and covered in splints has in fact sustained serious injury. They easily become angry if a defence lawyer tries to prove otherwise. Defence lawyers have learned their lesson and tend to avoid the risk of taking such cases to court. In court, damage awards could go into the millions, so defence lawyers usually opt to settle out of court for more moderate amounts.

Gorman and Winograd describe such a case in which discretion seemed the better choice.[53] A hollow fibreglass natural-sized mannequin fell from 30-inch-high table in a big department store and struck a 25-year-old woman on the head. Examination in the ER showed a superficial 2-cm bruise on the back of the head. She sought damages from the store.

Personal injury plaintiffs usually have a pre-accident history of medical problems, and this plaintiff was no exception. Before the mannequin incident, the woman had been investigated in and out of hospital for innumerable conditions, and all tests had been normal. Prior to the mannequin incident her medication for pain relief included Dilaudid (a morphine product) every three hours. Her previous diagnoses included *hysteria* and *factitious disorder*. Following the hit on her head, the plaintiff complained of respiratory and general weakness, along with diminished sensation below the neck. A diagnosis of possible quadriplegia was made. She was given a wheelchair and urged to diminish her medication intake. Despite her alleged difficulties, the woman continued to drive her car, and four months after the mannequin event, while in the process of parking, was involved in a collision. Further extensive orthopaedic, neurological, and laboratory examinations again demonstrated no physical abnormality.

Two years later the plaintiff was medically examined on behalf of the defence, with both her mother and lawyer present. The mother briefly removed her daughter's oxygen mask, revealing an alert young woman. Apart from weakness of all four limbs and a finding of diminished sensation over the trunk and limbs (which are not objective signs of injury), all neurological tests were normal. A drug screen was impossible because the mother had spilled the urine specimen and, as all available veins had been thrombosed by numerous previous venipunctures, no blood could be taken. The examiner made a diagnosis of factitious disorder, probable chronic intoxication with prescribed medications, and probable malingering. The defence counsel, who had believed that the exposure of this young woman in a motorized wheelchair wearing an oxygen mask would prejudice a jury toward her, arranged a settlement.

I have presented this case in full because I wish to make the point that anyone who is determined to adopt an invalid lifestyle usually manages to do so. Such pseudo-invalids frequently manage to have their chosen lifestyle generously financed through successive injury litigation suits. The severity of this young women's injuries was feigned, but the accoutrements of illness – wheelchairs, braces, and oxygen masks, however unneeded, can influence outcomes.

Are the persistent symptoms of whiplash intentionally concocted or are they unconsciously engendered? When awarding compensation this may be the million-dollar question. Are the symptoms malingered or are they somatoform? Even with all the cooperation in the world, it is difficult to know what happens in another person's mind, and it is much more difficult when that person is determined to prevent you from finding out. The examiner himself may have strong conscious or unconscious motivations that bias his judgment about what he finds. However, does this impossible diagnostic problem really have to be a problem?

The only theoretical difference between malingering, factitious disorder, and the somatoform disorders is the degree of conscious intentionality involved in the production of symptoms. But how significant is conscious intentionality? Traditionally, psychiatrists, immersed in Freudian doctrine, have perceived repression as the pathological mental mechanism by which disconcerting material is banished from the conscious mind. Most often this disconcerting material is, of course, sexual. Yet do concepts derived from hypothetical anxieties about sexuality really provide an appropriate basis on which to award compensation for injury?

If the evolutionary psychologists are right, then for millions of years our ability to deceive and detect deception has provided us with a reproductive advantage. Telling lies is difficult and there is evidence that a liar is more likely to be believed if he first deceives himself.[54] If this is so, some of us have evolved as better self-deceivers than have others.

Perhaps the essential difference between malingering, factitious disorder, and somatoform disorders depends upon how well Nature has done her work – the effectiveness with which the victim of whiplash can deceive himself and therefore others. Whether the plaintiff's intentions are conscious or not, the results are the same. The plaintiff, by his behavioural strategies, manipulates his world to get what he wants.

Perhaps Jonas and Pope are right; malingering, the factitious disorders, and the somatoform disorders should be blended into a single entity. No longer would experts, judge, and jury be assigned the impossible task of determining the degree of intentionality of symptom generation. It is not usually difficult to separate the primary effects of an injury from the illness behaviour associated with secondary gains. A competent physician can realistically estimate the time of recovery from an injury uncomplicated by secondary gain. The plaintiff would then receive compensation payment only for the injury, but none for the secondary gain, be the gain intentional or not. Such a change would certainly soon take the sting out of whiplash and other related conditions. It would also put a lot of lawyers and healthcare practitioners out of work.

I cannot leave the topic of diagnosis without a mention of skulls. Judges use skulls to assign responsibility for the effects of injury. The *thin skull* (sometimes called the *fragile skull*) rule goes like this. If you hit someone on the head and he happens to have a thin skull so that it breaks and you thereby cause him serious injury, you are responsible for the injury, even though it was a very little hit that would not ordinarily have damaged a skull.

This longstanding legal principle worked well when confined to physical injury. The troubles started when the law became concerned with injury to the mind. Lawyers and judges just applied their thin-skull guideline to the mind. It landed defendants in a horrible mess. Take the woman upon whom the fibreglass mannequin happened to fall. Any worthy defence medical expert would find out that the plaintiff habitually reacted catastrophically to the smallest of accidents – she was, in fact, *an accident waiting to happen*. "Ah," says the plaintiff's lawyer, "If she was an accident waiting to happen, then she is indeed a thin skull. There is no difference between an egg-shell skull and an egg-shell personality."[55] "Yes," says the judge to the storeowner, "The evil-doer must take his victim as he finds him." The storeowner finds himself supporting the woman in her expensive invalid lifestyle for the rest of her life, and perhaps even more painfully, covering the plaintiff lawyer's huge fee for having successfully saddled him with the responsibility for the woman's incompetence.

There is all the difference in the world between a thin skull shattering and a thin mind doing the same thing. A thin skull straightforwardly breaks in pieces, but a thin mind goes to pieces in a way that suits its owner, and what suits its owner is that the other person pays.[56]

The Supreme Court of British Columbia, by disallowing psychologists' opinions on a plaintiff's credibility, seems hell-bent on escalating British Columbia's already booming whiplash industry. However, Mr Justice Gow, one of BC's Supreme Court judges, did somewhat redress the balance. He espouses the concept of the *crumbling skull,* and thereby gave some protection to inoffensive defendants. I quote the judge's own words:

The issue becomes, therefore, is this a "thin skull" case or a "crumbling skull" case? The difference is this. In the former the skull, although thinner than the average skull, is before the accident in a stable condition and, but for the accident, would have remained so. The defendant cannot be heard to say that as his victim did not have a skull of average thickness the amount of compensation for which he is liable must be calculated on the basis of imputing to his victim a skull of average thickness. The latter is where the skull, whether thick or thin, is not before the accident in a stable condition, but in a state of continuing deterioration and the accident has accelerated the process of that deterioration. In the latter the defendant is not saddled with responsibility for the whole of the pre-accident condition of the skull. His negligence is not treated as having been the sole cause of the post-accident condition, but an aggravating cause. Depending upon the circumstances the aggravation may range from the very substantial to the very slight.[57]

With the crumbling skull line of argument, the falling mannequin can be perceived as having caused a little crumble in a fast crumbling skull. The damages that the storeowner pays are reduced to more manageable proportions. Justice is perhaps a little better served!

"Cured by a Verdict?"

Conflicts of interest are inherent to the human condition, and we are apt
to want *our version* of the truth, rather than truth itself, to prevail.
– Steven Pinker (1997)

Lawyers spend a great deal of their time shovelling smoke.
– Oliver Wendell Holmes, Jr

If there is money to be made from something, someone will probably
make some. Do people claim injury and even remain disabled because
they can make money from compensation? The people who go to the
trouble of jumping onto crashed buses, making *paper accidents,* and
staging crashes certainly do, but what about the ordinary person in the
street – you and me? If we were in a car accident, would we complain
of symptoms simply because compensation was available? I have presented enough information about whiplash to make the answer to this
question, at least for most of us, an unhesitating, "Yes!"

An epidemiologist looking at whiplash symptoms cannot but conclude that there is a direct relationship between the persistence of
whiplash symptoms and the availability of compensation. However, as
epidemiologists are low down on the medical totem pole, their insightful opinions are usually ignored, especially when their insights stand
in the way of remunerative clinical practice. It is clinicians who capture
the limelight about health and disease, but clinicians speak from the
limitations of their own perspective. Like the blind men who, when
feeling the elephant, all obtained their own particular impressions of
the pachyderm, clinicians, each with their limited view of whiplash,
come up with very divergent opinions about the role that compensation plays in the genesis of its symptoms.

It was in Prussia that the compensation problem all started. In 1871,
seeking to provide protection for injured civilians, Prussia enacted the
world's first accident insurance laws, which made it possible to collect
for injuries sustained on its national railway system (see chapter 7).
Claimants were disabled by apparently trivial injuries and, as with
whiplash today, many physicians were soon bogged down in their
attempts to explain the nature of these perplexing injuries.[1] Were they
due to the physical *shock* of the collision, which caused invisible micro-

scopic damage in the nervous system, or were they due to psychological shock from the unexpected collision? When faced with such an
enigma of human behaviour, the French advise "cherchez la femme,"
but the journalist's standard advice of "follow the money," is perhaps
more realistic. Rigler, a Prussian physician, went straight for the
money.

In his book on the effects of railway collisions, written seven years
after the enactment of the first insurance law, Rigler coined the much-
disputed term "compensation neurosis."[2] Since then other sceptics
have come up with similar terms – litigation neurosis, greenback neurosis, compensationitis, American disease, entitlement neurosis, Greek
disease, Mediterranean back, unconscious malingering, and whiplash
neurosis, to mention but a few.

These terms all emphasize the part that money plays in the persistence of symptoms that follow a minor compensable injury. I will stick
to "compensation neurosis" as the generic for all these terms. Not only
are they all pejorative but they are also inaccurate for, while financial
considerations are indeed a major motivation for the development of
symptoms, other motives, such as the need for a dependency role, may
sometimes be as cogent as the money – perhaps even more so.

While financial enticement undoubtedly initiated the epidemics of
railway spine and whiplash, once these conditions gained general
acceptance as legitimate medical conditions, many people in psycho-
social distress adopted them as a fashionable illness with which to
justify a variety of personal difficulties. Myre Sim, a professor of psychiatry at Birmingham in Britain, in his thoughtful book *Compensation
Claims: Insurance, Legal and Medical Aspects* provides a clear vignette of
such a situation: "The Plaintiff may already be suffering from a psychiatric disability, usually of a depressive nature, and the accident
provides a Heaven-sent opportunity for an honourable and even lucrative escape from a situation which was becoming unbearable."[3]

Also, of course, accidents are accidents, and people can be genuinely injured in them. The unfortunate victim then has to contend
not only with the lure of compensation, but with the effects of the
injury as well. Over 100 years ago H.W. Page, the English physician
who introduced the concept of *nervous shock,* wrote: "The anticipated
compensation can hinder the convalescence of the truly sick person,
so the legal order itself slows the healing process."[4]

Resentment for a real or imagined injustice can also keep an injury
going forever. Ernst Kretschmer, a German psychiatrist, now remembered by psychiatrists as the first person to study the association
between different body-builds and mental illness, wrote eloquently
about such feelings of disgruntlement. I will let him make the point:

"Resentment is the complex attitude of mind in those who, in fact, have suffered injustice, or deem themselves to have been injured. It is to see life in perspective from below; it is a constant gnawing feeling of rebellion, the many-sided attitude of the weak in relation to the powerful, of the poor towards the rich, of the sick, the degenerate, and the disintegrating toward health and youth – in a word, the attitude of all malcontents who are constantly ready, in their "life envy," to revenge themselves or to continue in their state of malicious resentment."[5]

Acrimony fostered in the workplace or the road rage of frustrated and resentful drivers demands atonement. Resentment expands and the victim soon is holding his employer or the auto insurance company responsible for all his woes; in no way will he be prepared to recover until restitution has been made. Staying ill, especially when the designated culprit is paying for it, can be sweet revenge.[6]

Many physicians have avoided a diagnosis of compensation neurosis out of honest uncertainty as to the cause of their patient's symptoms. Doctors, lawyers, and union leaders may have been genuinely perplexed by the unexpected complaints that occurred during the earlier stages of the mysterious psycho-social epidemics that have flourished in our communities. Later, once the causes of a new epidemic have been more fully evaluated, the paramount role that compensation plays in the genesis of symptoms becomes apparent – at least, to anyone willing to see it. However, by then there is a problem: lawyers, doctors, chiropractors, and physiotherapists are making their livelihood from the epidemic; the last thing they want to hear is that they are the cause of it.

"Compensation neurosis" is too accusatory of everyone involved in the process. "Traumatic neurosis" proved a more acceptable term. But if compensation neurosis is an inaccurate term, traumatic neurosis, with its uncompromising verbal linkage of symptoms to the accident, is even more falsifying, since its symptoms usually have little or nothing to do with any actual trauma. Inaccurate as it may be, however, traumatic neurosis won out as the accepted name for conditions like railway spine and whiplash.

Hermann Oppenheim, the aforementioned influential neurologist from Berlin, first coined the term to indicate the supposed but invisible damage to the nervous system caused by the perturbation of a railway collision. Plaintiffs and their medical and legal advisors readily accepted "invisible damage" to be the cause of railway spine's various debilitating symptoms.[7] In train collisions the brain and spinal cord of the unfortunate passenger had suffered shock, but this shock did not imply a psychological condition. When World War I came along, shellshock was at first also attributed to similar microscopic physical injury (see chapter 20). Then psychiatry became more in touch with human feelings, and it was accepted that being the target of exploding shells could be an upsetting experience in itself. Shock began to acquire a psychological connotation.

"When I use a word it means just what I choose it to mean – neither more nor less," said Alice "in a rather scornful tone." In the Alice-in-Wonderland world of awarding huge compensation for minor or non-existent injury, "traumatic neurosis" meant just whatever anyone wanted it to mean. Some plaintiff experts used the term to cover symptoms arising as a psychological reaction to an accident, others continued to use the term to describe the behavioural manifestations of a supposed brain injury, and others just left it up to the judge and jury to guess what they meant.

Of course, "traumatic neurosis" left lawyers, doctors and plaintiffs all in a state of cherished confusion. More thoughtful physicians were disenchanted with the term. In 1927 a group of distinguished British neurologists meeting at the Royal Society of Medicine debated the problem of "traumatic neuraesthenia," an alternative name for traumatic neurosis. Sir Farquhar Buzzard opened the discussion: "The use of the term *traumatic neurasthenia* has led to much confusion in the minds of doctors as well as of lawyers, and until the medical profession adopts a clear conception of its meaning it is impossible for our legal brethren to adjust its proper relationship to the law of the land. Perhaps it would not be regrettable if, as a result of this discussion, the term were to receive its deathblow and be decently buried."[8]

In the ensuing discussion, the speakers noted the frequent occurrence in their practices of plaintiffs with traumatic neurasthenia following railway accidents who, having escaped without a scratch, subsequently developed "delayed shock" and sued for compensation. The neurologists agreed that, since, in many cases, no possible physical injury could have occurred, traumatic neurasthenia must be a psychoneurosis – a condition that develops for psychological reasons especially in situation where compensation is due.

The British neurologists had an enlightening discussion, but in no way did they deliver a deathblow to traumatic neurosis; it remained as lucratively confusing as ever, though traumatic neurosis gradually came to be viewed more as a psychological illness due to the psychological shock of the accident than a physical injury due to any physical trauma. Once this change occurred it fell to the lot of plaintiff psychiatrists to present a scientifically acceptable psychological explanation for the symptoms of traumatic neurosis. With their predilection for unconscious impulses, psychiatrists soon turned traumatic neurosis into an even more perplexing condition.

Psychiatrists had the challenge of distinguishing between traumatic neurosis and compensation neurosis, both of which they held to be unconsciously induced. Gordon R. Kamman, a psychiatrist from St Paul, Minnesota, nicely demonstrated the mental agility required to define and differentiate these two neuroses. It is not easy being a psychiatrist.

Kamman perceived a traumatic neurosis as a reaction to a symbolic stimulus, to an idea. He emphasized that the size of the reaction to an idea has no relationship to its method of delivery: "To whisper quietly in a person's ear that he is sitting next to a rattlesnake can produce just as dramatic a reaction as when the person actually perceives the snake himself. It is not the trigger that sends the bullet on its way; it is the powder charge inside the gun: it is the reaction that the stimulus sets off inside the recipient ... Dynamically speaking, the traumatic neurosis is a narcissistic regression in which the ego instincts, rather than the psychosexual instincts, are affected."[9] (This is a difficult concept and you have to be clever indeed to understand what Kamman means.)

Compensation neurosis is an entirely different kettle of fish. "The disorder is precipitated by certain environmental factors acting on personality defects ... This is the principal reason that the symptoms shown by people suffering from compensation neuroses (often miscalled 'traumatic neuroses') almost invariably disappear within a short time after legal and financial settlement has been made."

Although insisting that the unconscious mechanisms of formation of these two neuroses are quite different, Kamman noted that both these neuroses are indicative of genuine suffering. "People suffering from a compensation neurosis are just as sincere in their belief that they are sick as are those with traumatic neurosis."

The unconscious is an ill-defined realm; how do ideas get into it? Kamman clarified: "Fear is engendered in many cases by injudicious remarks on the part of physicians and attendants who are with the patient: 'My, but that is a tremendous laceration,' or 'He's lucky his brains aren't bashed in.' This type of suggestion seeps into the patient's unconscious mind and perpetuates the anxiety which helps mask the desire for financial gain."

Again, although these two neuroses are different, Kamman points out that there is no clear-cut dividing line between them: "We should recognize the existence of a spectrum between these two absolutes." He points out that it is "one of the most difficult medico-legal tasks to determine how much of the post-accident syndrome is due to traumatic neurosis (narcissistic regression) and how much to compensation neurosis (fore-conscious or unconscious desire for money)." I doubt if any lawyers or doctors ever really managed to do so, but in the end it did not matter anyway because both neuroses were perceived as beyond the voluntary control of the plaintiff, so both entitled the plaintiff to compensation.

For a discipline aspiring to be scientific, psychiatry found traumatic and compensation neuroses an embarrassment. In 1980, with the publication of *DSM-III*, the American Psychiatric Association tidied up these neuroses into their well-defined components:[10]

- *Brain injury:* actual physical injury to the substance of the brain;
- *Post-traumatic stress disorder* (PTSD): the effects, physical and mental, of the psychological horror of the accident;
- *Somatoform disorders:* the symptoms are ostensibly attributed to the accident, but are in fact generated unconsciously as an expression of ongoing psychological distress;
- *Malingering:* the patient intentionally exploits the accident for the purpose of financial or other consciously perceived gains.

Commendable as this housekeeping was, it had the unfortunate effect of providing yet more diagnoses for physicians to make and more disorders from which accident victims could suffer – and suffer they did ... though not, of course, from "malingering."

Arguments about compensation neurosis continue, but they now take place within the format of the *DSM*. Are the symptoms intentionally or unconsciously produced? Is the plaintiff malingering or does he have a somatoform disorder? Although the terms have changed, the obfuscation surrounding these diagnoses persists; indeed, it is most carefully nurtured. Many authors have jumped into the fray.[11]

Foster Kennedy reported the effects of the different compensation packages paid by Denmark and Germany to their injured workers prior World War II. Germany paid ongoing compensation while Denmark provided a lump sum that could not be followed by further benefit. In Germany 95 per cent of injured workers remained sick, while in Denmark, a mere 30 miles away across the border, 93 per cent of Danes recovered from what in Britain would have been known as "traumatic neurosis."[12] Kennedy's famous description of a compensation neurosis is a veritable Satan's credo to plaintiff lawyers and their experts: "A compensation neurosis is a state of mind, born out of fear, kept alive by avarice, stimulated by lawyers, and cured by a verdict.[13] A great deal of energy still goes into gainsaying Kennedy's famous observation.

Other authors have also pointed out the effects of compensation on accident rates and disability. In Britain, the Workman's Compensation Act of 1906 substantially increased employers' financial responsibility for employee's injuries. It also increased the number of industrial accidents. In the six years following the Act, the number of reported accidents rose 44 per cent, from 326,701 to 472,408, despite the fact that the number of people at work remained the same.[14]

Some years back, Sweden's welfare state was the envy of the world. A sick Swede received 96 per cent of his earnings. But, despite Sweden's excellent and universally available medical services dedicated to keeping Swedes well, it was not long before there were huge numbers of sick Swedes. Sweden's medical absenteeism rate was by far the highest in the world. Out of financial necessity, Sweden reduced sickness benefits to 65 per cent of earnings and its absenteeism rate sharply dropped.[15]

Although on a smaller scale, financial incentives work much the same way with whiplash. Earlier I pointed that the Australian province of Victoria, while having similar rates of rear-end collisions to New Zealand, had eight times the number of whiplash claims (chapter 3). Because of its high rate whiplash claims, the Victoria government changed its auto insurance law in 1987 so that a would-be claimant had to report the accident to the police and also bear the first A$317 of the medical expenses himself. Two years later, despite an increase in traffic density, whiplash claims had fallen by 68 per cent.[16] Awerbuch, the Australian rheumatologist, comments that there are no data to support the notion that the non-claimants nevertheless had whiplash symptoms.[17]

Numerous authors have commented on the deleterious effect on people's actual health of paying them to be sick. "No stratagem could have been developed with greater bias against a person's getting well than the system which so generously awards a person for staying sick."[18] To Eugene Bleuler, continuing to be sick under such circumstances is normal behaviour. Indeed, Bleuler suggests that a person who does *not* claim for persistent symptoms after a compensable injury may well have had an unrecognized brain injury that has affected his judgment.[19]

Subsequently, numerous studies and observations have also widely confirmed the detrimental effects of compensation upon disability rates. Patients receiving compensation do less well in rehabilitation programs, have poorer response to treatment, and, in general, recover less quickly.[20]

The issue of the relationship between settlement and recovery has been a particular bone of contention. Henry Miller, the lawyers' bugbear, took the position that after settlement claimants recover and return to work, while Mendelson, an Australian psychiatrist, advances the position that settlement does not affect recovery; that the plaintiff is *Not Cured by a Verdict*.[21]

Australian, British, and North American plaintiff expert psychiatrists quote Mendelson's views as incontrovertible evidence that the plaintiff will never recover after settlement and so will require enough compensation to last his lifetime. A corollary to Mendelson's contention is the argument that, since the symptoms do not disappear after settlement, the desire for compensation cannot have been their cause in the first place.[22]

Despite the overwhelming straightforward evidence that compensation promotes disability, ingenious arguments to the contrary are unendingly produced. A recent English whiplash study nicely demonstrates how the obvious explanation that compensation promotes whiplash claims is denied, and implausible explanations are offered in its stead.

Professor C.S. Galasko and his colleagues at the Department of Orthopaedic Surgery, University of Manchester, England, studied the increasing incidence of traffic-accident patients attending emergency departments with neck sprains, at various intervals from 1982 to 1990.[23] During these eight years the percentage of neck sprains compared to other road traffic accidents rose from 7.7 per cent to 45.5 per cent. How did the authors explain this "relentlessly increasing epidemic"? By "poor driving habits or/and changes in traffic patterns." But could these two factors really account for an almost six-fold increase in the number of people visiting the emergency department with neck sprain? There was no remarkable increase in the number of cars on the English roads over this eight-year period, and there is no evidence that English driving habits had taken an appreciable turn for the worse.

The obvious reason for this dramatic increase in the number of neck sprain patients attending the emergency department is that during these years the whiplash epidemic was spreading throughout Britain. The English became whiplash-sophisticated; by 1990 anyone involved in a collision knew of the need to register the accident before submitting an insurance claim. The authors, however, dismiss this simple explanation on the grounds that the patients surveyed denied it. Of the 389 whiplash patients seen in the year 1990, only 0.36 per cent stated they had attended the emergency department for "insurance reasons." But what patients say and what they do are by no means the same. At the 24-month follow up, 49 of these 389 patients had settled an insurance claim, while 230 patients still had a claim pending. What prospective whiplash claimant would be stupid enough to admit the real reason for visiting the emergency department? Are these surgeons really soft-headed enough to believe that the English are so soft-headed?

In the face of massive evidence to the contrary, whiplash interest groups around the world (Ontario, Switzerland, England, and Australia), still maintain that whiplash symptoms are directly caused by injury due to the accident and have little or no relationship with compensation. They mutually reference each other's work in support of the position that whiplash claimants are wronged and misunderstood victims.

Shapiro and Roth (University of Western Ontario) write: "Media stereotypes depict the patient with whiplash limping into the courtroom, attired in cervical collar and grimacing in pain. At the conclusion of the proceedings, the plaintiff wins a large settlement, casts off the collar, and lives a healthy, wealthy, and pain-free life. This common misconception, shared by most laypersons, has its counterpart in the scientific community, where it is known by the pejorative term *compensation neurosis.* "[24]

Mayou (England) and Radanov (Switzerland) teamed up to refute the position that compensation worsens whiplash symptoms: "It had frequently been alleged that psychological factors and social variables (especially the influence of possible compensation) are major causes of persistent physical complaints and disability."[25] They quote Barnsley, Lord, and Bogduk (Australia) in support of the position that whiplash symptoms are due to physical injury: "Between 14 per cent and 42 per cent of patients with whiplash injuries will develop chronic neck pain and that approximately 10 per cent will have constant pain indefinitely.[26]"

In turn, Bogduk[27] (Australia) quotes Shapiro and Roth[28] (Ontario) in support of his position that whiplash pain is physical in origin and that patients continue to suffer pain long after settlement. Bogduk cites the Radanov (Switzerland) position that whiplash patients have normal personalities, to support his contention that whiplash pain is not psychogenic but is caused by injury to the zygapophyseal joints.[29]

Merskey (Ontario) references Mendelson (Australia) and writes in relation to whiplash: "Even the bare facts indicate that compensation is rarely a sufficient cause of continued complaints of chronic pain."[30] Merskey quotes the extremely dubious findings by Radanov et al (Switzerland) that continuing whiplash pain is related to the severity of the initial injury. Merskey comments: "Many seemingly trivial collisions with little damage to vehicles can cause greater damage to people." In turn, Radanov (Switzerland) supports Merskey's position: "These results highlight that patients' psychological problems are rather a consequence than a cause of somatic symptoms of whiplash."[31]

Barnsley, Lord, and Bogduk (Australia) take the same position: "There is no real evidence, therefore, that either malingering for financial gain or pre-existing psycho-social factors contribute in any significant way to the natural history of whiplash injury. The unavoidable conclusion is that the overwhelming majority of whiplash injuries result in organic damage."[32]

Harth and Teasell (Ontario), referencing Bogduk (Australia) write: "It is hard to deny in the light of [this] evidence that injuries to the zygapophyseal joints are an important cause of the chronic whiplash syndrome, and account for half to two-thirds of the cases."[33] Moldofsky (Ontario), one of the progenitors of fibromyalgia and an advocate of its application to whiplash pain, cites Mendelson (Australia) in support of his statement that "litigants do not complain more that non-litigants."[34]

Finally, Wallis, Lord, and Barnsley (Australia) dismiss and ignore all the results of the formal studies of the effects of litigation and compensation on the perpetuation of symptoms: "The argument for compensation neurosis is based only on single cases or anecdotal evidence and is unsupported by any valid epidemiological or sociological studies. Indeed, formal studies and reviews have shown that financial compensation does not effect a cure and that despite settlement, a substantial proportion of patients suffers persistent pain and distress."[35]

This self-reinforcing loop of whiplash misconception provides the supposedly scientific basis on which ubiquitous whiplash clinics justify their interminable treatment of alleged whiplash injury. A patient whom for purposes of anonymity I shall call Mr W provides a routine example of just how profitable these ongoing treatments can be. Mr W's case finally settled at the time of writing this chapter. He had been a patient at a nearby whiplash clinic.

Mr W, a taxi driver, was rear-ended in 1990 while sitting in a stationary taxi; no objective evidence is available to substantiate an injury sustained in this accident. However, Mr W subsequently complained of ongoing headaches, neck and back pain, along with a TMJ disorder. He had been in two previous small motor vehicle accidents both of which were followed by a prolonged absence from work.

Mr W denied having had any significant problems after the two previous accidents or having any other health problems. He refused ophthalmoscopic examination of the eyes on the pretext that the bright light of the ophthalmoscope made his headache worse. Even an extremely experienced Toronto neurologist had overlooked Mr W's cataracts, which were impeding his ability to drive and therefore earn a living.

Three surgeons examined Mr W and found no significant signs of neck injury. Nevertheless, a whiplash clinic provided Mr W with extensive treatment for neck injury. In his ten-inch-thick medico-legal brief there was a signed mimeographed form from the clinic stating:

The above patient is being treated for injuries sustained in a motor vehicle accident.

It is my professional opinion that the above patient requires a series of occipital steroid blocks as part of his/her medically necessary treatment. These blocks involve injections into several different locations at the base of the skull. Each treatment requires the use of large amounts of local anaesthetic. The blocks cause distension of the tissue, and make each treatment an extremely painful process for the patient.

The patient feels that the occipital steroid block would be very difficult to tolerate without some form of anaesthesia.

Please be advised that I am therefore going to proceed with the performance of the above-noted procedure under [general] anaesthesia, as is our practice with a large proportion of our patients.

Between 1992 and 1994, Mr W received 85 injections, each requiring a general anaesthetic. The average cost of each treatment was about $400.

The whiplash clinic was by no means the only healthcare facility to profit from Mr W's supposedly injured neck. The Ontario Health Insurance Plan records show that payments were made to at least 67 practitioners, some of whom also provided extensive services to him. The cost of the taxicab fares required to take Mr W to his various medical appointments alone amounted to over $60,000. Despite all this treatment, Mr W continued to complain vehemently of neck pain and was still doing so when his case came up for settlement in 1998. Although Mr W's cataracts have been removed and his vision is now normal, he has become so entrenched in his invalid lifestyle that he will probably join the many other whiplash litigants who do not return to work after settlement. Since the settlement (after the lawyers have had their fill) is seldom sufficient to provide long-term support for such claimants, they inevitably become dependent upon the state. Mr W will no doubt live out an impoverished life on a rather ungenerous Canada Pension benefit.

A letter to the *Medical Journal of Australia* from Rob McMurdo, a family doctor from Greenwich, New South Wales, asks the apposite questions: "The financial reward of the compensation system is less of a gamble for the medical and legal professions than for the patient/claimant. Why do some doctors continue active therapy when they state there is no detectable disability? Why do solicitors foster and encourage disability and delay return to work?"[36]

PART FOUR

Treating the Treatment

22

Making Victims of Ourselves

Will 1995 be the year of the Universal Suing? Policemen, I read,
are resorting to the courts because of the state of their nerves after horrid
things they have seen at football matches; and a lot of soldiers want
compensation because they have discovered that war is beastly.
Oh, sceptred isle set in the polluted sea, where are we heading?
– Alec Guinness[1]
When you encourage a man to see himself as victim of anything –
crime, poverty, bigotry, bad luck – you are piling bricks on his chest.
– David Gelernter, *Drawing Life: Surviving the Unabomber*[2]

The alacrity with which we now seek to turn ourselves into victims
has made victimhood a contemporary epidemic. *Time* magazine
writes that the United States has become "a nation of finger pointers" and that "twin malformations are cropping up in the American
character: a nasty intolerance and a desire to blame everyone else
for everything." Cry-babies pronounce themselves victims of anything from the Universe down. "The cry-baby is the abject, manipulative little devil with the lawyer and, so to speak, the actionable dia-
per rash ... Victims become addicted to being victims: they derive
identity, innocence and a kind of devious power from sheer, default-
ing helplessness."[3]

We have looked at the financial rewards of victimhood, but the
incentives are often less clear and sometimes incomprehensible. Some
people are incorrigible victims who exalt in their ill-used status.
George Cruickshank, a nineteenth-century English cartoonist, rev-
elled in attacking both quacks and their determined victims. His car-
toon, set in front of the Royal College of Physicians in London, immortalizes the triumphal satisfaction of duped patients as Dr Fox with his
universal vegetable pills leads them goose-stepping to their doom (Fig.
22–1). There is an intractable streak of gullibility in the human soul.

Victimhood can bring much gratification. Real or imagined it serves
a multiplicity of social functions. The commiseration with other self-
proclaimed victims can bind families and communities together.
Victimhood justifies any amount of bad behaviour; it permits unrestrained indulgence of anger at the alleged perpetrator of the real or
imagined wrong.

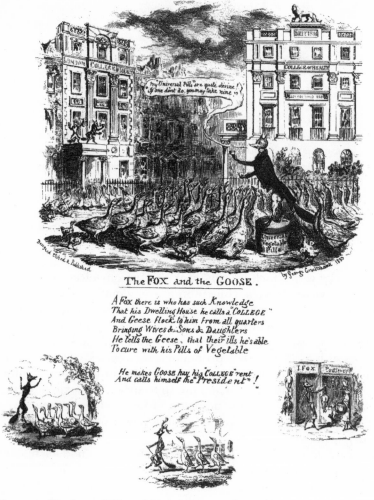

The FOX and the GOOSE .

A Fox there is who has such Knowledge
That his Dwelling House he calls a COLLEGE "
And Geese flock to him from all quarters
Bringing Wives &... Sons & Daughters
He tells the Geese , that their ills he's able
To cure with his Pills of Vegetable

He makes GOOSE hay his COLLEGE "rent
And calls himself the "President" !

Fig. 22–1   The foxes of this world are always sure of a meal

Robert Hughes, in his bestseller *The Culture of Complaint*, writes that the all-pervasive claim to victimhood tops off America's long-cherished culture of therapeutics. To seem strong may only conceal a rickety scaffolding of denial, but to be vulnerable is to be invincible. Complaint gives you power – even when it's only the power of emotional bribery, or of creating previously unnoticed levels of social guilt.[4] Any explanations as to why a person opts to become a victim of a copycat illness – fashionable or occupational – are necessarily speculative, but it is perhaps possible to speculate intelligently. The exigencies of illness can give power and control; sickness compensates for a lack of social clout. Disgruntled workers and soldiers use illness to demonstrate their discontent. In the competitive politics of family and society, sickness is a winning card. The needs of sickness are imperative. Sickness gains attention; often the sick member of the family hogs it all. The sick person is in control. Florence Nightingale, "the patron saint of ME" and hailed as its first and most distinguished victim, from her sickbed had the power to successfully overcome male resistance to the much overdue reform of the medical services in the British army.

I have repeatedly emphasized the disproportionate numbers of women who develop fashionable illnesses. I am not misogynistically picking on women and I wish to make the point that men have picked on women. The Western world may be shocked by the way that the Taliban treat women, but until the coming of the *scientific* age the ways in which members of Christendom treated *their* women were certainly no better and sometimes worse.[5] For millennia patriarchal Western civilization has exploited, belittled, abused, and disempowered women, a collective bullying that had grave consequences for women's health. Actually, even the coming of the *scientific* age only slowly improved women's lot. To bolster their gender superiority, secular and insecure patriarchs merely substituted the authority of *science* for the authority of the Bible. While Thomas Aquinas had perceived women as "misbegotten men," Freud and his followers perceived her as "castrated male," a lesser man, who lacking the phallic addendum, was destined to a life of "passivity."[6] The developmental task of girls was to adjust appropriately to the painful realization of their dependent social status.

Nineteenth-century craniometrists measured the size of human skulls and, after much dickering with the figures, established that a woman's small brain justified the male dominance over her.[7] Gustave LeBon, a highly influential psychologist and the acknowledged founder of social psychology, wrote in 1879 of the female brain:

There are a large number of women whose brains are closer to those of gorillas than to the most developed male brains. This inferiority is so obvious that no one can contest it for a moment; only its degree is worth discussion. All psychologists who have studied the intelligence of women, as well as poets and novelists, recognize today that they represent the most inferior forms of human evolution and that they are closer to children and savages than to an adult, civilized man ... Without doubt there exist some distinguished women, very superior to the average man, but they are as exceptional as the birth of any monstrosity, as, for example, of a gorilla with two heads; consequently, we may neglect them entirely.[8]

Sociobiology, the latest biological movement for the understanding of behaviour, perceives "woman as the lesser man," physically weak and genetically programmed to be passive and dependent.[9]

Disempowered women are inevitably dependent upon men and, in an odd way, men become dependent upon women to do their chores and to massage their artificially inflated egos. Neediness and dependency easily slip us into the role of victim or victimizer. The victim entices a rescuer to provide the wanted care and protection, and the rescuer has the gratification of helping someone yet more vulnerable than himself. Co-dependent relationships are fraught with pitfalls, and it is always difficult to disentangle who is doing what to whom.

A traditional marriage may be skewed by co-dependency but professional relationships, whether between priest and parishioner, lawyer and client, or doctor and patient are often just as bad and sometimes worse. The troubled person hands over his uncomfortable problems to a trusted saviour. Such trust is extolled as a virtue, but the helper, of whatever calling, easily slips into the exploitation of the needy person's helplessness. Few human interactions are as vulnerable to psychopathology. Co-dependency presents a huge barrier to constructive and adult relationship.

Disempowered Victorian women, as we have seen, manipulated their world with neurasthenia. In their invalided state, they required supervision, and helping professionals, along with fathers and husbands, were quick to offer their services and advice. In the 1890s, when women began riding bicycles, doctors and ministers of religions became frantic. It was a subject "much 'cussed' and discussed."[10] Perennially concerned with women's delicate physique and the possible impropriety in sexual behaviour, they feared that unregulated bicycle-riding would lead to moral and physical decline.[11] Bicycles were a ride to freedom and women's many professional advisers did what they could to curtail it. Even James Prendergast, an American gynaecologist who argued that the exercise of riding was beneficial to women warned that bicycle-riding could, "at times, [give rise] to friction and heating of the parts where it is very undesirable and may lead to dangerous practices," though he went on to comment that this danger was not nearly so great as the laity believed.[12] In the *Georgia Journal of Medicine and Surgery,* a doctor complained that young girls learn to masturbate on the saddle. He gave the example of Miss M, "a strong, healthy country girl" who purchased a bicycle. "The bloom of youth faded from her former rosy cheeks, and her health failed." After numerous visits to the doctor and the administration of various tonics the truth about the bicycle came to light. "In her rides on the wheel, it was no uncommon thing for her to experience a sexual orgasm three or four times on a ride of one hour." On the doctor's advice she gave up the wheel and "without further use of medicines the young lady rapidly regained her health."[13] An English vicar warned that on no account must the saddle be tilted upwards.[14]

Apart from a concern that these "bifurcated bloomers" might surreptitiously self-abuse on the saddle, doctors worried that the jarring and jolting would cause spinal shock and fatigue; they doubted that the female physique could tolerate such strenuous activity. Besides causing moral ugliness, bicycling caused physical ugliness as well. Too much cycling could cause *bicycle face*, with its strained expression, projecting jaw, and "general focusing of all the features towards the centre, a sort of physiognomic implosion."[15] In a ten-part report on cycling in the *British Medical Journal* of 1896, E.B. Turner, an English surgeon, warned that no woman should cycle before acquiring a certificate from her doctor stipulating that she was fit to do so.[16]

It was imperative for their own well-being that women, and especially women from the middle classes, know their place in life. They were raised to be obedient, pleasing and feeble. Lydia Becker, a leader of suffrage struggles of nineteenth-century England, captured their predicament: "*A great lady* or a factory woman are independent persons – personages – the women of the middle classes, are *nobodies*, and if they act for themselves they lose caste!"[17] Writing in the mid-1950s, Annie Reich, a distinguished New York psychoanalyst, remarked that a woman's self-esteem was often equated with her complete annihilation.[18] Virtually all the words for women are words containing the root word men, and that "in culture and language, women under patriarchy were erased."[19] And *nobodies* women were. As late as 1929, the Supreme Court of Canada ruled that women were not *persons* within the meaning of the British North American Act.[20]

There is wide recognition that historically women have channelled their resentment into illness. Ellen Showalter speculates in *The Female Malady* that the physical symptoms of fashionable illnesses are, in body language terms, a desperate, and ultimately self-destructive, rebellion against patriarchal oppression.[21] Robert Bly, the American poet and author of *Iron John*, well known for his attempts to raise male consciousness, writes of women's anger and physical symptoms: "Women's anger is long-standing; it didn't begin flowing yesterday. And yet during the hundreds of years in which Western women were economically dependent on their husbands, anger had to be expressed primarily unconsciously through bodily diseases, hysteria, depression, and early death. The act of speaking anger could put a woman on the street."[22] Robert Woolsey, professor of neurology at St Louis University, perceives somatoform symptoms as a "protolanguage – a code used by [women] to communicate a message which, for various reasons, cannot be verbalized."[23]

When the possibility of straightforward negotiation of wants and needs is blocked, manipulation inevitably becomes its substitute. Once a language is learned it is not easily unlearned, especially when it is one that seems to work. Being a victim of circumstances or of illness can be a rewarding form of manipulation. It would indeed be out of keeping with human behaviour if women, finding themselves blocked in a one-down situation, did *not* use helplessness or a fashionable illness to get what they want.

Pregnancy can be another example of the manipulative powers of victimhood. The knowledge and means of contraception are widely available in all developed countries, yet social services are overburdened with a seeming epidemic of teenage pregnancies, and women who are dissatisfied with their lives are more likely to have unprotected sexual intercourse. A study from the University of Surrey examined the secondary gains obtainable from the victimhood of "unplanned pregnancies." The authors divided subjects from a North London family practice into three groups: women with planned pregnancies, those with unplanned pregnancies, and non-pregnant women. The women with unplanned pregnancies were significantly more likely to benefit from the secondary gains provided by motherhood than were women with planned pregnancies or non-pregnant women. Escape from the labour market, cementing a precarious relationship, and a passport to better housing were among the secondary gains made accessible through the victim status of an unplanned pregnancy.[24]

Childhood sexual abuse, real or imagined, is a quick ticket to victimhood. Undoubtedly, sexual abuse, along with physical, emotional, and mental abuse and neglect, and unrelenting parental control, are all cruelties we commonly impose upon our children. However, the legitimacy of singling out sexual abuse from all the other adversities of childhood as the central cause of widespread and long-lasting suffering is less certain.[25] Children dread rejection and the psychological scars left by real or imagined abandonment blight many people's lives. Rejection carries with it the deep shame of feeling unlovable. It is perhaps less painful for an adult to blame his psychological difficulties on childhood sexual abuse than on the humiliation of being unwanted. He was at least a wanted child – if only sexually.

Difficulties previously attributed to self-abuse are now attributed to sexual abuse inflicted by others. In the early 1980s, when childhood sexual abuse became a possible route to victimhood, any would-be victims were served up an easy explanation for their problems and, into the bargain, a perpetrator to hold responsible for them.

Psychologists quickly published an orgy of books linking childhood sexual abuse to adult problems.[26] Many American states removed statutes of limitations making it possible for adult children to sue for decades-old alleged sexual abuse, and insurance companies paid out hundreds of millions of dollars for the treatment of adults alleging such abuse.[27] As with whiplash, healthcare professionals and lawyers soon turned sexual abuse into a flourishing industry, leaving in their wake many thousands of distraught women and fractured families.[28] Margaret Hagen, a well-known American psychologist, likens the scientific basis for such abuse claims to astrology. She cites cogent examples of the evidence presented by self-serving healthcare practitioners under the guise of science, examples so appalling that they make even *Whores of the Court*, the title of her book, an egregious slur on the world's oldest profession.[29]

An initial problem for healthcare practitioners poised to exploit the effects of childhood sexual abuse were the relatively small numbers of adults who remembered any actual incident of abuse; this obstacle was quickly surmounted by the claim that all such memories are repressed. If a woman has problems, then childhood sexual abuse should, it is claimed, be suspected. Susan Blume, a self-appointed expert on the effects of childhood sexual abuse, provides a checklist of thirty-four common human difficulties and suggests that if these are present then incest may be their cause.[30] In *Secret Survivors: Uncovering Incest and Its After-effects in Women*, she reports that unremembered sexual abuse is the most common reason why women seek psychological treatment. She notes that these women are often mislabelled as "promiscuous, disturbed, psychotic, borderline, or suffering from a chemical imbalance."[31]

Psychologists encouraged unhappy women to enter therapy and work at recalling memories of their abuse.[32] Ellen Bass and Laura Davies's book *The Courage to Heal: A Guide for Women Survivors of Child Sexual Abuse* has sold over 800,000 copies. It promises: "If you are willing to work hard you cannot only heal but thrive."[33] According to their thesis, the more memories recalled, the greater the healing. These therapists encourage their patients to become incompetent victims, insisting that "the courageous act of recovering memories of sexual abuse" is so traumatic that inevitably few women can expect to continue their normal lives during the course of therapy.[34]

Thousands of therapists set to work, some with the use of hypnosis, to help their clients recover memories. They came up trumps –

horrendous memories of sexual abuse were recovered. Into the bargain, the therapists discovered that some of their clients, unable to absorb their distressing sexual experiences, had severed the material from consciousness and in the process developed multiple personalities, or *alters*. "These split-off alters then conspire with the victims of sexual abuse in the denial of their painful secrets."[35] While some of the recalled "painful secrets" may be genuine enough, most are certainly not; there are just too many alters and too many horrific memories to be credible.

Here is Bass and Davies's example of a woman who developed "multiples," a middle-aged academic with a doctorate in biological chemistry from Yale University. She recalled that her seemingly normal parents were associated with a ring of criminals for profit, she was forced to torture animals in kindergarten and was made to stick a knife in a baby, the children in her school were auctioned off to buyers who immediately tortured and sexually abused them, one girl was killed, stripped of her polka-dot dress, and her dead body dumped in a field.[36]

With this sort of case history template, women all over the Bible belt of North America soon remembered being forced to participate in satanic rituals, seeing children dismembered, boiled and burned.[37] In 1986 therapists at an international conference in Chicago reported that 25 per cent of their patients with multiple personality disorder recalled memories of being raped with crucifixes, forced to kill and eat babies, and, as adolescents, forced to become serial breeders of babies for use in ritual sacrifices. Psychologists held more conferences on child abuse, and the reported cases multiplied.[38]

A 1991 survey of members of the American Psychological Association found that 12 per cent of the members had treated adults who claimed to be the victims of satanic ritual abuse. Some psychologists had treated dozens of such cases. The majority of respondents reported that they believed their patients' stories were true.[39]

Bass and Davies, along with the other writers on recovered memories, took the position that, after recovering the memories of abuse women would start feeling better and increase their self-esteem. But do they? A woman remembers that her father had touched her in the bath, but there is no improvement. Obviously more memories lie hidden and more therapeutic exploration is required. Then comes a memory of father forcing intercourse upon her, but still no improvement in self-esteem. A few more months of work and the woman recalls she had her father's baby – still no improvement in self-esteem. Then comes the memory that she was forced to kill, dismember, and eat the baby. Memories flood back of her being forced to masturbate in public with a crucifix and having to drink urine or blood and eat faeces.[40] Damn it, even after years of work with her therapist on recovering all these memories, the woman still feels no better, and her self-esteem is worse than ever! Treatments, as you must know by now, are often counter-productive.

Inspired by these recalled memories, concerns grew about the widespread presence of ritual satanic abuse in the community at large. Therapists hypothesized that underground satanic cults had existed for centuries, but that just as individuals had turned a blind eye to sexual abuse of children so had society ignored the widespread presence of ritual satanic abuse.[41] It was ignored no more. Charges of such abuse were laid against suspected individuals and organizations. In 1983, California, with its gift for drama, produced the McMartin preschool case, the best known of the many allegations of satanic ritual abuse.

Fashionable illnesses spread. Memories of ritual satanic abuse were soon recovered in European and other countries, and allegations of such abuse became widespread.[42] In Canada and Britain police investigations continued for years. In the peaceful Orkneys, remote islands off the coast of Scotland, nine children were removed from their homes when a villager reported strange practices by Jews and Quakers, and the children reported satanic rites performed by people dressed as Ninja Turtles.[43]

While the accusations grew more fantastic, the objective evidence for any such rituals remained non-existent. Seven years and $15 million later the charges were dismissed in the McMartin case for lack of evidence.[44] After a £6 million inquiry, the charges against the Orkney Jews and the Quakers were dismissed, with the judge criticizing the social workers involved for their use of suggestive questions.[45] The FBI has now studied 300 satanic ritual abuse allegations but found no evidence to corroborate them.[46]

In Canada, extensive investigations by the RCMP have not produced one shred of evidence that organized satanic abuse exists.[47] Jean La Fontaine, professor of social anthropology at the London School of Economics, in a three-year inquiry conducted for the British government, investigated another 84 cases of alleged ritual abuse; she found no evidence of its occurrence.[48] In the British case, the epidemic was clearly set off by enthusiastic therapists, social workers armed with sexually equipped dolls, children's sexually active imaginations, all helped along by popular films and TV shows. Of course, the children in the end did get abused. Social workers removed them from the security of home and, in an effort to substantiate their stories, over-zealous police doctors performed vaginal and rectal examinations on them.

Insightfully, a decade or so before recovered memories of sexual abuse became fashionable, Michel Foucault, in his *History of Sexuality*, had suggested that the perversity of sexual abuse lies more with the inquisitorial investigators than with the subjects of the abuse.[49]

Multiple personality disorder (MPD) is "the presence of two or more distinct identities or *personality states* that recurrently take control of [a person's] behaviour."[50] The disorder was once a rare oddity and before 1980 only about 200 cases had been reported in the medical literature, most of which were linked to spiritualism and incarnation.[51] Then in 1973 a New York psychotherapist published an account of 2,534 hours of psychotherapy with a woman with multiple personalities. The story of Sybil hit the world. Sybil was allegedly sexually abused as a child, though in this instance by her mother. The story of her sixteen alters became a best selling-novel and was later made into the famous film.[52] Minds began to come apart.

When the International Society for the Study of Multiple Personality Disorder and Dissociation was founded in 1982, Multiple Personality Disorder, or, as the *DSM-IV* now lists it, Dissociative Identity Disorder (DID), had arrived.[53] In the early 1990s, Colin Ross, the Canadian psychiatrist and president of the International Society for the Study of Multiple Personality Disorder, estimated that one per cent of the population of the United States (over two million Americans) met the *DSM* criteria for the diagnosis of DID.[54] As with most other epidemics of fashionable illnesses, the cases occurred in the areas in which the doctors or other therapists who treated and wrote about the condition were located.

Healthcare practitioners were the principal vectors of the epidemic. A social worker who had worked with satanic abuse victims at a rape crisis centre in a Southern Illinois University moved to Britain and organized a conference on child abuse at Reading University, spreading theories about child abuse among British social workers.[55] Again, as with other fashionable illnesses, it is argued that the symptoms must be genuine, for how else would all the cases have such similar complaints. Healthcare practitioners are remarkably obtuse to the fact that patients develop the diseases and symptoms in which the practitioner shows interest.

The numbers of alters were at first small. Dr Jekyll had only Mr Hyde; Eve, with her three faces, had just two. Following Sybil's publicity, double digit numbers of alters became common, even occasionally stretching to three digits. Not only were more North Americans splitting, they were splitting into smaller pieces. As in many other fashionable disorders, women were in the lead. The *DSM-IV* notes that the disorder is three to nine times more frequently diagnosed in women and that "females tend to have more identities than do males, averaging fifteen or more, whereas males average [only a measly] eight identities."[56]

For people who want victim status, but who are bereft of molesting relatives, cannot recall any childhood sexual trauma, or failed to be delivered up by their parents to satanic abuse, there remains the possibility of alien abduction.[57] Although aliens are reported to abduct earthlings to impart spiritual wisdom to them, these abductors seem not averse to some sexual interference as well.

Barney and Betty Hill were the first to be taken. Their abduction occurred in 1966 at a time of intense public interest in UFOs. They were driving through the White Mountains of New Hampshire when they fell into the hands of aliens. Subsequently, the Hills also fell into the hands of a psychiatrist who examined them under hypnosis. As every member of the public suspects, psychiatrists see the world in terms of sex, and this psychiatrist ran true to form. The couple recalled that, once on board the spaceship, the aliens took a sperm sample from Barney and examined Betty for pregnancy.[58] Following the Hills's excursion into space, reports of aliens taking humans onto spaceships came thick and fast. Like the Hills, all the alleged abductees lost their memories and required hypnosis to recall the sexual things that the aliens had done to them. Characteristically, the aliens come at night, usually in a spaceship. They are bathed in light and can walk though walls. The aliens supposedly do gynaecological examinations on women and use attractive females to collect sperm specimens from males.[59]

In the United States, in the fifteen years between 1975 and 1990, the number of practitioners involved in mental health increased from 72,000 to 198,000 thousand, the biggest jump being in social workers who went from 25,000 to 80,000.[60] Like work-hungry lawyers, social workers and other mental health practitioners needed work. It came. Susan Blume: "Most survivors [of sexual abuse] need many years, and often many therapists, before they can face the truths of their past."[61] With vast numbers of women needing help recalling their forgotten sexual abuse, patching together their numerous alters, and dealing with the shock of abduction by aliens, sexual abuse therapists are kept gainfully employed. It apparently takes several years to identify all the alters and assign them names, and even longer to fuse all these alters together into one patient.

Tana Dineen, the Canadian psychologist author of *Manufacturing Victims*, adds another dimension: "Whereas the medical profession had been unwilling to acknowledge the expertise of non-medical and untrained psychologists, lawyers were eager to find 'experts' who could be employed to support their clients' cases."[62] However, the charges of satanic murder were singularly unsuccessful in court because, without a body, it is difficult to get a conviction and, dig as they might, the police could find no bodies. Allegations of sexual abuse were another matter. With the junk science of "memory recall" lawyers were in their element. On the strength of "recovered memories" often obtained through hypnosis, many men, especially fathers, were sent to jail.[63] More profitably, lawyers initiated civil suits for the lifelong psychological damage the accused had inflicted upon their daughters.

Over the last few years I have seen many people who claim to have PTSD on account of small collisions, but I have seen only one person who actually had it. He was a man who, while going through an acrimonious divorce, was unexpectedly arrested on a charge of sexually abusing his daughter some fifteen years previously. He had been held in jail where he was threatened and assaulted by the other inmates who took him for a paedophile. I have seldom seen anyone so bewildered and frightened. The courts eventually found that the charges against him were fabricated.

Of course, parents resented these out-of-the-blue sorts of accusations. The *memory wars* began. In the mid-1990s the adversaries of *recalled memory syndrome* organized to fight the accusations. Responsible medical associations in the United States, Canada, Britain, and Australia issued warnings about the unreliability and uncertain significance of recovered memories.[64]

Some healthcare practitioners began to have second thoughts. Lawyers again did well. They had more lawsuits. Parents now sued their children's therapists for the alienation from their children caused by the *false memories* they had elicited, and the adult children, having retracted their accusations, sued the therapists for loss of support from their resentful families. Not that the accusations are finished. In Ontario, lawyers use advertising posters and intensive letter campaigns to locate ex-pupils of residential schools and, it is alleged, offer them $50 in cash to make a sexual abuse claim: the lawyer will keep 25 per cent of any future settlement.[65] Lawyers are above the law and are never held responsible for the mischievous lawsuits they so enthusiastically whip up. The therapists, of course, claim they are victims of the system.[66]

Healthcare practitioners are "anxiety makers." We have undoubtedly caused our patients much harm with our unwarranted concerns, and never more so than when it comes to sex.[67] In Victorian times, the doctors' attribution of sickness to masturbation not only blighted many people's lives with the burden of guilt but it also helped spread sickness. Sanctioned against finding normal sexual relief by masturbation, men turned to prostitutes, making syphilis and gonorrhoea rampant in the community.

Just how harmful is our present day iatrogenically induced fixation on childhood sexuality? Adults, especially men, are easily frightened off from providing intimate care to their own and other people's children. Children are given a clear, if often unspoken message, that any sensual or sexual feelings for another person are unacceptable. Perhaps as a substitute for feelings of attraction, children concentrate on the outward manifestations of perfect "attractiveness" – weightlessness for girls and "macho" aggressive behaviour for boys. Nearly two in five American children are raised in homes without fathers, whose absence is strongly linked to two social nightmares: boys with guns and girls with babies.[68] Children are hungry for masculine attention but they are now less touched and hugged by male teachers, other guardians, or even their own fathers. With affection from *normal* men in short supply emotionally needy children are more likely to accept attention from paedophiles, and maybe affection from a paedophile is sometimes better than no affection at all.[69] Socially and iatrogenically induced "paedophobia" is probably not a sensible way to solve such pressing social problems.

Once it was women who were the victims of witch hunts, but perhaps in some ways they remain the victims. Ian Hacking, a professor of history at the University of Toronto, in his thoughtful book *Rewriting the Soul: Multiple Personality and the Sciences of Memory*, suggests that the current theories of abuse, trauma, and dissociation are part of another cycle of oppression of women, all the more dangerous because the theorists and clinicians represent themselves as being so entirely on the side of the "victim" – whom they thereby construct as helpless, rather than an autonomous human being."[70] Once professionals, be they priests, lawyers or doctors, have committed their integrity to a belief system upon which their livelihood depends, the process is difficult to halt.

It is also difficult to halt our propensity to set ourselves up as victims, since victimhood has many uses. Lawyers, often aided by psychologists and psychiatrists, lose no time in helping clients to exploit illness. Multiple personality disorder quickly became an ingenious explanation for undesirable behaviours. A man, charged with leaving a string of murdered women on a hillside, claimed he had MPD: it was not he but one of his alters who was responsible for the killings.[71] A Wisconsin man, having had sexual intercourse with a women with 21 alters was charged with sexual assault; three of the alters had apparently not given consent. By the time of the trial, the medical experts claimed that her alters had increased to 46, giving her even more dissenters to the intercourse.[72] Clearly this sort of group sex is best avoided.

Fashionable illnesses have much in common with the factitious disorders. Both conditions are a solicitation for emotional sustenance. Feldman and Ford write: "Studies of prevalence consistently show that many factitial patients work in healthcare settings, holding jobs as nurses, physical therapists, and nurses' aides. It is thought that their jobs as caregivers may be so emotionally draining that they begin to feel a desperate need for nurturance and use illness as a way of getting it."[73] In the American epidemic of neurasthenia, ten per cent of Beard's patients were physicians, and today both physicians and nurses are disproportionately represented amongst the victims of ME and CFS.[74]

Another incarnation of a fashionable illness in our times is the stress experienced by today's "supermums." Supermums are proverbial for the onerous expectations they place upon themselves. They struggle to dovetail their two or more roles – a struggle well observed by social commentators. Anson Rabinbach, in *The Body without Fatigue: A Nineteenth Century Utopia* suggests that fatigue and exhaustion are less the result of overwork than of the work ethic itself, the the drive to succeed.[75] Simon Wessely, the English psychiatrist interested in the fashionable disorders, characterizes supermums as perfectionists and overachievers. "One sufferer told the journalist that 'until my symptoms started I gave 120 per cent to every aspect of my life.' Sufferers 'work until they drop, whilst everyone else creeps to bed with the slightest headache or sniffle ... Lazy people don't get ME.' "[76]

John Balla, the Australian neurologist who described the "late whiplash syndrome," suggests that its development may correlate with discrepancies between a person's expectations and achievements.[77] People who, for whatever reason, feel they are a failure may adopt the sick role, frequently formulising the symptoms into a fashionable illness.[78]

The fact that many more women (at least in peacetime) become victims of fashionable illnesses has perplexed observers. Several possible explanations are proposed. Women take to patienthood more easily than do men. They make two-thirds of all visits to conventional physicians; and women (especially with a college education) are more likely than men to consult alternative practitioners.[79]

The freedoms that women have earned over the course of the last hundred years or so have come at a price. In addition to their jobs, women are still saddled with many undiminished responsibilities, the care and emotional sustenance of children, husband, and elderly relatives, and housework. Even helpful husbands seldom do anywhere near an equal share of either housework or parenting.[80] A recent Scandinavian study of catecholamine levels demonstrates the degree of stress to which career women are subjected.

Catecholamine is a breakdown product of adrenaline (epinephrine). High levels of catecholamine in urine indicate psychological stress, and the study shows a dramatic gender difference in these levels. In male managers returning home from work, the levels decrease rapidly; the levels in women who go home to a house full of family chores increase.[81]

Women still have a raw deal in our society. Despite years of discussion of equal pay for equal work, pay equity remains mostly a good intention. Able professional women bang their heads against the glass ceiling. By the very fact of being physically smaller, women are more easily bullied and abused. The prudent employment of a fashionable illness can help redress this social and biological imbalance. While a fashionable illness may do little to restore genuine self-esteem it does, at least, provide emotional and social leverage, and even a sense of purpose and camaraderie.

Sometimes the judicious use of a fashionable illness is the only practical way to juggle conflicting obligations. Titbits of statistical evidence indicate that women use the fashionable illnesses in this way. RSI increased in frequency in Australian mothers just before schools broke up for the summer vacation. The same happened in fruit pickers as the picking season drew to a close.[82]

Like Sisyphus, condemned forever to push a boulder up the hill only to have it roll down again, perhaps men and women, driven by disparate needs, are condemned to remain in perpetual struggle. Conflicting gender roles may always be a problem, but when it comes to whiplash and other such similar illnesses, problems with gender roles prove disastrous. Women patients are locked into the role of inadequate victims, while the patriarchal professions exploit their victim position.

Would-be victims have the "me-too syndrome" and are quick to adopt any hallmark of suffering; concentration camp survivors now serve as a role model. There are now incest survivors, chronic fatigue survivors, alien abduction survivors, Gulf war survivors, even psychiatric survivors (people who have survived treatment by a psychiatrist), and last, but not least, whiplash survivors. Unlike many of the victims of concentration camps, the thing that the new survivors have in common is that their victimhood, real or imagined, leaves them dejected, unproductive, and dysfunctional.

Victimizers and would-be-victims both lose some of their humanity, but while victimizers often flourish (at least in this world), would-be-victims, retaining a hurt and resentful stance towards the world, seldom do. Habitual victims get victimized. Much of this book is about the re-victimization of whiplash victims by the legal and helping professions. Victims of fashionable illnesses are not just geese ripe for exploitation by the purveyors of today's nostrums, they are sitting ducks for victimization; on one occasion, even literally so. A psychiatrist, Kenneth Olson, diagnosed a former nurse's aide as having a multiple personality disorder. He found she had 120 alters, one of which was a duck. Olson billed each alter for group psychotherapy, the total cost coming to $300,000.[83] One wag, noting that veterinarians' fees are now higher than those of physicians, suggested that Olsen should have charged more for the duck!

It is easy to feel morally superior about our victimhood, but to the reasonably impartial observer, it is often difficult to determine who exactly is the victim: the person with the fashionable illness, or the person or institution that is arbitrarily accused of being its cause and is therefore held morally and financially liable. We may no longer be possessed by demons, but fibromyalgia grabs us by the scruff of the neck. We no longer get hysterical paralysis so that we cannot walk, but we get such terrible chronic fatigue that we are too tired to do so anyway. Someone else has to look after us, we let ourselves off the hook.

"History is a parcel of party tricks played with the dead," and in the histories of individuals the tricks can be particularly ingenious. An inventive psychologist can always help a client to unearth explanations for ongoing disappointments with life. But for anyone who faces the future with vision and courage, the past, however awful it may have been, is accepted as the precious bedrock from which the child became a *person*. It is not so much the past that determines the future, but the future that determines the past. Death and taxes are assuredly not the only two certainties in life, for life and other people will undoubtedly do bad things to us. Societies developed spiritual ways to accept inevitable misfortunes gracefully. For Buddhists, adversities are Karma. God sends Muslims, Jews, and Christians trials by which to test them. However many boils and other tribulations God sent Job, he steadfastly refused to curse his maker. A Victorian Englishman, requiring amputation for a prolonged and painful tubercular arthritis of the foot, remained unbowed:

In the fell clutch of circumstance,
I have not winced or cried aloud:
Under the bludgeonings of chance
My head is bloody, but unbowed...
It matters not how strait the gate,
How charged with punishments the scroll,

I am the master of my fate:
I am the captain of my soul.[84]

Punitive gods and stiff-upper-lipped Englishmen are, perhaps thankfully, somewhat out of fashion. Nevertheless, we continue to live in a precarious world. It is risky going to work. It is risky having children. It is risky sending them to school. It is risky taking a new medicine to make us feel better or having surgery to make us look more beautiful. If we are bored on the weekend, we take to the dangerous roads for an outing. When the roads are made safer, we drive faster, intuitively calculating an acceptable level of risk. Life without risk becomes dull, and many of us find ways to make it more exciting. When something goes wrong, which it inevitably will, perhaps it is unreasonable to hold society or someone else totally responsible. I, for one, would prefer to live in a caring society, one that helps pick up the pieces when things go wrong. But is it really necessary always to make super-amends, especially when in doing so, much of the benefit goes to lawyers and healthcare practitioners?

One of the worst transgressions against good behaviour these days is to blame the victim for his own predicament. Victims scream that they are doubly abused. Nevertheless, victims are sometimes the authors of their own plight. A complicated interrelationship exists between victim and abuser. Surrendering one's status as victim means accepting responsibility for one's own faults and failures. Although I know of no controlled study to confirm that this is so, one of the more useful functions of psychotherapy is to help victims who are repeatedly trapped in abusive relationships to break their habit of always appearing hurt. Once a person gives up the victim role, he is much less likely to be victimized.

In the arena of fashionable illnesses, as in national politics, the insistence of victimhood has an uncanny knack of blocking creative solutions to pressing problems. Well-nursed grievances keep conflicts brewing forever. All the fashionable illnesses that I have discussed in this book are associated with problems that are in dire need of solutions – humanizing the workplace, making roads safer, reducing environmental pollution, and last, but not least, giving women a fairer deal. The fashionable illnesses consume the very resources that might be used to remedy at least some of these outstanding problems. Women carry a heavy burden and it is not surprising that many women ache and are fatigued, but to attribute these symptoms to a mysterious disease process surely avoids the need for women to claim a more comfortable place in society.

Perhaps society is changing. Men may have thought women's brains too small for intellectual work, but Maria Montessori, herself a gifted anthropologist, recalculated her male colleagues' sums and found that women's brains, in proportion to their body size, are, in fact, larger than men's. Montessori founded her schools so that women's superior intelligence could be allowed to blossom.[85] Perhaps the media's current preoccupation with women taking up the majority of university places proves Montessori right. In Ontario, boys lag so far behind girls in literacy rates that remedial classes are to be held to help boys catch up. Women are bright and they are on the march, and they are starting to take the lead as healthcare practitioners themselves.

23

Treatment Exuberance and Serendipity

The learned have their superstitions, prominent among them a belief
that superstition is evaporating.

– Garry Wills, *Under God*

Healthcare, as you must certainly realize by now, has much to do with
providing its practitioners with a living, and nowadays patients have to
support many more of them. In the early years of the eighteenth century, Boston (then North America's most populous city) had six physicians per 100,000 inhabitants.[1] There are now 240 physicians for
every 100,000 Americans, a figure that is expected to rise to 290 in the
next seven years.[2] The numbers of alternative practitioners are
expanding even more quickly. Healthcare practitioners, conventional
or otherwise, have always created new illnesses from which their
patients can suffer, but now, with the proliferation of practitioners, illness creation is increasing by leaps and bounds.

The provision of sensible and effective healthcare has always been
difficult. To protect their citizens from unscrupulous practitioners,
governments seek to license and regulate healthcare practitioners.[3]
While such measures are no doubt necessary, they inevitably create
healthcare monopolies that soon lead to stultification and renewed
exploitation of the public. To give a related example, a Canadian who
takes a cat to the vet for a dollar's worth of distemper shot that only
veterinarians can buy will, after an hour or so's wait and an unnecessary full examination of his cat, be charged $40.00 for his cat's care.
Not surprisingly, many cats go without their shots. Much of human
healthcare works the same way.

Illness expands to meet the treatments available. To avoid too much-
finger pointing, here is an illustration from my own specialty. Over the
last four decades the pharmaceutical industry has introduced many
antidepressant drugs. To prescribe these drugs, psychiatrists need
depressed patients. We found them. In the 1950s the rates of depression were considered quite low. Now it is claimed that depression
affects 100,000 per million people and that depression leads to more

disability than any other disorder.[4] I don't suppose that my colleagues or I deliberately upped the prevalence of depression; we just sort of unconsciously did it. We began seeing human problems in terms of depressive illness. (The actual amount of each antidepressant that we and other doctors prescribed correlated not with its demonstrated effectiveness but with the money its manufacturer spent on its advertising.[5])

The world is full of medical Messiahs creating patients to cure.[6] In jurisdictions where medical billing practices encourage it, some doctors even create make-believe patients for whose treatment they then bill exorbitant sums. One Ontario doctor, although his office is usually rather empty of patients, is reported to have billed for 136 items of service in one day including 25 hours of psychotherapy – and he is not even a psychiatrist. When his patients were contacted by fraud investigators, they found they were being treated for illnesses they knew nothing about.[7] One apparently healthy but unfortunate patient, on applying for life insurance, discovered that for years his doctor had been treating him for alcoholism, various mental illnesses, and a brain tumour – his prospective insurance company was unhappy. It is generally estimated the cost of such medical fraud is about 10 per cent of the annual $4 billion that the Ontario health service pays its doctors.[8]

Like whiplash claimants, most doctors are probably either too honest or too cautious to perpetrate such obvious fraud, but finding unnecessary illnesses to treat is another matter. Whether or not an illness actually requires treatment is often a judgment call and when faced with an illnesses that doesn't really need treatment it is easy for a doctor to convince himself and probably everyone else that in treating it he is just being particularly conscientious. Even the World Health Organization (WHO) with its one sentence definition of health seems intent on obtaining more territory: "Health is a state of complete physical, mental and social well-being and not merely the absence of disease or infirmity." Since most of us have physical, psychological, and social problems much of the time, WHO manages to make patients of us all. You might imagine that WHO already has enough sick and starving people on its hands without wanting more patients, but bureaucrats also like to expand their empires.

"Medicine has fostered a profoundly dependent public which searches for cures that do not exist."[9] Canada's Sir William Osler, regarded as the world's most able physician of the early years of the twentieth century, observed that "Man has an inborn craving for medicines," and Beatrice and Sidney Webb, socialist saints whose "children" were erudite papers for social improvement, argued that the doctor would be unable to resist "the patients' prevailing passions for bottles of medicines," and so opposed Britain's Lloyd George's 1911 National Insurance Act.[10]

Humans have always held bizarre ideas about the sanctity of treatment, and there seems no limit to what we will do in its name either to ourselves or to our loved ones. *Giving someone the treatment* has an obvious meaning; many historic remedies – the cautery, bleedings, and disgusting concoctions delivered by mouth, inhalation, ointment, or enema – were the kind of care most of us would prefer to forgo. When illness was regarded as retribution for sin, the nastier the remedy the better the cure! Treatment is also the giving of *treats*. Delicious fruit-flavoured syrups containing opium were a staple for the Victorians; nowadays we mostly prefer Valium.[11]

For centuries the management of hysteria has kept doctors well-heeled. In the Victorian pandemic of hysteria, three-quarters of all medical practice was devoted to diseases peculiar to women, and hysteria was the most common chronic illness from which women suffered.[12] Hysteria provided ample opportunities both for *the treatment* and for *treats*. *The treatment* was often surgical. Osler described the then popular surgical cycle in women: "Appendix removed, right kidney hooked up, gall-bladder taken out, gastro-enterostomy [joining the stomach to the gut], clean sweep of uterus and adnexa [tubes and ovaries]."[13]

Treats also were much in demand. Doctors commonly viewed hysteria as an illness caused by blockage of the womb consequent upon sexual deprivation. An orgasm was required to release the womb's pent-up juices, but unfortunately many ill-informed and indolent husbands or lovers proved inadequate to the task. In Britain it was even illegal to state in print that a wife could or should derive sexual pleasure from intercourse. Both the church and the medical profession prohibited women from providing such relief for themselves. In fact, in the 1850s, Isaac Baker Brown, a gynaecologist from Guy's Hospital (my own medical school) made a fortune by the surgical removal of the clitoris to ensure that they did not.[14]

While Brown was cutting off clitorises, many other physicians were busy rubbing them. The womb needed to be unblocked, and genital massage was a standard treatment. Though lucrative, genital massage was described as "the job that no one wanted."[15] It was hard and time-consuming work. A century later such services might well have caused an epidemic of repetitive stress injury amongst doctors, or at least amongst their assistants, since the self-employed rarely suffer such illnesses. In 1883 British physician Joseph Mortimer Granville invented the vibrator, which eased the physician's task – reportedly often reducing the time required to unblock the womb from one hour to ten minutes.

In her recent book, *The Technology of the Orgasm,* Rachel Maines gives a well-documented account of fifty kinds of medical vibrators in use up to the end of the nineteenth century. There were electric machines for the doctor's consulting room, foot-driven portables for home visits, and large steam-driven models for multiple simultaneous servicings at health spas.[16]

Genital massage was not regarded as sex, for sex, from the andro-centric Victorian doctor's viewpoint, required penetration by the penis. Neither, mysteriously, was it considered to be masturbation – a practice far too proscribed to be used as treatment. The doctor's genital massage induced "hysterical paroxysms" and it was these paroxysms that allowed the female juices to flow and so provide a cure.

Health practitioners have always viewed self-treatment with mixed feelings. Victorian physicians were worried lest their vibratory equipment fall into the hands of women themselves, which, of course, it eventually did. Women obtained their own vibrators and by the 1960s they had few reservations about using them. By then, however, physicians had long since discarded genital massage. In the 1920s porn flicks featuring vibrators broke the illusion that vibrators were simply a treatment device. Vibrators quickly disappeared from medical practice, and nowadays no sensible physician would provide such intimate relief for his patients, though *playing doctor* remains a popular pastime with the laity.

Much desexualized, hysteria metamorphosed into the present-day fashionable illnesses including, of course, whiplash. For these illnesses, orthodox medicine now favours *scientific* treatments such as *radio-frequency neurotomy,* treatments more in line with today's therapeutic expectations.

Other issues aside, genital massage was at least harmless, for Victorian treatments often did more harm than good.[17] Cleansing the body through vomiting, purging, and increasing urination was central to medical practice. The customary regular ingestion of Spirit of Wormwood, antimony, mercury, and other toxic heavy metals, prescribed to induce cleanouts, must have hurried many of our ancestors to an untimely end.[18]

As with Daniel Palmer's chiropractic realignment of vertebrae, any alternative to the practice of conventional medicine, however bizarre, was likely to have been an improvement. Christian Hahnemann also helped. He founded homeopathy in the early years of the nineteenth century with the conviction that a drug gains in *spiritual and curative powers* as it becomes less *material.* Hahnemann made drugs less material by diluting them. Homeopaths still do – often to one *decillionth* (i.e., a millionth of a millionth of a millionth, up to ten of these millionths) of a single grain.[19] However noxious the treatment, diluted to this degree, it is rendered totally safe.

"Patients," Osler pointed out, "are more often damaged than helped by the promiscuous drugging that is only too prevalent ... One of the first duties of the physician is to educate the masses not to take medicine."[20] It was perhaps discriminatory of Osler to pick on the masses, for the *somebodies,* on whom we have much more information, were also frequently harmed by medical treatments.[21]

Sir William Gull, a nineteenth-century English physician (the first physician to describe hypothyroidism) was, like many other scientifically minded doctors, irked by his profession's unthinking acceptance of unsubstantiated treatments. He decided to teach his colleagues a lesson. There were innumerable treatments for rheumatic fever. Gull introduced a new one – mint water – the first innocuous substance that came to mind. He demonstrated that patients recovered just as well on mint water as on the other treatments. Misunderstanding the point of Gull's experiment, doctors enthusiastically prescribed mint water, turning it into yet another fashionable cure for rheumatic fever.[22]

Oliver Wendell Holmes, a nineteenth-century American physician, famously summed up the case against Victorian medicine: "The disgrace of medicine has been that colossal system of self-deception in obedience to which mines have been emptied of their cankering minerals, the vegetable kingdom robbed of all its noxious growths, the entrails of animals taxed of their impurities, the poison bags of reptiles drained of their venom, and all the conceivable abomination thus obtained thrust down the throats of human beings suffering from some default of organization, nourishment, or vital stimulation."[23]

Holmes, having made exceptions of opiates and the "miracle of anaesthesia," continued his attack: "I firmly believe that if the whole materia medica [the drugs that doctors prescribe], *as now used,* could be sunk to the bottom of the sea, it would be all the better for mankind – and all the worse for the fishes."

While doctors had no shortage of treatments, few of their treatments actually worked. Up to the early 1930s, the only really useful medicines that doctors had in their black bags were pain relievers, insulin for the treatment of diabetes, thyroid extract for hypothyroidism, some medicines for anaemia, salvarsan (Ehrlich's treatment for syphilis) and barbiturates for epilepsy. For most patients the honest doctor had nothing to offer but kind attention.

Then the sulphonamides arrived. Sulphonamides prevent the growth of certain bacteria and, by so doing, enabled doctors to cure some dreadful infections which previously had been rapidly fatal. The pharmaceutical industry followed up the sulphonamides with the antibiotics and a legion of wonder drugs all of which added enormously to medicine's prestige. The medical profession had come into its own. Some of these new treatments were miraculous, and treatment, which had always had a special place in the human heart, became doubly sacrosanct.

Politicians would win or lose elections according to their commitment to provide us all with the new wonders of healthcare. But while treatment received respectability, treatment's longstanding craziness did not abate. The witchcraft of medicine was practised under the guise of science. The use of pointless medical interventions escalated, but few people thought to question their value.

Along with treatment, investigations were "in." The number of laboratory tests, x-rays, and other clinical investigations rocketed, greatly increasing the cost of medical care.[24] The beneficial effects of many of these new tests were dubious. For instance, Samuel P. Martin and his colleagues from the Department of Preventive and Social Medicine at Harvard examined the changes in coronary care for the 30 years from 1939 to 1969. They found there had been a huge increase in the use of investigations, sedative medication, and oxygen, but there was no significant change either in the duration of the hospital stay or in mortality.[25] By 1982 the cost of tests and procedures in the United States accounted for as much as one-quarter of all hospital costs. Unnecessary tests continued, "the false positives often leading to costly and sometimes harmful interventions."[26]

It was not only financial incentives that pushed up the use of these tests. In the 1950s and 1960s, while British doctors had no financial incentives to order tests, the number of investigations grew by 6 per cent annually.[27] Why? Doctors like to keep up with the Joneses. If one hospital gets a new investigation, doctors in all the other hospitals want it. "Without it there may be unnecessary deaths and our patients will stay in hospital longer." Even though there is often no evidence that the patients in the hospital with the new investigation are actually any better off, doctors will still order it. Gerald Sandler, a physician working in the Britain's National Health Service, found that routine blood and urine tests contributed to a diagnosis in less than 1 per cent of 630 outpatients, but the cost of these tests was "soaring as their technical complexity grew."[28] By the mid-1980s hospital doctors were ordering so many blood tests that an editorial in the *New England Journal of Medicine* called them "medical vampires."[29]

Indeed, some hospitalized patients had so much blood taken from them that they became anaemic and needed transfusions to treat their anaemia.[30]

Laboratory tests are not the only problem. The alimentary canal has orifices at both ends, and with improvements in endoscopy, gastroenterologists were enthusiastically inserting endoscopes into these convenient openings. Diagnostically, many of these insertions were and are unnecessary but, as Clark, writing in the *Lancet*, pointed out: "Doctors are trained to act, not to think. It is easier to perform an endoscopy than to think about the problem."[31] This is particularly true when doctors are well paid for performing these kinds of investigations and poorly remunerated for taking time to think about the patient and his illness.

Indeed, most gastroenterologists were so busy with their endoscopes that for years they overlooked the cause of peptic ulcer, one of the most common complaints which they are called upon to treat. These ulcers were rare at the start of the twentieth century but by the early 1960s they weren't. About one in ten males suffered from a duodenal ulcer. The ulcers were attributed to the psychological stresses that weighed upon the shoulders of these family breadwinners. Then peptic ulcer cases suddenly declined and by 1972 they were down by almost 50 per cent.[32] The gastroenterologists, sliding their well-lubricated endoscopes into their patients' orifices, paid little attention to the significance of this unexpected decline.

Then in 1983 Robin Warren, a pathologist at the Royal Perth Hospital, Australia, reported the presence of large numbers of small, curved, almost unknown bacterium (later called "*Helicobacter pylori*") in about half his gastric biopsy specimens.[33] Barry Marshall, a young Australian gastroenterologist paid attention. One of his patients, whose gastric biopsy specimen had contained Helicobacter, was given antibiotics for an incidental chest infection. His gastric symptoms disappeared. Marshall did another gastroscopy; the Helicobacter, along with the symptoms, were gone.

No one else shared Marshall's enthusiasm about his patient's unexpected recovery. Once he knew what to look for, Marshall gastroscoped nearly 200 more patients and he found Helicobacter present in every patient with an ulcer. But Helicobacter were reluctant to grow in the laboratory. Then by a serendipitous mistake, over the Easter holiday, the laboratory staff left the culture plates in the incubator for four extra days. The Helicobacter grew. Marshall swallowed the culture. Unlike most people, he was delighted to develop the symptoms of gastritis, a diagnosis confirmed by a friend with an endoscope. Marshall treated himself with the appropriate antibiotic; he recovered.

With his simple clinical observation, Marshall stood the gastroen-
terological world on it head. He overturned years of medical misconception about the cause of peptic ulceration. Once they are located in
the lining of the stomach, Helicobacter remain in place, causing
ulcers and other trouble until they are eradicated by antibiotics.[34]
Now, peptic ulcers are curable by a two-week course of antibiotic; they
do not require ongoing treatment with expensive acid-suppressing
drugs.[35]

Second to prescribing treatments, giving health advice is the doctor's next stock in trade. Our treatments are often hit or miss, but
what about our advice? The story of coronary thrombosis will illustrate the problem. Perhaps the tale of coronary thrombosis is not so
different from the story of peptic ulcers. The first case of this
twentieth-century epidemic was reported in 1925.[36] Then gradually
coronary thrombosis became a dreadful killer, especially of middle-
aged men. The epidemic peaked in the 1950s and by the mid-1960s
the numbers of cases declined.[37] As with ulcers, the cause of coronary thrombosis was often attributed to the arduous responsibilities
faced by the modern male. By the end of 1970s, excellent evidence
accumulated implicating a high animal fat diet, smoking, and lack of
exercise as the culprits behind the epidemic. Doctors sensibly
advised patients to stop smoking, exercise more, and avoid foods
high in animal fats and cholesterol.[38] Perhaps, though, these three
identified culprits were not the only killers. In fact, there was some
uncertainty about the animal-fat-containing foods. In two large controlled trials, men at high risk for heart attacks were divided into two
groups. The men in one group were prevailed upon to forgo their
culinary pleasures of meat, eggs, and all other fatty things, while the
men in the other group were allowed to live their lives in peace.
There was no difference in the death rates between the men in the
two groups.[39]

However, by this time much medical credibility, along with drug and
food manufacturing fortunes, had been invested in the conviction that
animal fats and cholesterol were paramount causes of heart disease.
Business often wins out over science. Doctors continued to spread the
gospel, and their teachings about fats and cholesterol hit home.[40]
Surveys show that North Americans still believe a low cholesterol and
animal-fat intake are the most important factors in the prevention of
heart disease.[41]

Animal fats are *saturated fats*, meaning that their molecules have no
room for any additional hydrogen atoms. Vegetable oils, in contrast,
are *unsaturated fats* and, unlike animal fats, they contain little or no
cholesterol. Doctors recommended replacing butter with *margarine,*

and lard with vegetable-made *shortening*, on the rationale that these substitutes were safer.

In giving this advice we overlooked a simple fact: in order to make vegetable oils spread like butter, their manufacturers "hydrogenated" the vegetable oil – a chemical process that saturates the molecules of the vegetable oils with hydrogen atoms. Not only does this manufacturing process make the treated vegetable oils similar to animal fats but it also produces "trans" bonds, a molecular structure that is not normally present in nature.[42]

Whether a pudding contains butter or margarine, its proof is in the eating. Human dietary investigations are difficult to perform, but two studies on the effects of processed vegetable oil consumption were published in 1997, one involving men and the other women. Both studies indicated that these chemically altered fats cause trouble.[43] Ascherio and Willett, from the Harvard School of Public Health, "conservatively" estimate that 30,000 premature deaths occur in the United States each year due to the consumption of trans fatty acids from foods containing processed vegetable fats. It takes an enormous amount of competent doctoring to save 30,000 lives.[44]

Doctors are usually too busy investigating and treating patients to worry overmuch about the causes of a disease or even about preventing it.[45] While massive resources are allocated to the surgical and medical treatment of coronary heart disease, relatively few are directed towards understanding its causes or studying the validity of medical advice to reduce its incidence. Perhaps we should have had misgivings about advising patients to exchange the delights of butter for the insipidity of margarine. During the first quarter of the twentieth century, a number of countries had introduced margarine as a cheap substitute for butter. Terry Anderson, an epidemiologist at the University of Toronto, observed that death rates from heart disease rose in each of those countries. But epidemiologists' findings are often ignored and Anderson's interesting observation was overlooked.

Something else was also wrong with the heart attack story. As with peptic ulcers, the incidence of coronary thrombosis had already begun to fall before any substantial changes occurred either in people's animal fat consumption or in their smoking habits.[46]

Then a new idea hit the heart scene. In 1988 Finnish investigators found high serum antibody titres to chlamydia, a disease-causing bacteria, in men with coronary artery disease. Besides causing some atypical pneumonias, chlamydia has become the most common of sexually transmitted diseases. Could a chlamydial infection play a role in the aetiology of coronary thrombosis?[47] Four years later, South African investigators reported chlamydia in the atheromatous plaques of the coronary arteries.[48] Then in 1997, researchers in a pilot study at St George's Hospital in London identified heart-attack patients with high chlamydia antibody titres and treated half of them with an antibiotic while leaving the other half untreated. The treated group had fewer subsequent adverse cardiovascular events than the untreated group.[49]

In another pilot study, investigators from Buenos Aires randomized 200 men with angina (heart pain due to narrowing of the coronary arteries) into two groups. The men in the treatment group were given antibiotics, while the men in the control group were not. During the six-month follow-up, the men in the treated group had significantly fewer heart attacks and deaths.[50] In 1999, researchers from the College of Dentistry in Gainesville, Florida, noting that there is an association between periodontal disease and the incidence of coronary heart disease, showed that bacteria from the gums can invade the cells of the coronary arteries.[51]

None of these studies permit any definitive conclusions. But did doctors, with their generous prescriptions of antibiotics, fortuitously eradicate bacteria from the walls of the coronary arteries? Or did fluoride in the water supply so improve the health of people's teeth that gums are no longer an entry site for bacteria? Many hopeful leads in medicine turn out to be wrong, but it is easy for doctors, in their exuberance for treatment,[52] to disregard important and sometimes easily implemented preventive measures. There is much to be said for pre-empting the illness in the first place.

If a drug is powerful enough to do good, it is powerful enough to do harm. The rate of drug-induced iatrogenic illness has always been high. In the 1960s, an American study showed that an adverse drug reaction was a major factor in 4 per cent of all patient admissions to hospital and, for a patient once in hospital, the dangers of an adverse drug reaction increased.[53] Twenty per cent of all patients admitted to an American teaching hospital had an adverse reaction to a medical intervention – in 5 per cent the reaction was serious enough to be life-threatening or fatal.[54] Contemporaneously in Britain, Sir Derek Dunlop, chairman of the Committee on Drug Safety, estimated: "Probably ten per cent of our patients suffer to a greater or lesser extent from our efforts to treat them."[55]

Forty years later, the problem of drug-induced illness has not gone away. Studies still show that adverse drug reactions (not including deliberate overdoses or the illicit use of drugs) account for about 3 to 11 per cent of hospital admissions in the United States.[56] The danger from in-hospital drug adverse drug reactions also remains high. A recent survey of American hospitals found the incidence of adverse drug reactions was 6.7 per cent.[57] In 1996, 106,000 hospitalized patients died of a drug reaction, ranking adverse drug reactions as the fifth cause of death in the United States.[58]

Hospitals may be the cathedrals of modern medicine but they are unhealthy places in which to be sick. Added to the adverse effects of drugs are the dangers of acquiring serious infections. Like teenagers to pop stars, virulent and often antibiotic-resistant bacteria congregate around the hospitalized sick. Hospital-acquired infections kill more Americans than auto accidents and homicide combined.[59] The results of a preliminary review indicate that over 10 per cent of patients admitted to British hospitals experience an adverse event. "A third of these events led to moderate or greater disability or to death. Half of them were judged to be avoidable by ordinary standards of care."[60]

To a hammer, everything is a nail. Hospitals are for treatment; they treat. The 1978 congressional subcommittee investigating the excessive use of surgery in the United States reported that two million unneeded surgical operations were performed annually at a cost of $4 billion and more than 10,000 lives.[61] More recently, the 1997 National Confidential Enquiry into Postoperative Deaths in Britain found that some 20,000 patients who had died during or shortly after surgery should not have been operated upon in the first place.[62] Unlike surgeons of many countries in the world, most British surgeons are salaried, and so they are not driven by financial incentives to operate. Neither are they in cutthroat competition for patients. In 1970 John Bunker from Stanford University, in comparing both the number of surgeons and the number of operations performed in Britain and the United States, found that in proportion to the population, Americans had twice the number of surgeons and they performed twice the number of operations.[63] Since Bunker's survey, the number of American surgeons in need of work has increased.[64]

When doctors have a work slowdown or go on strike the death rate in the affected communities falls.[65] In response to rising malpractice premiums, doctors in Los Angeles County withdrew all but emergency medical services for thirty-five days; the death rate steadily declined to nearly half its usual level, leaping up again when full medical services were resumed.[66] The 60 per cent reduction in elective surgery accounted for most of this dramatic fall. When Israeli doctors went on strike, bringing all elective surgery to a halt, the country's death rate plummeted by 50 per cent. A 52-day-doctors' work stoppage in Brazil led to a 35 per cent decline in the mortality rates.[67]

Some surgical deaths are inevitable. Risky surgery may be performed in an attempt to prevent an otherwise inevitably fatal outcome, but other deaths are caused by unwarranted surgical intervention. The authors of the Los Angeles study, having considered other evidence concerning elective surgery, conclude: "It would appear, therefore, that greater restraint in the performance of elective surgery might well improve U.S. life expectancy."[68]

Surgeons and psychiatrists are at opposite ends of the medical spectrum, but my criticism is not an internecine attack on surgeons. Psychiatrists have an insalubrious record as well. Anxiety and insomnia are ubiquitous and irksome conditions that psychiatrists and family doctors attempt to cure with sedatives and hypnotics often doing more harm than good. Pharmacologically, sedative and hypnotic drugs are really the same, the difference being that in small doses these drugs relieve anxiety while in larger doses they induce sleep. At first these drugs work like a charm; an insomniac gets the best night's sleep ever and the miserably anxious person starts to feel quite human.

There is, however, a snag. The body's chemistry adjusts to the presence of these drugs and within a few weeks the sleepless become sleepless again and the anxious become anxious again. Once tolerance has developed, the dose needs increasing. Stopping these drugs, even in normal volunteers who have been on them for a few weeks, induces withdrawal anxiety and insomnia.[69] The patient is easily hooked; addiction to these drugs is a major problem.

To help themselves sleep, the Victorians poisoned themselves with bromides, but in 1903 barbiturates arrived. While barbiturates were useful for treating epilepsy, as a treatment for anxiety and insomnia they caused medical mayhem, and they remained a major social problem until the 1980s.

The epidemic of barbiturate misuse hit Europe with full force after World War II.[70] America quickly caught on, and American doctors were soon prescribing 250 tons of barbiturates each year.[71] In addition, by 1951 half the barbiturates produced in the United States were earmarked for the illegal market. The FDA regarded the illegal distribution of barbiturates as its biggest problem in drug control. These drugs were proving more dangerous than heroin.[72] By 1960 Americans had sufficient barbiturates in stock to supply every resident with 18 doses annually.[73]

Britain often has difficulty keeping up with the States, but by 1970 half a million Britons were regular users of barbiturates, and 2 per cent of the population had become addicted. The typical barbiturate user was a middle-aged woman, though teenagers often got in on the act.[74] Over half of all poisoning deaths in Britain were due to barbiturates, with 12,000 of such deaths occurring between 1965 and 1970.[75]

Doctors create fashionable illnesses and in the developed countries they also created the dangerous fashion of making suicidal gestures by barbiturate overdose. Neil Kessel, professor of psychiatry in

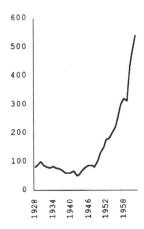

Fig. 23–1   Doctor-encouraged suicide
Annual admissions of patients with self-poisoning to the Edinburgh Royal Infirmary
1928–63. Doctors prescribed increasing amounts of barbiturates and patients increasingly overdosed with them.

Manchester, England, during the early stages of this iatrogenic epidemic examined the admission rates to the Edinburgh Royal Infirmary
of patients with barbiturate overdose. His results are shown in Figure
23–1 above. Such increased hospital admission rates for barbiturate
overdose were repeated throughout the developed world. It is easy to
miscalculate the non-fatal dose of medication, and what was meant as
a harmless-attention getting suicidal gesture sometimes turned into
the real thing.

Barbiturates were selling well. Clearly, pharmaceutical companies
were not going to stop manufacturing them, neither were patients
going to stop demanding them nor doctors prescribing them.
Something had to be done. The Campaign on the Use and Restriction
of Barbiturates (CURB) was begun in the early 1970s and by 1974 prescriptions for barbiturates had fallen by 50 per cent and barbiturate
deaths had also begun to fall.[76]

Health campaigns are all very well, but what really sounded the
death knell for barbiturates was the introduction in the early 1960s of
the benzodiazepines, the Valium group of drugs. The benzodiazepines
were more costly, so the pharmaceutical industry preferred them; they
had all the nice effects of barbiturates, so patients liked them too, and
since a benzodiazepine overdose is about 70 times less likely to be fatal
than is a barbiturate overdose, doctors did not have to worry so much
about prescribing them.[77]

The benzodiazepines were regarded as wonder drugs and soon became the new "mother's little helpers." Psychiatrists and family doctors handed them out like Smarties. In fact, they often still do. The effects of these minor tranquilizers are not unlike those of alcohol. After a massive investigation of prescribed-drug use associated with traffic accidents, Fabio Barbone and his colleagues from the Medicine Monitoring Unit at the University of Dundee estimated that in Britain benzodiazepines are responsible annually for 1577 traffic accidents, of which 110 are fatal. As those drugs do not show up on breathalyser tests, the police usually fail to realize that the driver at fault is drunk on pills.[78]

These traffic accidents are only the tip of the iceberg when compared to falls and other household injuries induced by benzodiazepines. Like alcohol, the benzodiazepines are also a cause of family disruption. They are highly addictive and, as with barbiturates, withdrawal from them is difficult.[79]

Although street drugs are a great concern, prescription drug addiction remains a much greater medical problem. In Canada there are five times as many prescription drug addicts as there are people hooked on heroin or cocaine. The figures are much the same in the rest of the developed world.[80] In comparing numbers of deaths due to unwarranted surgical intervention to deaths due to unwarranted prescriptions, the pen probably remains mightier than the sword.

Besides facilitating the indiscriminate prescription of very potent drugs, medicine's new progress contributed to dehumanizing the relationship between patient and doctor; "medical achievement" began taking precedence over patient care. *Clinical science* produced the wonders of transplant surgery, but only after untold numbers of patients (not to mention laboratory animals) died miserable deaths in the name of medical progress. Sir Heneage Ogilvie, my teacher of surgery at Guy's Hospital Medical School, succinctly stated the problem: "The science of experimental medicine is something new and sinister, for it is capable of destroying in our minds the old faith that we, the doctors, are the servants of the patients whom we have undertaken to care for and the complete trust that they can place their lives or the lives of their loved ones in our care."[81]

Britain's Maurice Pappworth, another great teacher of clinical medicine, in his book *Human Guinea Pigs* exposed the extent to which patients were being used to expand the treating skills of the medical profession. Hospital ethics committees now vet all medical research in an effort to minimize such patient abuse.

A case in point is the story of the three-month-old conjoined twins, Mary and Jodie, unfolding as I write. Britain's St Mary's Hospital,

Manchester, offered to treat the twins for free. Their Maltese parents brought Mary and Jodie to Britain but, being Catholic, when they learned that Mary, the smaller of the twins, would die on separation, they refused consent for surgery. After a protracted legal battle, the hospital obtained a court order permitting the surgeons to separate the twins against the parents' wishes. Mary indeed died during the twenty hours of surgery, while Jodie faces more surgical intervention. While such dramatic surgery enhances the power and prestige of the hospital and surgeons, it seems to have left the family members and their community with a resentful sense of defeat. It also hugely drains the healthcare resources that are urgently needed for the everyday care of many ordinary children. It is this sort of *clinical science* that also recently enticed a woman to sell her healthy grandchild as spare parts for transplant surgery.[82]

By promising so much, clinical science raised everyone's expectations of enjoying a lifetime of good health. "God our help in ages past" had clearly performed a somewhat second-rate job in taking care of us, so we quickly turned to doctors as "Our hope for years to come."[83] At least in statistical terms doctors were doing a somewhat better job, but they too have failures, and while God can be cajoled or cursed for His therapeutic inadequacies, He remains safe in His heaven. Doctors can be taken to court and held financially accountable for theirs.

Sarah Boseley, writing in Britain's *Guardian* under the headline "Bad Medicine" asks what happened to the doctors "with an air of comforting authority whom we have admired and trusted from the first time they laid a hand on our feverish forehead?" She notes that the "most caring of doctors can be flawed by arrogance," and asks whether "doctors have disavowed their Hippocratic oath which bars them from doing harm?" Doctors, she writes, must be honest about their mistakes.[84]

The *Guardian* then provides a sampling of headlines on doctors in disgrace taken from British national newspapers for the previous month – sixteen in all. These include: "Hospital errors killing hundreds of new babies." "Girl 11 was awake as surgeons pinned bone." "Doctors face record number of complaints." "Seventy-seven deaths probed in GP murder enquiry" (a seemingly caring GP was subsequently found guilty on 25 counts of murder and is suspected of killing some 275 more of his patients.[85] He injected elderly women with fatal doses of morphine and appears to have profited financially from their deaths).[86] "Fatal blood blunder" (patient died after receiving the wrong blood). "Struck off for seven years of blunders" (a gynaecologist was found guilty of serious professional misconduct). "Cerebral palsy boy wins £3.3 million damages" (an obstetrician was found to have damaged the boy's brain "in a botched delivery"). "Father awarded £300,000 damages for Down's baby shock" (it was claimed that doctors failed to detect the congenital abnormality in early pregnancy, at which time the foetus could have been aborted). "GP who had an affair with married patient is struck off."

Patients can be exasperating and, although doctors must sometimes be sorely tempted to do away with a particularly vexatious one, medical murder, still less mass murder, is, I hope, uncommon. The other improprieties and mistakes that the *Guardian* itemizes are a different matter; they are recurrent events. Of course, it is desirable that physicians should demonstrate a high standard of competence and ethical behaviour, and Boseley is correct in her suggestion that doctors should be more open with their patients and more prepared to own up to their treatment mistakes.

There is, however, a difficulty. As the *Guardian* article so amply illustrates, the public has developed zero tolerance for doctors' mistakes but doctors make a great many of them. In the United States, the Commission on Medical Malpractice, on reviewing a random series of medical charts for medical mishaps, estimated that mistakes of sufficient severity to warrant the payment of compensation were made at a rate of one in every seven hospital-patients.[87] In the interest of equal justice for all, perhaps this compensation should be paid to these injured patients, although, in view of the huge sums involved, our healthcare services would then jolt to a very sudden halt. No doctor or medical institution could afford the insurance premiums to protect against such claims.

In all fairness to doctors, our shortcomings are probably no worse than those of other workers; they may well be a lot less so. People inevitably make mistakes, but unlike physicians, most people, when they do so, are not singled out for public humiliation. A thoughtless slip can fetch a damage award against the doctor of an amount that he could hardly hope to earn in a whole lifetime of exemplary service. Few people relish owning up to their mistakes and, with the disincentive of a vast damage suit against him, it requires particular saintliness for a doctor to come clean.[88]

Again, the *Guardian* asks, can doctors be trusted? In any other large unselected group of people there are some scoundrels, some saints, and lots of people somewhere in between; there is no reason for doctors to be any different.[89] Patients are also often of two minds about their doctor's honesty. They may demand immediate honesty about the mistakes he makes, but expect him to lie like a trooper when completing sickness certificates, injury reports, or insurance application forms. *Caveat emptor.* Anyone seeking a reliable physician needs to use all the criteria normally employed to check an unknown person with whom one hopes to do business.

In normal life, "Trust me" is an indication that one is about to be duped; it works every time. Honest people know that we live in a dishonest world, and they understand the need for objective confirmation of reliability. Boseley's trusted doctor "with an air of comforting authority" is pretty much a mythical character. Doctors probably should be knocked off their pedestals and brought down to human size, but whether, on failing to live up to unrealistic expectations, they should also be flung into the cesspit is debatable. It would perhaps be more useful to develop a greater understanding of the many pitfalls involved in the treatment of illness and to evolve sensible ways by which treatment can be made more useful and less risky.

24

Medical Decision-Making: Getting It Right

The art [of medicine] is long, and life is short.
– Hippocrates

The real revolution in medicine ... began with the destruction of dogma.
It was discovered, sometime in the 1830s, that
the greater part of medicine was nonsense.
– Lewis Thomas, *The Medusa and the Snail*[1]

The practice of medicine has always been full of pitfalls and it is getting worse as an ever-increasing number of medical interventions becomes available. How do doctors decide which one of these interventions to choose when so many of them are likely to be wrong? Essentially, a doctor has four basic criteria for deciding on a treatment:

- Personal habit and the practices other members of the profession customarily use;
- The blandishments of the pharmaceutical industry;
- Scientific or pseudoscientific speculation;
- Evidence-based medicine and the findings of randomized controlled trials.

We are all creatures of habit and doctors often continue to do what they were taught to do, sometimes decades previously, in medical school. They also do what patients expect them to do, which is based upon what other doctors do. Once a treatment is established, it remains in the treatment repertoire, with neither doctor nor patient stopping to consider whether it is actually useful.

Just as some people like to try out the latest gadgets, some doctors like to use the latest treatments. Such novelties are often inserted into the doctor's repertoire by samples dropped off by a "drug rep."[1] About 10 per cent of healthcare budgets is spent on drugs, and much time and effort is spent on encouraging doctors to prescribe even greater amounts. In Canada, the pharmaceutical industry keeps track of doctors' prescriptions and in 2001 the drug companies are scheduled to spend an average of $20,000 per Canadian doctor to persuade them to prescribe their particular products – not only with drug samples but with office refrigerators and expensive trips also.[2]

Over the centuries, doctors and scientists, with increasing sophistication, have observed how nature and the body works. Each new observation leads to suggestions for new treatments, most of which do not work and some of which do more harm than good. Occasionally such observations produce a lucky break. Two and a half centuries ago, an English country parson, observing that the willow "delights in wet and moist ground where agues [feverish aches and pains] chiefly abound," supposed that willow trees must provide a remedy for the ague. He gave bark from the *Salix* (the Latin name for the willow) to his aching parishioners.[3] The active drug in the bark was later named salicylic acid and in 1887 Bayer successfully synthesized a derivative of this acid and called it Aspirin, the first and subsequently the most successful drug to be made in the laboratory.[4] As the acquisition of knowledge speeds up, the observations used to inspire new treatments become more sophisticated. Scientists know enough about the simpler parts of the chemistry of life to hazard educated guesses about what will happen if they either facilitate or hinder a particular chemical process. They can even design drugs for specific purposes, though the results are often surprising.

Even the most carefully thought-up drugs may have all sorts of unexpected side effects. Occasionally, the unexpected side effects are even useful; indeed, many of our new wonder drugs were discovered not by thoughtful design but by good fortune. For instance, veterinary surgeons used phenothiazine as a worm killer and noticed that it calmed frightened animals. It *tranquilized* humans as well. Largactil, the best known of the anti-psychotic drugs then revolutionized the treatment of schizophrenia and much of psychiatry. An anti-tuberculosis drug was found to cheer up consumptives and in this way the antidepressant drugs were discovered. Sildenafil provides a recent invigorating example of such an unexpected useful side effect.

In the late 1990s Pfizer Pharmaceuticals developed sildenafil for the treatment of angina. Clinical trials of its safety and effectiveness were performed. Although apparently safe, sildenafil was not particularly effective against chest pain, but then something unusual happened. At the end of the clinical trials, when the investigators, as is customary, arranged to collect the left-over pills, the men in the trial were reluctant to give them up. Sildenafil was working wonders for their sex lives. So was born Viagra.

Evidence-based medicine and the findings of randomized controlled trials are the fourth basis on which a doctor makes treatment decisions. Because the effects of a drug are often unexpected and complicated, the usefulness of a drug is difficult to assess. In addition to these difficulties, many patients, believing that a drug will help, show improvement, while conversely, anxious patients develop negative placebo effects – effects that are then unfairly blamed on the drug.

The only reliable way to uncover both the useful and the harmful effects of a drug (or any other medical procedure) is by the use of a randomized controlled trial (see appendix 2). This approach to determining the effectiveness of any medical procedure has become central to the practice of good medical care. It is time to look more carefully at this newer way of making treatment decisions.

The big change started with mothers and babies. In the late 1970s, obstetricians Iain Chalmers and Murray Enkin, the one British and the other Canadian, examined the studies on which routine childbirth procedures were based, and found that only about 20 per cent of these procedures were based on any study that justified their use. Their findings so shocked the medical world that investigators began organizing randomized controlled trials (RCTs) on these commonly used procedures.

About half of the 226 care procedures used in obstetrics have now been partly or fully evaluated. On the basis of these evaluations, Chalmers and Enkin divided these forms of care into four categories. One hundred forms of care were shown to reduce the negative outcome of pregnancy and childbirth, 36 showed promise of doing so, and 86 were of uncertain value, whereas 61 were found useless or worse.[5] These forms of care were given up.

Lesley Page, professor of midwifery practice at Thames Valley University, in England, writes of the "dark ages of maternity care of the 1970s and 1980s, particularly in North America," before routine obstetrical procedures had been submitted to RCTs: "These were the days of routine purging with enemas in labour, sterilization of the pubic area, shaving and episiotomy rates of over 90 per cent.[6] Images of women, shaved, draped in sterile green, flat on their backs, hands manacled to the table so they would not unsterilize the area or reach out to take their new born into their arms, with foetal monitors and intrauterine pressure catheters in place are with me still. All these invasive, highly uncomfortable, and harmful procedures were introduced into routine practice without benefit of evaluation, on the basis of untested theories."[7] Doubtless, a charismatic obstetrician had suggested an improvement on the process of childbirth, or some electronic gadget manufacturer had sweet-talked obstetricians into accepting the marvels of foetal-heart monitoring, but no one bothered to conduct the appropriate studies to see if such innovations were useful.

A group of doctors at McMaster University, in Hamilton, Ontario, impressed by Chalmers and Enkin's findings, pointed out that, as with obstetrics, most of the traditional treatments and procedures used in medicine have also not been subjected to scientific evaluation. In seeking to improve medical decision-making, the McMaster doctors introduced the concept of evidence-based medicine (EBM). They suggested that the traditional reliance on sporadic observations and the opinions of individual physicians should be replaced by systematized observation.[8]

Canadians have a reputation for being non-controversial, but seldom have Canadians, inadvertently or otherwise, managed to open up such a can of worms. Demanding evidence that a treatment actually works upsets a lot of people. Drug companies do not like it when an RCT demonstrates that their cold cure, worth many billions annually in sales, works no better than a placebo.[9]

Although RCTs were actually introduced into medicine just over half a century ago, it is only within the last few years that they have come into their own. In 1948 Britain's Medical Research Council, as part of its investigation into the effectiveness of streptomycin in the treatment of tuberculosis, asked the gifted statistician, Sir Bradford Hill, to design an appropriate methodology to use in its investigation. Hill created the first sophisticated RCT.[10] Fifty years later the *British Medical Journal*, in a special edition commemorating this event, comments that while some people still scoff at these trials others see their introduction as "the most important development in medicine of the century."[11] Sir Richard Doll, another renowned medical statistician, refers to the Medical Research Council's RCT study into the effectiveness of a treatment for tuberculosis as "the 1948 watershed" in medical care.[12]

Only occasionally are treatments developed (penicillin, for instance) with such incontrovertible efficacy that no doubt remains as to their usefulness. The effects of most treatments are far less clearcut. The decision to use Aspirin to prevent a reoccurrence of a stroke or myocardial infarction illustrates the usefulness of this kind of treatment evaluation.

As we have seen, a useful purpose for a drug is sometimes discovered through an unexpected side effect, and aspirin's ability to prevent blood clots was such a windfall. Following tonsillectomy, children have sore throats for which they were often prescribed aspirin. Lawrence Craven, a family physician from Cleveland, observed that the aspirin-treated children were more likely to bleed – sometimes to death – from their tonsillectomy wound than the children who had been given no aspirin.

On the strength of his observation, Craven suggested that aspirin be used to prevent intra-arterial clotting, a common cause of strokes and coronary thrombosis.[13] Would aspirin be useful? A particularly tricky point since another of aspirin's side effects is to erode the lining of the stomach, a not uncommon cause of fatal gastric haemorrhage. Do the useful effects of aspirin win out over the bad?

Several large RCTs showed that a daily aspirin tablet following a myocardial infarction or stroke reduces the patient's chances of dying in the subsequent months from 10 per cent to 9 per cent or even down to 8 per cent. No single practitioner would ever see a large enough number of such cases to detect the presence of so small an improvement, since, at most, Aspirin would only save one in fifty of his patients. This small success rate may seem no big deal, but, since strokes and myocardial infarction are common events, the number of lives saved by Aspirin soon adds up – 10,000 to 20,000 for every million patients treated.[14] No small success, especially if you happen to be one of the beneficiaries. Small benefits derived from multiple medical interventions soon become substantial but RCTs are still needed to determine what these interventions should be.[15] When subjected to an RCT, some neglected treatments are found useful, while some commonly used treatments are revealed to be harmful – killing more patients than they cure.[16]

Evidence-based medical studies have been divided into two kinds. "Disease Oriented Evidence" (DOE) interprets the results from the doctor's viewpoint, while "Patient Oriented Evidence that Matters" (POEM) interprets them from the patient's point of view.[17] Their results can be very different. The use of cholesterol-lowering drugs for the prevention of heart attacks serves as an example.

As heart attacks (coronary thrombosis or myocardial infarction) are often associated with high blood cholesterol levels, doctors try to lower these levels in an attempt to prevent heart attacks. Various drugs can accomplish this reduction. RCTs of the effects of three such drugs contrast the findings of DOE and POEM.

RCTs show that these drugs reduce the number of heart attacks by as much as 29 per cent, as well as death from heart disease.[18] From the DOE viewpoint the drugs are a success. Cardiologists can rejoice that they are reducing deaths from heart disease, and drug manufacturers can claim that their products work. From the POEM viewpoint, things are not so rosy. Although fewer patients in the treatment groups died of heart disease, more patients in these groups died of cancer, violent death, and suicide. The added deaths equalized the total number of deaths in the treatment and the control groups.[19]

Why more patients on cholesterol-reducing drugs die of cancer remains unclear. The suicides and violent deaths are easier to explain. While these drugs may be good for the arteries they are not so good for the mood. They make some people so depressed that they kill themselves, while others, feeling angry and upset, behave in such a way that they manage to come to a violent end.[20] DOE and POEM are not the same thing.

The McMaster Evidence-Based Medicine Working Group writes of its work: "The new paradigm puts a much lower value on authority. The underlying belief is that physicians can gain the skills to make independent assessments of evidence and thus evaluate the credibility of opinions being offered by experts."[21] Sensible as this advice may be, it has drawbacks. Busy physicians are often in no mood to look favourably upon the arduous task that is thrust upon them of assessing RCTs.

When it comes to treatment, people have all sorts of personal axes to grind. Physicians are quick, and sometimes with good reason, to point out RCTs' long list of faults: trials may be "poorly managed" and "methodological inadequacies distort the results"; "random" selection is often far from random;[22] trials are "unethical" since they use patients as guinea pigs, and "politics hijack the conclusions of these trials"; "marketers use them to further their own profit-making ends"; junior doctors in search of accomplishments to swell their résumés often conduct the trials; and trials are mostly performed on hospital patients, often making the results irrelevant to family practice.

Last, but not least significant, in view of the huge material resources and much personal conviction invested in the results of these trials, the investigators may be more blind to the faults of the trial than to the participants who are its subjects and controls.[23] Even Sir Bradford Hill, the father of the RCTs, comments: "I am faced with trials [of drug treatment] on such an ill-defined or undefined pot-pourri of patients that I can but hopelessly speculate on who got what, when and usually why. These poorly conducted trials not only tell us nothing but may be dangerously misleading – particularly when their useless data are spuriously supported by all the latest statistical techniques and jargon."[24] One irate English doctor writing in the *Lancet* asks, "How often have the double-blind led the blind into a cul-de-sac?"[25]

Paranoia is never far under the surface. Many healthcare practitioners see evidence-based medicine as a government and insurance plot to ration healthcare.[26] Practice guidelines derived from these trials can be rigid and peremptory, making doctors feel that *cookbook medicine* is arrogating their art.[27] People seldom like losing their cherished beliefs, and doctors, like the rest of the world, may well prefer to let sleeping dogmas lie. Despite these concerns, RCTs undoubtedly help make medical decisions more rational and sometimes more humane.

Although the effectiveness of new drugs is now routinely subjected to RCTs, the risks and benefits of the many hundreds of traditional treatments still used in medical practice have still to be investigated by this stringent method.[28] The future for the effective use of information obtained from RCTs looks brighter. Around the world various scientific organizations collect, collate, and assess the reliability of the results of thousands of RCTs, and make their findings readily available, either in print or electronically.[29]

Physicians can access the best medical knowledge currently available. Likewise, patients can research their particular illness and vet the sources from which the information comes. Armed with such knowledge, patients need no longer be in a one-down position when discussing the risks and benefits of possible treatments with their physicians.[30] Although physicians have a reputation for being control-freaks about making treatment decisions, the evidence suggests that patient-physician collaboration and information-sharing leads to the best illness outcomes.[31]

Never before has the medical profession been in a position to offer such competent care to its patients, yet something odd has happened. When conventional doctors began to lose confidence in the magic of their treatments, the public lost faith in its doctors.[32] Many people have now turned away from conventional medicine to consult alternative healers.

Faith, Magic, and the Search for Alternative Care

Every profession is a conspiracy against the laity.
– Bernard Shaw

Every woman ought to be filled with shame
at the thought that she is a woman.
– Clement of Alexandria, an influential early Christian patriarch

Turf wars between competing factions for the spoils of questionable-but-lucrative occupations are inevitable, and the healing professions are no exception. Nowadays fights over which profession can have the right to prescribe treatment and then to bill insurance or government health plans for doing so are particularly acrimonious. For instance, my own discipline is particularly exercised over clinical psychologists who are seeking to prescribe psychotropic drugs.

For years there has been little love lost between the medical profession and chiropractors and osteopaths. Such alternative practitioners have always encroached upon the doctors' realm, but in the last decade or so, new rivals have appeared over the horizon. Women! Gender politics is a healthcare issue that cannot be ignored, though the trouble started some 500 years ago.

For thousands of years, women were the traditional healers of mankind, and countless generations of "wise women" had acquired experience in the care of the sick, including surgery. Even in women-despising Christendom, women healers had established a niche of competence for themselves.[1] But as times changed, the church became preoccupied with women's promiscuous behaviour for, among other things, women were said to be visiting men in their dreams. Pope Innocent VIII appointed the monks Henry Kramer and James Sprenger to punish these "abominations and enormities, lest the souls of the multitudes face eternal damnation."[2] Kramer and Sprenger set to work finding the offending witches. They did so by demonstrating areas of reduced skin sensation (the very activity that Dr Keith Pearce at Mrs M's damage suit trial compared to the rheumatologists' hunt for tender points in fibromyalgics.) Sprenger and

Kramer's "witch-prickers" found many anaesthetic spots, and the church consigned the thus-identified "witches" to the flames. Not surprisingly perhaps, the church feared female retaliation and healers were the women with power. If a woman could heal she could also hex. She could make the crops to fail, the neighbours to fall sick and die, and men to droop in impotence, and she could certainly undermine the authority of the church and menace the lives of priests.

The power of the women healers had to be curtailed. Healing practitioners are often viewed with dissatisfaction so it was a convenient time to tidy up medieval "healthcare." Only the university-educated were now allowed to practise the healing arts. While to our modern ears this may seem like a straightforward attempt to protect the public against untrained practitioners, it was not. It was intended to put women healers out of business.[3] As women were not allowed to attend universities, they were automatically unable to practise.

The church's recipe for health was somewhat self-serving. Possession by demons and God's punishment for sins were its all-embracing explanation for illness. The university-trained physicians were dependent for their healing powers upon this medieval theology to which they added much garbled nonsense handed down to them from ancient Greece and Rome. The new doctors were expensive and mostly unavailable, and were likely a poor substitute for the "wise women" who had centuries of practical experience behind them.[4] With the exception of the asexual Virgin Mary, the only females who could be involved in the healing process were the safely dead female saints whose relics could be used to drive out disease-causing demons.[5]

Some present-day women healers claim that the new physicians used the burning times to further their own ends. Perhaps they are right.[6] How many "wise women" were eliminated in this way remains a matter of considerable gender contention.[7]

Ideas are power. For millennia a male god served men's interests well, while women were, and often still are, turned into second-class citizens. Some feminists have had enough of a Father God who keeps them girls and creates men in his own image. They are tired of His perceived petulance, rigidity, despotism, and self-righteousness. "God is a woman!" The ancient earth goddesses – from the virgin of the hunt to the canny old crone weaving life's threads in its eternal cycles of birth and death – are more akin to their souls. New Age healers return to these neglected goddesses and invoke their healing powers.

Perhaps, as some New Age women maintain, they remember the burning times from their past lives, or perhaps some more conformist women have read the results of the random controlled trials of male-dominated medicine's birth procedures. On many grounds women have had good reason to be suspicious of patriarchal and conventional medicine. Other kinds of healthcare are less tainted. What about these alternative methods?

Diane Stein, the author of several New Age books on alternative healing, claims that Asian healing (acupuncture, for one) "has been found in countless studies to be as effective as Western medicine."[8] I have no idea if acupuncture works better than placebo, but Stein is probably right. "Have faith, though it be only in a stone, and you will recover" is an old Arabic proverb, which is likely to be right about ninety-nine times out of a hundred, though you would probably do just as well without the stone. Mother Nature, being the marvel she is, cures most of our illnesses and injuries without the need of any medical or magical intervention, but few of us have the forbearance to allow her to do so. The doctor's traditional job has been to amuse the patient while nature begets a cure.

When treatments are shown to be no better than placebo, doctors move on to more active and powerful methods. Their "amusements" become both potentially more harmful and certainly more expensive. There is a perplexing paradox about treatment. Patients want doctors to be honest, yet honesty about treatment does not always seem the best policy. In fact, the more the practitioner embellishes the effectiveness of his treatments, the more effectively they often appear to work.

Reliable information about treatment outcomes is an essential part of good healthcare, but such information can also be stark and unkind. Evidence-based medicine may tell you that treatment "A" offers a 30 per cent 5-year survival rate and treatment "B" a 45 per cent 5-year survival rate. Such information may increase the probability of your 5-year-survival by 15 per cent which, for an imminently fatal disease, is no mean accomplishment. But you probably do not feel too happy. Such inexorable exactitude provides little room for miracles. Few of us have the courage to await with tranquillity an uncertain outcome; we need input – to take charge – we want to feel in control.

Alternative practitioners offer greater solace – the recently acclaimed Italian doctor with his special herbal remedy for breast cancer is said to have remarkable results, though he is "too busy to keep records."[9] But he was not alone in his faith in a natural treatment. A Canadian survey found that 67 per cent of women diagnosed with breast cancer reported using some form of alternative care.[10]

In looking to God for salvation, religions soon disagreed about how best to keep in His good graces. Now that we have pinned our faith on treatment, we cannot agree upon which healthcare denomination will serve us best. In the search for more *certain* salvation, patients have no shortage of unorthodox practitioners to choose from.[11] These practitioners, while using widely diverse methods of treatment, fit more or less into one of two overlapping groups – alternative and complementary.

Alternative practitioners, like their conventional counterparts, do things to patients, though not the same things that *stuffy* conventional physicians do. The alternative practitioners are chiropractors, homeopaths, osteopaths, naturopaths, acupuncturists, reflexologists, iridologists, clinical ecologists, aromatherapists, self-proclaimed *experts* in nutrition, astrology counsellors, and psychic healers, including experts in past-life regression.

The complementary practitioners, while usually respecting the tenets of science, work in areas neglected by conventional practitioners. When René Descartes separated mind and body, doctors took the body and left the mind. Oddly though, doctors never took much pleasure in the body, regarding it as a troublesome machine in need of constant repair. While they paid the body a great deal of attention and carefully sought to repair its breakdowns, doctors were careful to hold themselves aloof from it. Now, with the added threat of accusations of sexual abuse, doctors hardly touch a patient's body at all, preferring to examine it with x-rays and laboratory tests.

Unappreciated bodies hurt. Bodywork therapists – massage therapists, teachers of yoga and Alexander, Feldenkrais, and Tragor techniques – fill the gap by paying attention to the body's sensitivities. These therapists teach increased sensory awareness and the pleasures of physicality. Some bodywork practitioners seem to intuit the conversion of psychological distress into musculoskeletal tension and pain. In teaching their clients to release muscular tension, they perhaps help them to release emotional tensions as well.[12] In our touch-deprived society the bodyworker's hands can provide comfort and, frequently, relief from physical and emotional discomfort.[13]

Other complementary practitioners work with the mind. Doctors have not totally neglected the mind, but when they study it they often treat it like the body, objectifying it. They study it with questionnaires and make statistics of their findings.

What science cannot encompass, it discredits. Neither medicine nor science has ever been comfortable with subjectivity, though for most of us, such interiority provides meaning and significance to our lives.[14] Our search for subjective validation, while opening unlimited vistas to quackery, has concerned many thoughtful healers. Starting with the charismatic and notorious Madame Blavatsky (the co-founder of the Theosophy and mother of the New Age), writers and psychotherapists like Richard Bucke, Karl Jung, Alan Watts, Abraham Maslow, Aldous

Huxley, Mark Epstein, Thomas Moore, Ken Wilber, and Paul Davies, just to mention a sample, have sought to unite science with transcendence.[15] They seek to provide hope for the sick or searching soul. These practitioners are, of course, the antithesis of the *victimization psychologists*, for they place the responsibility for life's problems on sufferers themselves and not onto any outside cause. Whether such spiritual growth can ameliorate physical illness remains a hotly debated subject. There seems no doubt, however, that the insights gained through such experience can profoundly alter a person's assessment of an illness.

Healthcare practitioners, conventional or otherwise, often make extravagant claims for their treatments, but while physicians, chiropractors, homeopaths, osteopaths, and naturopaths are at least somewhat restrained in doing so by the dictates of their regulatory bodies, many unconventional practitioners remain exuberantly free from any such restrictions. In addition to their animal and vegetable treatments, they freely incorporate various psychological and electronic cures into their panaceas. If a treatment is foreign, mystical, *nutritional*, simplistically psychological, off-label (an orthodox drug put to unorthodox use), or even scientific-sounding, then some healer or other will likely exhort its therapeutic potential.

The media, in contrast to their condemnation of medical mistakes, errant doctors, and tragic hospital outcomes, nowadays often trumpet the successes of alternative healthcare.[16] The popularity of unconventional practitioners swells. Surveys show that 10 per cent of the population in Denmark, 33 per cent in Finland, and 49 per cent in Australia used *natural, holistic*, or other alternative treatments during the prior twelve months.[17] In the United States, the number of visits to alternative medicine practitioners rose from 427 million in 1990 to 629 million in 1997, thereby exceeding total visits to all American primary care physicians. Total out-of-pocket expenditures relating to alternative therapies are estimated at $27 billion, a sum about equal to the out-of-pocket expenditures for all American physician services.[18]

Some unconventional treatments are orthodox medicine's cast-offs.[19] Most of the medicines that Oliver Wendell Holmes deemed harmful even to the fishes in the sea are now long gone from the medical pharmacopoeia, but much-loved treatments, however useless or harmful, are not easily surrendered. Contemptuous of the pharmaceutical industry with its *artificial chemicals*, many unconventional healthcare practitioners are resuscitating these *natural cures*.

Some alternative treatments are based on sympathetic magic, the belief in a *sympathy* or causal connection between two similar objects or ideas – a perennially popular basis for treatment. In medieval times a saint's excruciating death often determined what diseases he or she was good at curing. St Felicia was beheaded; she was therefore good for headaches.[20] In the sixteenth century the doctrine of signatures held that the healing properties of plants were written into their nature. The aspen poplar with its trembling leaves was good for the shaking palsy, plants with chordate (heart-shaped) leaves were good for heart disease, and walnut shells for a head injury. In the seventeenth century, the long-preserved flesh of Egyptian mummies was a sure way to preserve life. During European epidemics of killing diseases, when the exigent demand for mummies outran the supplies in Alexandria, the flesh of freshly pickled slaves served as a substitute.[21] Gold and the elixir of life have long been linked together. The Chinese have the golden cure of consuming one's own urine, a long-cherished treatment for cancer and a great many other things besides. Westerners have now adopted the *waters of life* treatment as well. Amazon.com lists a dozen current titles on the virtues of urine therapy.

Impotence may not be as bad as death, but fearful enough for men to require magical treatments to prevent it. Powdered rhinoceros horn, deer antlers, seal and tiger penises, shark fin soup, sea horses, snakes, and turtles are all called into the service of keeping men horny.[22]

Using similar principles, psychic healers use gemstones to restore the damaged auras of the physically, mentally, and spiritually ill. The clarity of a crystal is needed to clear information. Red stones (rubies and garnets), giving energy and vitality, are required for problems of the uterus, menstruation, life force, red blood, circulation, leukaemia, and AIDS, while white stones (white opals or white chalcedony) encourage lactating mothers to let down more milk.[23]

Of course, magical cures are not confined to unconventional healers. Penicillin and the other antibiotics are perceived as powerful germ killers, so doctors prescribe them for viral illnesses against which they have no effect – a placebo use of antibiotics that is hastening the evolution of antibiotic-resistant bacteria, rendering one of medicine's most spectacular successes increasingly ineffective.[24]

North Americans have caught Europeans' enchantment with herbs and other untested treatments. Americans spent $2.5 billion on herbal treatments in 1996 and $4.3 billion in 1998.[25] While herbs, in contrast to the *chemicals* of the pharmaceutical industry, are championed as benign and innocent products of nature, they may be anything but! Plants, except when the consumption of their fruits aids in the dispersal of their seeds, no more want to be eaten than do you and I. To protect themselves from the voracious appetites of insects, plants are veritable factories of insecticides, creating enough to turn any self-respecting environmental sensitivity sufferer into an obligatory carnivore.[26] Similarly, plants produce chemicals that interact catastrophically with physiological processes of any large marauder that is thinking of eating them – perhaps a hungry human.

For the very reason that plant chemicals interact with our body chemistry, they can, in small quantities, be pharmacologically useful. A few berries of deadly nightshade will kill, but atropine, its deadly ingredient, prescribed in minute amounts, has many medical uses, some lifesaving. However, as every pot smoker knows, plants vary enormously in their content of pharmacologically active substances; soil, sun, rain, and the time of harvesting all exert their effects. Getting the right dose of a poisonous plant can be tricky.[27]

Herbal enthusiasts often cite the foxglove *(Digitalis purpurea)* as an example of the healing power of plants. Two hundred years ago, William Withering, an English physician, wrote of beneficial effects of the foxglove on dropsy (the massive swelling of legs and ankles associated with congestive heart failure). Digitalis entered the medical pharmacopoeia. As a young physician I happily prescribed *digitalis folia* (tablets of digitalis leaves) to my patients. There was a hitch.

The toxic dose of digitalis is only 30 per cent greater than its therapeutic dose, leaving little room for dosage error. Withering himself warned: "If inadvertently the doses of the foxglove should be prescribed too largely, exhibited too rapidly, or urged to too great a length; the knowledge of a remedy to counteract its effects would be a desirable thing."[28] A circumspect way of saying if the patient is dying of too much digitalis it would be nice if someone knew what to do about it.

The problem persisted. Nearly two hundred years later, Thomas W. Smith and his colleagues writing in the *New England Journal of Medicine* still complained: "Since Withering wrote his treatise, countless patients and physicians have had cause to concur with that judgment."[29] Several studies in the 1960s and 1970s report an incidence of digitalis intoxication ranging from 6 per cent to 23 per cent with a mortality rate as high as 41 per cent.[30] While for some patients digitalis was and remains a lifesaver, others were killed by it. Once the pharmaceutical industry had isolated and purified its active substance so that its dose could be controlled and its blood levels monitored, deaths from foxglove treatment dropped way down.[31]

There are many reasons to be suspicious of drug companies. Along with tobacco companies, they are often owned by multinational corporations whose concern is not our good health but their bottom line. Hoffman-La Roche, the Swiss pharmaceutical giant, topped the list of the leading corporate criminals of the 1990s. The company was fined

$500 million for conspiring to fix the price of vitamins.[32] It was not alone in its delinquency. Five other pharmaceutical companies were also involved in the conspiracy, bringing the total in fines up to $1.1 billion.[33]

Nevertheless, while government agencies monitor the activities of the pharmaceutical industry, the preparation, distribution, and use of herbal preparations has no such in-built controls, a lack of regulation that allows for untold skulduggery. Edzard Ernst, professor at the Department of Complementary Medicine at the University of Exeter in England, is unlikely to be biased against herbal medicine. In *Harmless Herbs?* he has reviewed the recent literature on adverse effects of herbal remedies, providing a horror story of fatalities and serious illness caused by these remedies. Besides the many adverse effects of the herbs themselves – including liver, kidney, and lung failure – some of the preparations are mislabelled, and some are contaminated by heavy metals, moulds, or pesticides. Herbalists, perhaps lacking faith in their natural products, sometimes add drugs from the pharmaceutical industry to their herbal preparations in amounts large enough to cause problems.[34]

Although plants are endowed with mystical properties, chemicals are chemicals whether they are *wildcrafted* from hedgerow plant or synthesized in an industrial plant. The essential difference between the two products is that the chemicals from an industrial plant are purer and their side effects, albeit usually inadequately, are systematically recorded.[35] When considering treatments, there is much to be said for the devil you know, but, to give a further example, many people who may be too apprehensive to risk Prozac, seem quite prepared to self-prescribe St John's Wort.

This little yellow-flowered herb is the alternative practitioner's substitute for the antidepressants of the pharmaceutical industry. A meta-analysis of 23 RCTs showed that St John's Wort is as effective as some antidepressants in patients with mild to moderate depression. It is also claimed to have fewer side effects.[36] This may be true, or perhaps just fewer of them have been reported. When a conventional treatment turns someone yellow, the jaundiced patient often happily tells the whole world about it, but when someone has self-medicated with camomile tea and turns yellow, he may not even tell his best friend.[37]

St John's Wort, like some of the conventional antidepressants, contains a monoamine oxidase inhibitor which, on occasion, can react with some common foods and drugs to induce such a catastrophic reaction that many American doctors, fearing lawsuits, hesitate to prescribe them.[38] Apart from such possible drug and food interactions,

St John's Wort in itself is not innocent of unpleasant effects. Cattle that feed on it become light-sensitive and may die of exposure to sunlight. Fair-skinned humans may get sunburn if they take twice the recommended dose, and it may not be easy to get the dose right. A sample analysis initiated by the *Los Angeles Times* of ten commercial brands of St John's Wort showed that seven of the ten had less potency than listed on the label and one brand contained 135 per cent of its advertised potency.

In treatment, the power of mystery often wins out over the transparency of science. The long list of plants and animals that stand in risk of extinction because they are so extensively culled as natural remedies provides ample evidence that our infatuation with treatment is little changed since Holmes wrote his diatribe against the Victorian pharmacopoeia.

Mystery has even been given a helping hand. Scientists have overwhelmed most of our imaginations with their quarks, black holes, ten-dimensional universes, and genetic engineering. Truth is now decidedly stranger than fiction, and most of us are incapable of telling the difference. Charlatans have never had it so good. Holistic healers rush in to fill the emptiness of mechanistic modern medicine. Dogmas and superstitions quickly substitute for the hard-earned scientific gains of the last three centuries. When evaluating healers it is often difficult to separate the wheat from the chaff.

Like their conventional counterparts, non-conventional practitioners range in trustworthiness from the unscrupulous to the impeccably upright. I will start with the smallest – literally so. Victor Herbert, a lawyer and doctor, and one of the founders of the National Council Against Health Fraud, found that to obtain a membership in some impressive sounding healthcare organizations only a fee is needed.[39] Herbert sent in his cat's name along with a cheque for $50.00 and a few weeks later received a certificate authenticating Charlie Herbert as a professional member of the International Academy of Nutritional Consultants. Buoyed by his success, he sent in another cheque for $50 along with his dog's name and received equally impressive credentials for Sassafras Herbert, certifying him as a professional member of the American Association of Nutrition and Dietary Consultants.[40]

Sparkling healthcare credentials can be fool's gold. Herbert's domestic pets may not speak with much authority, but Herbert, who is the editor of the prestigious *Mount Sinai School of Medicine Complete Book of Nutrition* and one of the world's experts on nutrition, does.[41] "The American public," he writes, "is ripped off to the tune of some $6 billion annually plus untold costs in human health and life by nutrition scams promoted by nearly all the radio and TV networks, newspapers,

magazines, and book publishers in the United States."[42] At the other
end of the trustworthy continuum are many helpful and upright complementary healthcare practitioners from various gifted psychologists
and yoga teachers, to hands-on bodyworkers.

Conventional treatments for colds, fatigue, and our ubiquitous
minor complaints, when subjected to the rigours of RCTs, often turn
out to be no better than placebo. Principled practitioners cannot use
them. In contrast, the alternative practitioners can nevertheless claim
success for their cures with an easy conscience. But for how long? In
keeping with alternative care's increasing popularity, its advocates
demanded a bigger slice of the healthcare pie. They got it. The
American federal government established the *National Center for
Complementary and Alternative Care* and endowed it with a $50 million
budget to support research into the effectiveness of its methods.[43]

Such research must eventually include RCTs, though, perhaps wise-
ly, its practitioners have been somewhat tardy in applying this acid test.
Some unconventional treatments have been tested and some, like St
John's Wort, were shown more effective than placebo; others have
not.[44] Either outcome may be a problem for alternative medicine. No
one will want a treatment that has been demonstrated not to work, but
any treatment endorsed by an RCT stamp of approval is ripe for the
picking. Conventional medicine may be elitist but it will certainly snap
up any alternative treatment that has been shown to be useful!
Alternative medicine and science do not seem destined to make comfortable bedfellows. Over the last century, patriarchal medicine, by
using the doctor's authority to certify sickness and disability, has
increasingly written people off as unable to cope with the ordinary
demands of life. Women healers are coming back. Equal numbers of
men and women are now entering medical school, and the majority of
alternative healers are women. Most women practitioners, conventional and otherwise, are feminists. Will they also leave a trail of disability? Some feminists see women (and sometimes even men) as
wounded victims of a patriarchal society of whom little can be expected, while others have a vision of women as competent persons fully
able to participate as responsible adults in a demanding world.
Patriarchal medicine has helped whiplash and similar illnesses to
flourish. It remains to be seen if feminist healers will turn the tide.

26

Medicine:
"A Disabling Profession"?

The medical and paramedical monopoly over hygienic methodology
and technology is a glaring example of the political misuse of scientific
achievement to strengthen industrial rather than personal growth.
— Ivan Illich, *Medical Nemesis*[1]

A race of hypochondriacs that concentrates all its attention on health
and an illusory security will achieve nothing but oblivion.
— Noel Poynter, *Medicine and Man*[2]

Healthcare practitioners with their treatment and advice loom large in
the subject of health, but in fact, their activity is only one of many factors that contribute to the level of our well-being. Healthcare practitioners have seldom shown much interest in these other factors.

The rampant killing diseases of the past had already stopped being
major killers before effective medical interventions were introduced
for either their cure or their prevention. You may find this difficult to
swallow since doctors and patients alike share a profound belief in the
decisive role that medical practice plays in keeping us alive and kick-
ing.[3] Evidence can be found in the relatively reliable statistics for
death rates for various diseases that have been kept in Britain going
back many years. Figure 26-1 shows the death rates for six major diseases from 1865 to 1965. I have superimposed upon these mortality
graphs averaged-out estimates made by university-educated subjects of
what they supposed these death rates to be. As you can see, these subjects grossly overestimated the effects of medical interventions on the
decline of these death rates.

By the time effective medical intervention was available for the five
infectious diseases that I chose to consider, the annual death rates
from most of them were already so small that they are hardly apparent
on the graphs. Why most of these diseases stopped being major killers
before doctors were able to prevent, cure, or ameliorate their severity
is open to speculation: chlorinated water, improved nutrition, refrig-
eration and safer preservation of food, better housing, proper sewage
disposal, and the pasteurization of milk are some of the many factors
that helped.

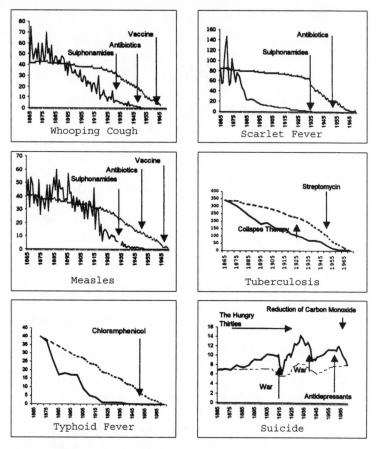

Fig. 26–1 Overvaluing the effects of treatment

Annual death rates per million from certain major killing diseases for the UK from 1865 to 1970 compared to mean values of the estimates of these death rates for the years 1866 to 1969 made by university professors (excluding physicians) and students. (See Appendix 4 for further explanation of this study.)

Knowledge gained through the advancement of science greatly improves disease prevention. Malaria, cholera, and AIDS may still harm and kill people by the millions, but death rates from these diseases would be vastly higher if we did not know their causes or have some ideas on how to prevent their spread.

Most well-fed and well-cared for children survive infectious diseases; underfed and poorly cared for children more frequently do not. The wealth generated by the industrial revolution raised people's living standards. When economic conditions improve, couples tend to have fewer children, and in smaller families children receive better care.[4]

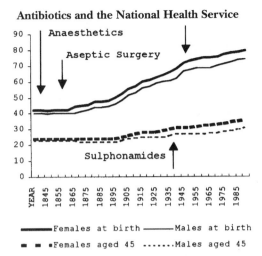

Antibiotics and the National Health Service

Females at birth ——————Males at birth

■ ■ ■Females aged 45 ·······Males aged 45

Fig. 26–2   Life expectancy of mid-lifers little changed by drugs
Life expectancy in years for males and females at birth and at age 45 for England (and Wales) from 1860 to 1995.

While the chances of a newborn baby surviving to middle age have increased enormously over the last 100 years, the increase in life expectancy for a 45-year-old has not risen nearly so dramatically, despite the wide availability of modern healthcare. Major innovations in healthcare were not followed by any obvious increase in the number of years the 45-year-old might expect to live.

Perhaps smaller families reduced mortality rates more than anything else, for it would have been impossible to improve social conditions in the developed countries had birth rates remained high.

Lastly, but certainly not least, although many children are now wanted, there are certainly exceptions. Judging from the expected gender ratios in world population figures, somewhere between 60 million and 100 million females are missing.[5] Unwanted children do not fare well, and in many parts of the world female babies are unwanted. While many of these babies are simply killed, others are less carefully nurtured than their wanted brothers and are therefore more likely to die. Contraception and safe medical abortion services (when actually available) enhance the likelihood of every child being a wanted child and so add to children's survival rates.[6]

It was social factors and not medical care that transformed our health statistics. I do not want to imply that medical intervention for these once killing diseases is without use, for while measles and other scourges from the past will probably no longer kill you, they may make you very sick.

Life expectancy is a useful statistical abstraction. It is the average number of years a person is expected to live in terms of the mortality rates calculated for the year in question. Figure 26-2 shows the increase in life expectancy in Britain over the last 140 years for males and females at birth and at age 45 years. You will notice two things: that there has been a steady increase in life expectancy to which the so-called "golden years of medicine"[7] (1945–70) made little discernible difference, and that while the outlook for a newborn has improved immensely over these 140 years, the outlook for the middle-aged, particularly the middle-aged male, is not much improved.

Why have the middle-aged fared so poorly? In developed countries the eight leading causes of death in middle age are: heart disease, cancer, stroke, accidents, diseases of the respiratory system (influenza, pneumonia, and bronchitis), adult onset diabetes, suicide, and cirrhosis of the liver. Many of these deaths are potentially preventable, for they are a result of our lifestyles. Smoking, obesity, and alcohol are major contributors to most of these causes of death.[8] While medical intervention reduces the death rates from some of these conditions, its effectiveness is puny compared to the results of non-smoking, exercising and staying trim, and avoiding an excessive alcohol intake!

Doctors can do little in the face of the social reality of a chosen lifestyle or destructive behaviour. For instance, it is often regarded as the doctor's job to prevent suicide and, apart from seducing or being seduced by our patients, failing to prevent a suicide is the event that lands psychiatrists in the most trouble. Much psychiatric effort is therefore devoted to the often thankless task of trying to prevent our patients from killing themselves – efforts that are mostly wasted and sometimes counterproductive.[9] Various psychiatric treatments for depression have not discernibly reduced suicide rates, whereas social conditions certainly alter these rates. Going to war will sometimes halve a country's suicide rate and a downturn in the business cycle will put it up.[10]

However, in Britain, in 1963 the suicide rate unexpectedly began to fall and within eight years it had plummeted by over one-third. The Samaritans, an organization devoted to offering telephone and counselling support for people considering suicide, had been founded ten years earlier and had steadily expanded its services. The Samaritans and the British psychiatrists both took credit for this amazing reduction in British suicides. Actually, neither had anything to do with it. The customary way of committing suicide in Britain at the time was to put one's head in the gas oven, but in the early 1960s the British Gas Board began changing the process for manufacturing domestic gas, and its new gas contained no lethal carbon monoxide.[11] It was the Gas Board and not psychiatric prevention that reduced Britain's suicide deaths (see Fig. 26–3).

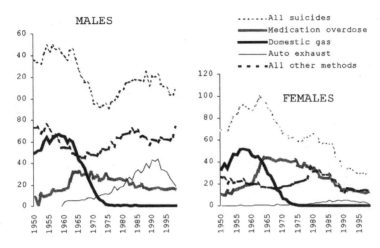

Fig. 26–3 Who prevents suicide?
Overdoses of medicines account for nearly half of all successful suicides. The British Gas Council was more successful than the medical profession in lowering suicide rates.

There was not one squeak of appreciation from British psychiatrists for the Gas Board's success. If only a fraction of this suicide reduction had been attributable to antidepressants, I promise you, you would never have heard the end of it. We doctors are not so much interested in a community's health indices as we are in our own therapeutic prowess – which is, after all, how we make our living.

In fact, doctors have often raised suicide rates. For instance, taking an overdose of medication was the second most common way of committing suicide in Britain, and the most common drugs used for this purpose were the widely prescribed barbiturates. By the mid-1960s medication overdoses accounted for almost half of British suicides. In the 1980s, when English doctors began prescribing benzodiazepines in place of barbiturates, suicide rates again fell, this time to their lowest recorded levels ever. The rates for women have remained low, but men's have crept up again, most of the increased suicide deaths being by car exhaust gases (see Fig. 26–3).[12]

In North America, household guns are the customary means of suicide. They are, of course, also widely used for killing family members and other people. Gun restriction, if politicians had the moral fortitude to impose it, would probably reduce American suicide deaths, at least for a while, and certainly reduce its phenomenally high murder rate. Any improvement in healthcare will have a negligible effect on gun deaths, but practical means to the betterment of health such as gun restriction are usually ignored in favour of more fanciful treatment solutions.

Perhaps medicine's recurrent claim that it is about to eradicate cancer will one day come true, but until then stopping smoking would
prevent more cancer deaths than anything doctors can possibly do.
Despite the hype about the effectiveness of cancer treatment (and
indeed some cancer cures are impressive), the overall success rate is
dismal, and total cancer death rates have remained virtually
unchanged for the last 50 years.[13] Forty per cent of people who develop cancer still die of it.[14]

Until recently, breast cancer was the number one killer cancer in
women. For several years medicine has waged a campaign for its early
detection. How useful has this campaign been? The screening tests for
breast cancer are regular breast examinations by a doctor or nurse,
self-examination by a woman herself, or mammography. About 80 per
cent of breast cancers are discovered by a woman herself, so teaching
women the technique of self-examination seemed a sensible way to go.

Some studies of the effectiveness of self-examination showed that it
reduced breast cancer deaths, but the results of other studies were disappointing.[15] Starting in 1989, over a quarter of a million women textile workers in Shanghai were randomly divided by factories into two
groups. The intervention group were given intensive instruction in
breast self-examination followed up by multiple reminders to keep
doing it, while the control were given instruction on low back pain prevention. The results of the first 5-year follow-up showed that while the
women in the group that used breast self-examination discovered
twice the number of breast lumps, surprisingly their death rate from
breast cancer was no lower than that for the women in the control
group.[16]

The results of breast self-examination have been so disappointing
that the position of the National Breast Cancer Center in the United
States is that the "evidence is not sufficiently strong to justify continued public health campaigns to encourage its use." The Center suggests the continued use of mammography instead.[17]

What about mammography? Stephen Feig, a widely published
American radiologist, claims it "reduces breast cancer deaths in
women aged 40 years and older by at least thirty to forty percent."[18]
The assertiveness of this claim might lead you to believe it, but mammography's effectiveness is also controversial.[19] What is less controversial about mammography is that it works better on women over fifty,
since the fuller breast tissue of younger women makes the results difficult to read, producing many false negative and false positive results.

Several authors now question the value of routine mammography.
Scandinavian authorities Gøtzche and Olsen even wonder about its
value in women over fifty as well.[20] Christer Rembold, writing in the

British Medical Journal, points out that even for women in the 50 to 59 age group it is necessary to screen 2451 women for five years to prevent one breast cancer death.[21] Questioning the value of mammography is like questioning the sanctity of the American flag, however. Angry letters, especially from American radiologists, have flooded the medical journals.

In the early 1980s the Canadian National Breast Screening Study enrolled nearly 40,000 women aged 50 to 59 and randomly assigned them to one of two groups. The women of one group received annual mammography along with regular physical examination of the breasts, while the women in the other group received only regular physical breast examination. The 13-year follow-up report has just been published. There was no difference in the deaths from breast cancer in the two groups.[22] Unfortunately in retrospect, the study did not use a control group of women who received no breast surveillance at all. Sadly it appears that no form of regular breast examination is particularly effective at reducing breast cancer deaths. Breast cancer is a slow growing cancer, often taking ten years or so before it becomes detectable, by which time the cancer has already spread to other places, so that its early detection adds little to women's chances of survival.

The campaign to diagnose breast cancer early has certainly increased women's anxiety about breast cancer. The statistic freely bandied about is that one in eight American woman have a lifetime chance of getting breast cancer, though it is usually not mentioned that this figure is only correct if she lives to be at least 100.[23] More realistically, a 40-year-old woman who does not have a mother or sister with breast cancer has a one in 200 chance of developing breast cancer in the next five years. With all the publicity for mammography, North American women have come to believe that their probability of dying of breast cancer is twenty times higher than it actually is and that the absolute benefit of mammography is 100 times greater than it is.[24]

The healthcare industry is not too keen on simple procedures, especially when there is an expensive high-tech procedure that can be used instead. Just as Victorian doctors did not approve of do-it-yourself genital rubs, present-day doctors are not over-enthusiastic about breast self-examination and, faced with its possible ineffectiveness, have been quick to drop their support of it. However, confronted with equal doubts about the effectiveness of mammography, there is no thought of dropping *it.* Rather, radiologists suggest the need to intensify its use. They now recommend that women as young as 25 be screened, and that the frequency of screening be increased from every two years to twice yearly.[25] The total cost of mammography in the United States is already about $3 billion.[26] Campaigns for breast self-examination may be allowed to go, but mammography seems here to stay. The *Economist*, in questioning the demands for more mammography in the face of its paltry successes, sums it up: "The blunt answer is that breast cancer is one of many diseases about which debate has been distorted by politics."[27]

Whereas, the results of breast screening have been disappointing, improved treatments have reduced breast cancer deaths in Canada, the United States, and Britain by about 15 per cent over the last 30 years. In all three countries, breast cancer has been demoted from being the number one cause of cancer deaths in women, though its demotion has nothing to do with its lowered death rates. Lung cancer in women has increased 300 per cent in the same time period. While attention was focused on expensively trying to reduce breast cancer deaths by medical means, lung cancer, which is easily preventable by not smoking, crept up almost unnoticed to become women's leading killer cancer. The rates of lung cancer deaths in women are now greater than they ever were for breast cancer.

In the United States, one of the most doctored of all countries, the Centers for Disease Control report that adult onset diabetes jumped 33 per cent between 1990 and 1998. The rise was sharpest in the 30- to 39-year-old age group; 6.5 per cent of the American population now has this form of diabetes. Besides being a potent cause of heart attacks and stroke, diabetes is the leading cause of adult blindness and amputation. Diabetes is scheduled to be the epidemic of the early years of the twenty-first century. "Virtual" sports don't burn calories!

It is half a century since Sir Austin Bradford Hill and Richard Doll (later Sir) demonstrated incontestably that smoking causes lung cancer.[28] Apart from reducing their own smoking, doctors showed little effective concern. Only in the last fifteen years in North America and the last ten years or so in Europe has the profession become vociferous about its dangers. Doctors in the underdeveloped world make little protest as tobacco companies, whose marketing activities are restricted by legislation in their home countries, shift their attention to these poorer countries. Increasing tobacco consumption will cause more people to die in the underdeveloped world than their doctors can ever hope to save.[29] Philip Morris, the makers of Marlboro, stung by the high level of publicity about deaths from smoking, recently had a dramatic change of heart. From adamantly denying that smoking was harmful, they admitted that tobacco does kill but that it does so usefully. Philip Morris prepared a cost-benefit analysis of smoking on the treasury of the Czech Republic. Balancing the costs of increased medical care for smokers and time lost through tobacco-related illness against income from tobacco taxes and the money saved to pension funds and housing costs through smokers' early deaths, Philip Morris reported a positive balance of US$224-million.[30]

It is certainly true that the viability of pension plans in the Western world is predicated on the fact that many smokers will not be around to collect their pensions. If smokers suddenly stopped smoking these plans would go bankrupt. Many pension plans are government-financed and since governments often seem more protective of their budgets than the health of their citizens, perhaps Philip Morris has a point.

Although most of us put good health high on our list of desirable assets, we often resist any changes that might bring it about. Edwin Chadwick, the nineteenth-century English engineer in charge of public health probably did more than any other person to improve health in England. He piped in clean water and insisted that the huge piles of human ordure be removed from the city streets. His clean-up was unpopular. The *Times* indignantly thundered that England would prefer to remain dirty than be bullied into cleanliness.[31] Similarly, fluoridation of water effectively reduces caries but some communities, with knee-jerk opposition, refuse to have their water supply "adulterated" with chemicals. Although wearing motorcycle helmets greatly reduces motorcycle accident deaths, many cyclists do not fancy wearing them. Under popular pressure, Florida has just rescinded the law that made their use mandatory. For another example, go to European medical meetings dedicated to the improvement of human health and observe the pall of tobacco smoke hanging over the heads of the participants. As residents of Toronto, we are constantly informed of the statistic that our polluted air is responsible yearly for 1000 premature deaths and 5000 hospital admissions, yet we somehow prefer to spend resources on direct healthcare than on making the kinds of environmental changes that would more effectively improve our health.

Acquiring good health can be an inconvenience, so it is tempting to hand the responsibility to someone else; and healthcare practitioners are often eager to jump in. Because doctors "usurp" health, Ivan Illich, the late philosopher and social activist, with considerable justification, described medicine as a disabling profession.[32] We can often do more to preserve our good health than doctors can, yet we continue to believe that without medical concern and attention our lives will be abruptly curtailed.[33]

Despite the convictions of clinical ecologists, the developed world, compared to times past, is a healthy place in which to live. Most of us (smokers excepted) can expect to survive comfortably into our 70s and 80s with little or no medical intervention.[34] Whether our world will remain a healthy place in which to live is a different matter. Countries, like people, have discretionary income. Should we fritter away our resources on often unnecessary healthcare, while the care of our environment, on which both our own health and the living world ultimately depend, gets short shrift?

27

Cutting Healthcare Down to Size

Medical care systems are the dinosaur of all institutions.
– Richard Carlson, *The End of Medicine*[1]

Despite nearly two decades of repeated intellectual efforts to redirect
health policy away from curative medicine to more fundamental
intervention, the task remains largely undone.
– T.R. Marmor, M.L. Barer, and R.G. Evans (1994)[2]

After World War II, when medicine began its first years of spectacular
success, many governments established publicly funded healthcare
services to bestow its benefits on all their citizens. These services were
created with great optimism. In Britain the authors of the Beveridge
Report, which fathered the National Health Service, finding the
health of the nation was poor, readily accepted that the initial cost of
the health service would be high. They assumed that once the "back-
log" of needy cases had been eliminated its cost would decline. They
assumed also that the savings accrued from anticipated reduction in
days lost through illness would help offset the cost of the service.[3]
Sadly, what seemed like the financial bargain of the century turned
into one of its more spectacular black holes; the cost of the service was
soon ten times greater than had been anticipated.[4]

In 1949, the first year of the National Health Service, it cost £433 million. Forty years later, in 1999, it cost £52,945 million; or more mean-
ingfully, the cost went from 3.5 per cent to 6.8 per cent of Britain's gross
national product. Its costs would have been even greater had not Britain
siphoned off doctors from its former colonies and, along with its own
junior doctors, exploited them unconscionably.[5] In Britain, as elsewhere, few people now want to relinquish these reassuring services, yet
they have left their creators disappointed, the recipients of care disgruntled, their healthcare practitioners unhappy, their sponsoring governments in a state of financial discomfort, and the number of work
days lost through sickness higher than before these services started.[6]

Britain is not alone in its healthcare dilemma. Speaking in 1991,
Hiroshi Nakajima, director general of the World Health Organization,
put the problem in a nutshell: "The health system is deteriorating
worldwide, in particular because of the continual rise in prices, both
in the rich countries and the developing nations."[7]

As governments and the insurance industry pour more money into healthcare, the healthcare industry both jacks up its prices and discovers an ever-increasing array of expensive treatments. No amount will ever be enough. In addition to having an insatiable appetite for money, much of modern medicine has been intrinsically disappointing. When compared to various social factors, medicine plays a relatively small role in keeping us healthy. However available treatment becomes, it cannot be expected significantly to improve our health indices.

René Dubos, in *The Mirage of Health,* in the early 1950s was the first modern writer seriously to question the belief that medicine was going to right our various ills.[8] By the 1970s other writers had followed suit. Ivan Illich argued in his best selling polemic *Medical Nemesis* that the medical establishment had become a threat to health, while various commentators showed in a more systematic way that there is little correlation between health and money spent on medical care.[9] Rich J. Carlson, an American lawyer, named his influential book *The End of Medicine.* Recognizing the diminishing impact that physicians and hospitals have on our health, Carlson predicted the gradual demise of modern medicine. [10]

But is Carlson wrong? Was he mistaken in his gloomy prognosis? Something big has happened in medicine. The Eldorado of new treatments is guaranteed to lever wads of research dollars from the coffers of science-ignorant politicians: the promise of the human genome has already done so. (George Bush, seemingly still stuck with the homunculus concept of conception, proudly announced his financial support of the Human *Gnome* Initiative.[11]) The initiative was a success. In a race to the finish, investigators have virtually succeeded in sequencing the 3 billion DNA molecules of the human genome. Will this deciphering of *God's manual for our creation* rescue medicine's declining fortunes?

Besides enlivening many areas of academic endeavour, the breaking of the genome's digital code is claimed to have great promise for medicine. Perhaps it does. Leaving aside the tricky possibility of splicing new genes into our genome,[12] the achievement opens up vistas of medical possibilities. The simplest of these possibilities, and one that is already in wide use, is the identification of disease-causing genes in the foetus, and its subsequent abortion. I doubt that either of the presidential Bushes would approve of the *gnome* initiative being put to such use but, for families aware that they harbour such genes, the potential avoidance of another family member's having a horrible hereditary illness is a godsend.

The extent to which such gene identification and abortion will lower the burden of hereditary illness remains to be seen. Couples are often lackadaisical about pregnancy and half of all pregnancies occur by accident. Even though the damaging effects of alcohol upon the foetus have been well recognized for nearly thirty years, the disaster of foetal alcohol syndrome (FAS) has not diminished. FAS remains the most common cause of mental retardation in the Western world and its victims add substantially to the population of North American prisons. It is not always possible to put knowledge into action.

Genes are the blueprints for the control mechanisms of the many thousands of chemical processes that comprise life, and the sequencing of DNA has made gene identification much simpler. Although we share about half our 30,000 genes with a one-millimetre-long roundworm, all but 300 of them with mice, and about 99% of them with chimpanzees, there is still sufficient gene variation among humans that individuals often respond differently to the same medication. What cures one person can be lethal for another. One day it may be possible to obtain a profile of a person's chemical processes. Doctors could then prescribe a useful rather than a harmful drug. How feasible will such measures be?

The pharmaceutical industry clearly believes that genes will be profitable. As pieces of chromosome are marked out and their genes patented, pharmaceutical companies are buying up huge tracts of these highly priced DNA estates. But owning a gene and knowing what it does, are two different things, especially as a gene may perform several totally unrelated functions. Instruction manuals are often the pits, but God's manual as to how we work is no exception; it is the most confusing ever. Will we ever make sense of it?

James Le Fanu, a respected English medical journalist, in his latest book, *The Rise and Fall of Modern Medicine,* argues that the "Golden Age of Medicine" that started after World War II had come to an end by the mid 1970s.[13] The *easy* or serendipitous medical discoveries had all been made, and chemists were running out of new substances to test. The cornucopia of new drugs is drying up so that the few drugs in the pipeline will be exorbitantly expensive. The antibiotics and anti-malarial drugs are losing their magic and mankind's old killers are reasserting their prowess. Le Fanu suggests that the "New Genetics," while keeping alive medicine's promise, has in fact contributed little of any practical value and is unlikely to do so for the foreseeable future.[14]

Perhaps the pharmaceutical companies are investing so heavily in the uncertainty of genes because, with so few fresh pharmacological ideas around, they do not know what else to do with their profits. Maybe we have just entangled ourselves in costly but unusable chains of DNA. Time will tell, but whatever else, such future medical care will probably be too expensive for most people to afford.

How much do our expensive healthcare services contribute to our good health? As part of a series of health insurance experiments, the Rand Corporation examined the effects of different levels of healthcare availability on people's health. Two thousand volunteer families were randomly assigned to one of several health insurance plans providing various levels of financial support for their healthcare needs. One plan provided all care free, while the other plans involved some cost sharing with the participants. Not surprisingly, the people who shared the cost of healthcare used fewer services, having about one-third fewer outpatient visits and hospital admissions than did the families with free care.

But what difference did the "one-third" additional make to the families with free care? After five years, the investigators compared the health status of people in the "free group" and in the "cost-sharing groups" and found two significant differences. People in the "free group" had a lower mean diastolic blood pressure and they could read smaller letters on the optician's vision-testing chart (Snellene's test). The hypertensives in the free group had their high blood pressure better controlled, and the short-sighted had their glasses renewed more often.

The Rand authors concluded: People, having specific conditions with well-established diagnostic and therapeutic procedures (myopia or hypertension), especially those in low income groups, benefit from increased availability of healthcare but, all other things beings equal, the greater availability of healthcare does not equate to better health.[15] A study by the Organization for Economic Co-operation and Development (OECD) into the health effects of the massive retrenchment in healthcare spending during the 1990s by its 29 member countries, found "paradoxically the effort to better contain cost led to more effective health care with better outcomes."[16] The World Bank reports that money spent on housing and better social services does more to improve health than money spent on building hospitals and direct healthcare.[17]

When one looks at healthcare spending and improved health in the developed countries, it seems that a "first shall be last" situation prevails. Japan spends almost the smallest proportion of its national wealth on health but in the 1980s its life expectancy caught up with, and now comfortably surpasses, that of the rest of the developed world.[18] The United States spends a greater proportion of its wealth on healthcare than does any other country but, when ranked with other countries in order of life expectancy, it stands only in thirty-seventh place – lagging behind such countries as Oman and Morocco.[19] As for infant mortality rates, the OECD 1998 Health Data for the 29 developed countries shows the United States near the bottom in the twenty-fifth place.[20]

We continue to work on the assumption that "if some medical care is useful, more would be better."[21] We have more of it. By 1998 Canada, for instance, spent more on healthcare than on education, and is scheduled to do so in increasing amounts. If we continue this way, we will be cooking the golden-egg-laying goose, for modern medicine is unsustainable without the affluence generated by a well educated community.[22]

While additional healthcare spending has diminishing returns, it creates an escalating problem. Entrepreneurs, big and small, prefer to go where the money is and the big money is now in healthcare. Illness expands to use the healthcare dollars available. Doctors and other healthcare practitioners seldom sit and wait for work to come their way, they make their own. Any healthcare practitioner who knows the rules of the game or any purveyor of latter day nostrums, from industrial chemists to backyard herbalists, can quickly convince the worried-well that they are sick or are about to become so, and doubtless need treatment. Into the bargain, because treatment is a motherhood issue, insurance companies and governments can usually be manipulated into paying for it. Any attempt to limit such payment is labelled the "rationing of healthcare" – the death knell to any government that tries to do it.

When suppliers of treatment determine its demand, we have an economic situation in which demand soon becomes unlimited.[23] The growth of healthcare costs in the United States demonstrates the results of such perverse economics. The Office of the Actuary of the Health Care Financing Administration reports that the annual per capita outlay for medical care has increased 200-fold over the past thirty years, from $204 in 1965 to $4,100 in 1995. If medical expenditures are allowed to increase at the same rate over the next thirty years the average annual per capita outlay by 2025 will be $82,000.[24] In 1998, 44 million Americans could not afford healthcare premiums, and each year another million are added to the list of the medically unprotected.[25]

Daniel Callahan, distinguished co-founder of the Hastings Center, the prestigious health research institute for bioethics in New York, in his book *False Hopes*, argues that America's hypochondriacal quest for perfect health has become an unsustainable impediment to normality.[26] The excellent becomes the enemy of the good. The huge costs of this enterprise both deprive people of basic healthcare and impose a heavy financial burden on the community at large.[27] Expensive medical care is counterproductive. It does little to reduce sickness but it certainly increases the number of *have-nots*.

Inevitably, in modern societies, as the numbers of our "kith and kin wither and thin," the state steps in as the all-providing care-giving surrogate parent. An effective parent, however, has two essential tasks: to provide care when it is needed and to withhold it when it is not. Failure to do either can create ever-deepening cycles of dependency. Spokespersons for the state, politicians and professionals, prefer to be perceived as caring providers: like the worst of parents, they promise the earth but deliver peanuts.[28]

As far as the economics of the healthcare industry are concerned, nurses are a dead loss. They neither prescribe remunerative treatments nor order expensive investigations. To cut costs, high-tech healthcare economizes on nurses' salaries. Also, for good or bad, young women are now much less prepared to be at the beck and call of the sick. Recruitment into nursing is falling and practising nurses are getting older. Professional healthcare administrators manage those nurses who remain in the system to distraction and nurses opt for early retirement.[29] Our healthcare services go from crisis to crisis. The officials who run them veer between trying to contain costs, and defusing the anger of patients and families for the inadequacies of the services they provide. Worse is yet to come. Half of all healthcare spending goes on the healthcare needs of people over 65, and the numbers of old fogies like me are mounting. When the baby boomers slide into decrepitude, they will be lucky to get even a bedpan.[30]

When healthcare is orchestrated by healthcare practitioners, it quickly becomes too expensive to be affordable.[31] We may choose to believe that healthcare is our right, but unless we make some changes in our healthcare delivery systems healthcare will not be there when most of us would like it to be.

Science, with its astonishing discoveries and inventions, has contributed enormously to our prosperity and hence to human health. It is science that has given us x-rays and all the other technologies that have made our medical miracles possible. While medicine has accomplished some remarkable feats in the last few decades, however, it has also remained distressingly static. While science in general has become greatly sophisticated in its understanding of uncertainty and complex events, medicine has boxed itself in with a simplistic pre-Copernican approach to the complex antecedents of illness.[32] It is stuck with a practitioner-centred model unsuited either for understanding the multifaceted antecedents of health, or for the effective provision of the community's healthcare needs. Just as the clergy once resisted the displacement of the earth from the centre of the universe (and, of course, the displacement of their own authority), the helping professions resist changes that displace them from the centre of human health. Good health requires more than good medicine.

It would be wonderful if our healthcare and legal services were as beneficial to us as they are to the professionals who provide them.[33] Fortunately for the survival of civilization, entrepreneurs will always be with us, though perhaps a sensible society would manage to put their skills to more constructive use. The huge upsurge of interest in alternative methods may not add much to health, but it demonstrates people's wide commitment to staying well when they are allowed to become active participants in the endeavour. Perhaps society's central healthcare question should be: how to encourage practitioners to collaborate with their patients to become better decision makers?[34]

It is one thing to pay practitioners well for work that needs doing and another to remunerate them for work that is unnecessary. The moguls of healthcare notwithstanding, it probably is possible to design healthcare systems that:

- are pleasant, humane, and effective;
- will not bankrupt the community;
- will not encourage practitioners to manufacture unnecessary illnesses;
- will not demoralize these practitioners so that they go elsewhere.

Designing such systems will require understanding, ingenuity, flexibility, and experimentation, combined with much public support.[35]

Maybe the critics of modern medicine are right that medicine with its determination to produce perfect health, has outworn its welcome. Health is not "a state of complete physical, mental, and social well-being," it is a capacity, despite the vicissitudes of life, to find "a place in the sun" and a chance to add to the rich panoply of life. Not all our ills require expensive treatment; some do better without. By relinquishing our hypochondriacal determination to find a cure (or a compensation) for every ill, we might succeed in designing healthcare services that are accessible when we need them and sufficiently solvent to allow us to incorporate and make available some of the exciting medical innovations that will result from our knowledge of the human genome.

Appendixes

Medical words confuse the laity and the proliferation of acronyms increases the comprehension gap between doctors and the non-medical public. I have done my best to avoid these abbreviations, but since acronyms are now an integral part of the medical literature, I have had to make exceptions. I have interpreted any acronym on first using it, but for any reader who overlooks this interpretation, I have provided below a list of acronyms accompanied by their meanings.

AIDS	Acquired immunity deficiency syndrome
ACR	American College of Rheumatology
BI	Bodily injury
BSS	Burning semen syndrome
CFIDS	Chronic fatigue immune dysfunction syndrome
CFS	Chronic fatigue syndrome
CPS	Chronic pain syndrome
CT SCAN	Computed tomography scan
DNA	Desoxyibonucleic acid (gene material)
DSM	Diagnostic and Statistical Manual of the American Psychiatric Association
EEG	Electroencephalogram
ENT	Ear, nose, and throat (surgeon)
ER	Emergency room
FAS	Foetal alcohol syndrome
FDA	Food and Drug Administration (U.S.)
GHQ28	General Health Questionnaire with 28 Questions
GWS	Gulf war syndrome
JAMA	Journal of the American Medical Association

ME	Myalgic encephalomyelitis
MMPI	Minnesota Multiple Personality Inventory
MRI	Magnetic Resonance Imaging
MVA	Motor vehicle accident
NHS	National Health Service (Britain)
OECD	Organization for Economic Co-operation and Development
OHIP	Ontario Hospital Insurance Plan
PLFS	Perilymph fistula syndrome
PTA	Post-traumatic amnesia
PTSD	Post-traumatic stress disorder
RCT	Randomized controlled trial
RSI	Repetitive stress syndrome
SPECT	Single photon emission computed tomography
SSRI	Specific serotonin uptake inhibitor (a group of antidepressants)
TBI	Traumatic brain injury
TM(J)(D)	Temporomandibular (joint) disorder
UFFI	Urea formaldehyde foam insulation
VA	Veterans Administration (U.S.)
WADS	Whiplash-associated disorders

APPENDIX 2:

THE USE OF PROSPECTIVE STUDIES AND RTCS

These two instruments are so central to the practice of sensible medicine that I will compare them to *retrospective* studies and provide an example of how they are used. It has to do with candies. Just in the way that many people are convinced that whiplash causes prolonged neck and other problems, so many parents, following some inspirational medical theories of a few decades back, are convinced that sugar causes children to become disturbed and unruly. Retrospective and prospective studies can be employed to determine if parents are right – if rambunctious children really should be deprived of candies.

In a retrospective study, the unruly children are matched as closely as possible with the docile and amenable. The consumption of sugar for each group is then estimated. If the unruly children are found to have eaten significantly more chocolate bars and jellybeans than the amenable children, then the parents are right, the candies must go. But then again, perhaps they needn't! There is a problem with retrospective studies. It is, for instance, not simple to measure retrospectively the consumption of sugar. What one parent considers a trifle, another considers a blow-out. Do the parents really know the amounts of "white poison" their children actually consume – what about the thriving trade in contraband jellybeans? Does behaviour live up to expectation? If a brainwashed child believes eating Mars bars will make him bad, will eating two of them make him worse?

In a prospective study, the study children are randomly divided into two groups (a randomized control trial), the one group being given sugar and the other an artificial sweetener; the children's behaviour is then assessed *double blind*. Double blind means that neither the children nor the assessors know which group has received the sugar or the artificial sweetener.

In point of fact, 16 such prospective studies on the effect of sugar on children's behaviour have been reported in the literature.[1] In some studies, the children chosen for the investigation were the very children whose parents complained of the disastrous effects of sugar consumption upon their behaviour. Often also, the parents formed part of the assessment teams. Fifteen of these sixteen studies showed that there was no significant difference in the behaviour of the children who had received sugar and those who had received an artificial sweetener. In the one exception to these 15 studies, sugar was found to have a mildly calming effect upon the children who had received it.[2]

Preconceived ideas die hard, and most parents will probably remain convinced that the candy bar slipped to Johnny that morning by an indulgent aunt is the cause of his obstreperous conduct. The "Twinkie defence," arguing that a violent criminal, because he had consumed a diet too high in carbohydrate, is not responsible for his actions may remain "legal junk science" (see chapter 17) but a doctor of scientific integrity can no longer maintain that sugar is a probable cause of disturbed behaviour.[3] Of course, such controlled experiments cannot rule out the possibility that sugar could cause disturbed behaviour since, unless everyone in the whole world is tested, there may always be the one exception. However, the combined weight of these prospective studies demonstrates that if sugar does cause disturbed behaviour it does so with such infrequency as to be immeasurable by ordinary scientific means.

Misconceptions take their toll on health. Parents seek to limit the deleterious effects of sugar; the occasional glorious chocolate binge is replaced by the more manageable unruly-behaviour-invoking dose of just one candy after meals. While children's teeth can cope with the occasional binge, however, it is the constant sugar coating of the behaviour-controlling regime that is likely to cause caries!

APPENDIX 3:
EVIDENCE AGAINST RESIDUAL BRAIN INJURY
BEING THE CAUSE OF POST-CONCUSSION SYNDROME
AFTER MINOR HEAD INJURY

Much is known about severe head injury and its outcome. Severe-head-injury patients frequently die, making their brains available for study. Furthermore, for either seizure prevention or control, surviving patients generally remain under ongoing medical care, making it logistically easy to monitor their progress. Many studies on outcome are available. In contrast, there are far fewer outcome studies of minor (mild) head injury. Those studies that are available mostly show that the prognoses of such injuries are good.

Many people with a minor head injury recover unobtrusively. Minor head injury is common, and most people are not particularly bothered by it. Herbert F. Crovitz (1983) and his team at the Veterans' Administration Hospital, North Carolina, in a retrospective survey of 1000 young adults, found that 24% of males and 16% of females reported a previous head injury with loss of consciousness.

Jess F. Kraus and Parovash Nourjah (1988), epidemiologists from the University of California, analysed the data on 2,435 San Diego County residents consecutively admitted to hospital with mild head injury. The median hospital stay of the mild-head-injury patients was 2 to 3 days. All but 15 of these 2,435 patients were discharged without further planned medical contact, and all but three were rated as having made a good recovery. The problem from a medico-legal point of view is that none of these patients were neuropsychologically assessed, so it is possible to argue that these mild-head-injury patients were left cognitively impaired but their deficits escaped the investigators' attention.

However, another study comes to the rescue. Robin Jacobson (1995), a psychiatrist at St George's Hospital Medical School in London, reviewed all the published studies on post-concussion syndrome in which the head-injured patients were neuropsychologically assessed. He found that most studies reported some disturbance of attention, memory, and information-processing efficiency during the first few days after injury, but this disturbance disappeared by the three-month follow-up. Of course, that most patients recover by three months puts joy into the plaintiff-personal-injury-litigation-lawyer's heart, for if only most patients recover by three months, then *most certainly* his was one of the few who did not.

The plaintiff lawyer should not rejoice too soon. The study has problems, and there are two reasons to suspect that the results of various post-concussion syndrome studies reviewed by Jacobson are biased towards the finding of a high incidence of ongoing problems. The studies that Jacobson reviewed included those in which the post-concussion syndrome complicated not only mild closed-head injuries, but moderate and severe injury as well.

Mixing minor and severe closed-head injury together is like doing an outcome study of the common cold but adding in some cases of pneumonia – it would be easy to get the impression that colds can be dangerous. Also, many studies did not include controls. In head-injury studies, the more controls used and the more consideration given to the pre-injury status of the patients, the less significant the head-injury symptoms were found to be.[4] The authors of two head-injury outcome studies were careful to choose appropriate controls.

Massimo Gentilini (1985) and his colleagues from the University of Modena, Italy, neuropsychologically assessed 50 patients with mild head injury. Each head-injured patient was compared to a control matched for age and gender chosen from amongst the friends and relatives of the patient's spouse. The psychometric assessments were made one month after the accident. The investigators found no conclusive evidence that mild head injury causes cognitive impairment one month after the trauma.

Freda Newcombe (1994) and her colleagues from the Department of Neurosurgery at the Radcliffe Infirmary, Oxford, neuropsychologically assessed 20 head-injured men (aged 16–30) and compared them to 20 controls of similar economic background who had been admitted for orthopaedic treatment. The PTA of these 20 subjects did not exceed 8 hours – a PTA which puts the head injury into the category of moderate. These subjects were assessed within 48 hours of the accident and again one month later. No significant difference was found between the two groups other than slightly lower scores on two of a series of tests at the 48-hour assessment. This study suggests that even in head injury of moderate severity, the measurable cognitive changes are slight and soon disappear. The authors comment: "It is suggested that the appropriate management and counselling of mildly head-injured patients may help to avert symptoms that are of psychological rather than pathophysiological origin." I doubt these authors would consider the management of head injury by a personal injury litigation lawyer as "appropriate management and counselling," yet this is exactly how many head-injured patients are now managed!

In life, we have choices. A minor head injury is the kind of event we can take in our stride or choose to make out of it an inordinate song and dance. People who opt for the former seldom seem to have problems with their "brains" while those who opt for the latter never seem to stop having them. Post-concussion syndrome frequently follows industrial and traffic accidents but seldom occurs after recreational accidents. Context makes all the difference to post-concussion syndrome.[5]

Clinicians, neuropsychologists, and lawyers mostly see only those minor head-injury patients who opt for the song and dance – a process of selection that no doubt colours their opinions about the possible after-effects of this injury. Lawrence M. Binder, a distinguished neuropsychologist from Oregon, after an extensive meta-analytic review of neuropsychological studies, considered the false-positive diagnosis of brain dysfunction so common that clinicians are more likely to be statistically correct with a diagnosis of "no brain injury" than with one of "brain injury."[6]

APPENDIX 4:

OVERVALUATION OF HEALTHCARE

Doctors and patients alike share a profound but mistaken belief in the decisive role that treatment plays in the maintenance of our good health. Some
years ago, two colleagues and I performed a study that illustrates that this is
so.[7] We selected six easily identifiable diseases, five of which were once major
killers but are now rare causes of death.[8] The sixth "disease" was suicide. As the
U.K. has for many years kept reasonably reliable statistics on the causes of
death, we used English data. We prepared graphs of the annual death rates for
each of our selected diseases but only put in the actual figures for the years
1865 and 1970, leaving the years in between blank. We wrote a short brief for
each disease containing information on when effective treatment and immu-
nization procedures became available. We stressed the importance of good
nutrition and a healthy environment in reducing the severity of many infectious diseases. In the brief accompanying the suicide graph, we noted that war
reduces the suicide rate and a downturn in the economic cycle increases it.

We selected three groups of subjects: final-year medical students, non-medical students and non-medical professors, all from the University of Toronto.
We gave each of our subjects the briefs and incomplete graphs, and asked
them to estimate the annual mortality rates by completing the graphs for the
years between 1865 and 1970. We then averaged out the responses for each
group. Although the non-medical professors were a little closer to reality than
the other two groups, the results for the three groups were so similar that for
simplicity's sake I have combined and averaged all the responses. (Malleson,
Eastwood, Moore 1977; also Figure 26–1.)

Notes

INTRODUCTORY EPIGRAPHS

1 Hodge (1971)
2 Wright (1994)
3 Evans and Stoddart in Evans, Barer, Marmor (1994) 55

HEALTH CARE ENTREPRENEURS IN SEARCH OF WORK

1 Insurance Research Council Inc. (1995)
2 Durr (1994)

CHAPTER ONE

1 Insurance Research Council Inc. (1995)
2 Deans (1986); Evans (1992); Hohl (1974); O'Neill, Haddon, Jr., et al (1972)
3 Evans (1992); Wiesel, Fetter, Rothman (1986)
4 Rogal (1987)
5 Barnsley, Lord, Bogduk (1994)
6 Livingston (1999)
7 Ommaya, Faas, Yarnell (1968)
8 Mandel (1992); Radanov, Dvorak, Valach (1992); Selecki (1984); Shapiro, Torres (1960); Varney, Bushnell, et al (1995)
9 Janjua, Goswami, Sagar (1996); La Rocca (1991)
10 Radanov, Di Stefano, et al (1994). These authors are the world's most prolific writers on whiplash and it is appropriate therefore to use their definition of common whiplash.
11 Teasell, Shapiro, Maillis (1993) are top Canadian whiplash experts. Strauss, Savitsky (1934), from the Academic University Hospital in

Uppsala, Sweden, warn, "Most physicians are unaware of the potential severity of the injury, and only a few patients are reassessed routinely for possible missed injuries after the initial examination. Emergency x-rays are usually normal and may contribute to the physician's perception of whiplash lesions as benign and self-limiting conditions." Hirsch, Hirsch, et al (1988) are orthopaedic surgeons from the University of Medicine and Dentistry of New Jersey. They write: "Whiplash injury is the most common cervical injury associated with rear-end impact motor vehicles, resulting in a complex injury, often associated with extensive soft tissue injury in the cervical spine."

12 Radanov, Di Stefano, et al (1994)

13 Teasell, McCain, et al (1991)

14 Barnsley, Lord, Bogduk (1993a)

15 Evans (1992); McKinney (1994); Milicic, Jovanovic, et al (1994); Rogal (1987)

16 Bingham (1968)

17 Algers, Pettersson, et al (1993); Balla (1980); Balla, Karnaghan (1987); Braaf, Rosner (1955); Carlow (1993); Di Stefano, Radanov (1993); Epstein (1992); Evans (1992); Foletti, Regli (1995); Lord, Barnsley, et al (1994); Magnússon (1994); Merskey (1986); Milicic, Jovanovic, et al (1994); Taylor, Cox, Maillis (1994); Weiss, Stern, Goldberg (1991); Wiley, Lloyd, et al (1986); Yarnell, Rossie (1988)

18 Kreeft (1993)

19 Braaf, Rosner (1958)

20 Barnsley, Lord, Bogduk (1993); Middleton (1956); Naf (1978); Selecki (1984)

21 La Rocca (1991), professor of orthopaedic surgery at Tulane University School of Medicine, New Orleans, reports that this syndrome presents with the most taxing and challenging features arising from the damaged sympathetic nervous system.

22 Christman, Gervais (1962)

23 Gennarelli, Thibault, et al (1982); Martinez, Wickstrom, Barcelo (1965); Ommaya, Faas, Yarnell (1968); Underharnscheidt (1983); Wickstrom, Martinez, Rodriguez (1967)

24 Burke, Orton, et al (1992); Daily (1970); Fite (1970); Gibson (1968); Haslett, Duvall-Young, McGalliard (1994); Horwich, Kasner (1962); Katano (Jul 1970); Kelley, Hoover, George (1978); Knight (1959); Middleton (1956); Roca (1972); Wiesinger, Guerry (1962)

25 Chester (1991); Compere, (1968); Grimm, Hemenway, et al (1989); Hart (1979); Oosterveld, Kortschot, et al (1991); Rubin (1973); Shapiro (1972); Toglia (1972); Toglia (1976); Woods (1965); Woods, Compere (1969)

26 Abdel-Fattah (1996); Braun, Schiffman (1991); Burgess (1991);

Capurso, Perillo, Ferro (1992); Epstein (1992); Frankel (1965); Fricton (1993); Levandoski (1993b); Levandoski (1993a); Mannheimer, Attanasio, et al (1989); Moses, Skoog (1986); Olin (1990); Pressman, Shellock, et al (1992); Roydhouse (1973); Schneider, Zernicke, Clark (1989); Weinberg, Lapointe (1987)

27 Braaf, Rosner (1955); Croft, Foreman (1988); Hildingsson, Toolanen (1990); Hohl (1974); Magnússon (1994); Wiley, Lloyd, et al (1986)

28 Merskey (1993); Teasell (1993)

29 Evans (1992); Magnússon (1994); McCain (1993); Percy (1994)

30 Kuch, Cox, Evans (1996)

31 Severy, Mathewson, Bechtol (1955); Williams, McKenzie (1975)

32 McKenzie and Williams (1971)

33 La Rocca (1991)

34 Seletz (1958)

35 Bingham (1968)

36 Maigne (1972)

37 Croft (1988)

38 Evans (1992); Schutt, Dohan (1968)

39 Dunn, Blazar (1987); States, Korn, Masengill (1970); Wiley, Lloyd, et al (1986)

40 Pearce (1989)

41 Nygren (1984)

42 Balla (1980)

43 Barnsley, Lord, Bogduk (1993a)

44 Spitzer, Skovron, et al (1995)

CHAPTER TWO

1 Marwick (1998); Spitzer, Skovron, et al (1995); Spitzer, Skovron, et al (1995)

2 Dunn, Blazar (1987); McIntire (1956)

3 Crowe (1964); Evans (1992).

4 Crowe (1964)

5 Davis (1945); Evans (1995)

6 Walz (1994)

7 William Gissane (1966,1967).

8 Gay and Abbott (1953)

9 Denny-Brown and Russell (1941)

10 Walz (1987,1994), a Swiss expert in biomechanics stresses, demonstrated that in ordinary traffic collisions even the second phase of the whiplash motion is insignificant. Grunsten (1989) and his colleagues from the Naval Biodynamics Laboratory in New Orleans studied the effects of rapid acceleration on 112 enlisted volunteers. Each volunteer, placed on

a sled, was tightly tied to the seat while the head and neck remained free. A piston delivered a sudden shove to the sled which delivered a thrust to the volunteer of up to 14 g – approximating an instantaneous acceleration to 40 mph. The movements of the head and neck were tracked with cameras and other sophisticated measuring equipment. It was observed that the muscular recoil brings the head back to approximately the initial neutral position.

11 Macnab (1971); Macnab (1982)
12 Alker Jr, Young, et al (1975); Allen, Barnes, Bodinah (1985); Bucholz, Burkhead, et al (1979); Cain, Ryan, et al (1989); Caldwell (15 Apr 1972); Davis, Bohlman, et al (1971); Deans, Magalliard, et al (1987); Jonsson, Bring, et al (1991); Jonsson, Cisarini, et al (1995); La Rocca (1991); Roydhouse (1985); Teife, Degrief, et al (1993); Tounge, O'Reilly, et al (1972); Twomey, Taylor, Taylor (1989); Caldwell (15 Apr 1972)
13 Sturzenegger, Di Stefano, et al (1994)
14 Barnsley, Lord, Bogduk (1993b)
15 Hirsch, Ommaya, Mahone (1970); Macnab (1966); Martinez, Wickstrom, Barcelo (1965); Ommaya, Faas, Yarnell (1968); Underharnscheidt (1983); Wickstrom, Martinez, et al (1970); Wickstrom, Martinez, Rodriguez (1967)
16 Macnab (1966)
17 Wickstrom, Martinez, Rodriguez (1967)
18 Ommaya, Faas, Yarnell (1968)
19 Gennarelli, Thibault, et al (1982); Underharnscheidt (1983)
20 Braaf, Rosner (1966)
21 Barnsley, Lord, Bogduk (1993b); Braaf, Rosner (1966); Burke, Orton, et al (1992); Croft (1988); Fite (1970); Fitz-Ritson (1991); Gibson (1968); Hirsch, Ommaya, Mahone (1970); La Rocca (1991); Larder, Twiss, Mackey (1985); Lord, Bogduk, Barnsley (1993); Merskey (1986); Pang (1971); Pennie, Agambar (1991); Sweeney (1992); Toglia, Rosenberg, Ronis (1969); Toglia, Rosenberg, Ronis (1970)
22 Hirsch, Ommaya, Faas (1970).
23 DM Severy is an orthopaedic surgeon at Yale who worked at the Institute of Transportation and Traffic Engineering at California. Severy, Mathewson, and Bechtol (1955), in their classic paper on controlled automobile rear-end collisions, provide figures for the size of the forces involved in rear-end collisions. Using Plymouths to rear-end other Plymouths at speeds ranging from 7 to 20 mph, they found that the acceleration of the front car ranged from 4 to 7 g, and the acceleration of the heads of the human volunteers in the car ranged from 3 to 12 g. Robert Ferrari and Anthony Russell (1997), from the Department of Medicine at the University of Alberta, estimate the forces used in the

animal experiments "were 10 to 50 times greater than the forces experienced in collisions producing whiplash patients."

24 Wickstrom, Martinez, Rodriguez (1967)

25 Norris (1991)

26 Barnsley, Lord, Bogduk (1993)

27 La Rocca (1996)

28 Macnab (1966); Martinez, Wickstrom, Barcelo (1965); Ommaya, Faas, Yarnell (1968); Wickstrom, Martinez, Rodriguez (1967)

29 Pennie, Agambar (1991)

30 Frankel (1959)

31 Seletz (1958)

32 Deans (1986)

33 Livingston (1998)

34 Porter (1989)

35 Lancet Editorial (1991)

36 An English pound roughly equals two American dollars.

37 Whiplash search http://www.lawtel.co

38 AMS v PAC, QBD 28/11/95 M0003439 Reading LTL 7/12/95

39 Livingston (1991); Livingston (1992)

40 Ratliff (1997)

41 Charles Galasko quoted by Livingston (1999)

42 Macnab (1971)

CHAPTER THREE

1 Parmar, Raymakers (1993)

2 Pearce (1994)

3 Melville (1963)

4 Henry Berry, Toronto neurologist: Absence of whiplash in demolition derbies. Personal communication (1995)

5 Castro and his colleagues (1997) from the Westfälischen Wilhelms-Universität compared the effects on the neck of collisions between standard cars and collisions between bumper cars of the type featured in amusement parks. Using 19 volunteers, the mean velocity of collision was 11.4 km/h for the standard cars and 9.9 km/h for the bumper cars. Electronic measuring devices showed the forces to which the volunteers were subjected in standard car collisions were in the same range as those in the bumper car crashes. Only one volunteer suffered any symptoms or was found to have any signs of injury after the collisions. The one volunteer with symptoms had a ten-degree reduction of cervical rotation that persisted for ten weeks. The authors point out that about half of whiplash injury claims made in Germany involve accidents in which the velocity of collision is less than 15 km/h.

6 Ferrari, Russell (1997); McConnell, Howard, et al (1993); Mertz, Patrick (1967a); Thomas, Ewing, Majewski (1979); West, Gough, Harper (1993)

7 Balla (1982); Schrader, Obelieniene, et al (1996)

8 Barnsley, Lord, Bogduk (1993)

9 John Balla (1982), the neurologist from Prince Henry's Hospital in Melbourne, compared the rates of chronic whiplash syndrome in both countries.

10 Mills, Horne (1986); Awerbuch (1992)

11 Spitzer, Skovron, et al (1995) See also Livingston (1999a)

12 Belli (1970)

13 Iceland, for instance, is a thinly populated country where it is still possible to drive for many miles without seeing another car. Working in Reykjavik, Magnússon and his Icelandic colleagues published the results of an occipital nerve release operation on thirteen whiplash patients. It must have taken a large number of whiplash patients to find 13 requiring this uncommon operation (Magnússon, Ragnarsson, Bjornsson 1996).

14 Partheni, Miliaris, et al (1999); Partheni, et al (1997); Backletter Editorial (1997): Two new studies question the basis for whiplash claims. The Backletter, 12, 133 and 142

15 Trimble (1981)

16 Schrader (1996)

17 Grady (11 May 1996)

18 Bjørgen (1996)

19 de Mol, Heijer (1996)

20 Freeman, Croft (1996)

21 Radanov (1997)

22 Merskey (1997): Merskey is playing fast and loose with Mother Nature. She has good reason for making women forget the pains and discomforts of childbirth for, without this amnesic anodyne, the human race might soon peter out. Conversely, if we forget how painful it is being charged by a rhinoceros, we might not take care to avoid rhinoceroses in future, and be less likely to survive and perpetuate our genes.

23 In reporting this study, I have substituted "average" for the statistical term "median." While "average" is not technically correct, it makes little difference to the import of the study's findings and it is likely to be more widely understood.

24 Obelieniene, Schrader, et al (1999)

25 See Deans, Magalliard, et al (1987). These authors list some of the many previous studies showing that whiplash is "disproportionately common after rear impact accidents."

26 Macnab (1971)

27 Macnab (1973)

28 Janecki, Lipke (1978)

29 Pennie, Agambar (1991)

30 Of these 30 patients, 6 had a fractured pelvis, 18 a fracture of the tibia, 15 a fractured femur, 3 a fractured ankle, and 3 more had fractures of a forearm, sternum or ribs.

31 Khan, McCormack, et al (1997)

32 Dunn, Blazar (1987); McIntire (1956)

33 Mertz, Patrick (1967b)

34 Irvin (19 Jan 1971)

35 O'Neill, Haddon, et al (1972)

36 Olney, Marsden (1986)

37 Haddon, Goddard (1962) found that 74 per cent of male and 56 per cent of female drivers had their head restraints improperly positioned, but even so it seems reasonable to suppose that head restraints should have made a bigger blip in the whiplash statistics. See also Olney, Marsden (1986).

38 Ferrari, Russell (1997); Malleson (1996)

39 Economist (27 February 1999)

40 Hirsch, Nachemson (1961)

41 Nachemson (1994)

42 Cassidy, Carroll, et al (2000)

43 National Highway Traffic Safety Administration (1998)

44 Toronto Transit Commission. Russell Hill Subway Train Accident 1995.

45 Talaga (1995)

46 The Cross Examination of Mrs O (1996). NO 95-CU-89529, NO 95-CU-89529. Ontario Court of Justice. Taken before Paul W Rosenberger, Official Examiner. TTC Subway Accident File.

CHAPTER FOUR

1 American Psychiatric Association (1994); Keaton, Ries, Kleinman (1984)

2 Keaton, Ries, Kleinman (1984)

3 Keaton, Ries, Kleinman (1984)

4 Leighton, Hughes, et al (1963); Strole, Langer, et al (1962)

5 Shepherd, Cooper, et al (1966)

6 Haller, Haller (1974), 195–234

7 Philippe Ariès (1962), Chapter 2: The discovery of childhood, 33–49, provides an excellent account of when, how and why the Church inculcating into its flock an abhorrence of masturbation.

8 The mental hospital attached to Britain's prestigious Institute of Psychiatry immortalizes his name.

9 Maudsley (1868)

10 Wool, Barsky (1994)
11 McWinney, Epstein, Freeman (1997)
12 Macfarlane, Morris, et al (1999); Nemiah (1975); von Korff, Ormel, et al (1992)
13 Epstein, Quill, McWinney (1999)
14 Lees-Haley, Brown (1993)
15 THM (1982)
16 Shorter (1992)
17 Quill (1985): Somatization Disorder: One of Medicine's Blind Spots.
18 Quill (1985)
19 Kral (1951)
20 FS Skey (1866): surgeon at St. Bartholomew's Hospital, quoted by S.A. Kinnier Wilson (1931)
21 Peabody (1927)
22 Peveler (1998)

CHAPTER FIVE

1 Marx (1928)
2 Ferrari, Russell (1997)
3 Ross (1999)
4 St Clare: The Gentleman's Magazine 1787, 268; quoted by Bartholomew, Sirois (2000)
5 Bartholomew, Sirois (2000)
6 Tyrer (1994)
7 Departmental Committee on Telegraphists' Cramp. (1911); Reilly (1995a); Tyrer (1994)
8 Bell (1989); Cleland (1987)
9 Raffle (1963)
10 Bell (1989)
11 Bell (1989)
12 Littlejohn (1989)
13 Bell (1989)
14 Bell (1989)
15 Littlejohn (1989)
16 American Psychiatric Association (1994)
17 Abrahamson, Pezet (1951); Ford, Bray, Swerdloff (1976); Fredericks (1969); Steincrohn (1972)
18 Ford, Bray, Swerdloff (1976)
19 Carson (1962)
20 ACOEM position statement (1999)
21 Stewart, Raskin (1985)
22 See the position statement of the American College of Occupational and

Environmental Medicine (ACOEM) 1999, for a reliable synopsis of their findings.

23 Terr (1986), from the department of immunology at Stanford, examined 50 disabled workers who attributed their illness to twentieth-century disease. He found no consistent physical, laboratory, or immunological abnormalities. Many other investigators have substantiated these negative findings. See also the ACOEM position statement.

24 Marco (1987)

25 Gots (1997) also provides a useful update on this condition.

26 McLaren (29 Apr 2000)

27 Fox (1985); Norman (1986); Olsen, Dossing (1982)

28 Gunby (1981); Norman, Newhouse (1986)

29 Gagnon (1985); Hoey, Turcotte, et al (1984); Norman (1986)

30 Pabst (1987)

31 Day, Lees, et al (1984); Gerin, Siemiatycki, et al (1989); Hoey, Turcotte, et al (1984); Norman (1986); Norman, Newhouse (1986); Norman, Pengelly, et al (1986); Sun (1986)

32 Beard (1869)

33 Beard (1880)

34 Beard (1880); Beard (1881)

35 Beard (1880); Beard (1881)

36 Beard (1881)

37 Nice (1908)

38 Nemiah (1975); Shorter (1992)

39 Nemiah (1975)

40 Wessely (1990)

41 The 1980 edition of *Diagnostic and Statistical Manual of Mental Disorders* did away with the diagnosis of neurasthenia.

42 Wessely (1997)

43 Johnson (1996)

44 Shorter (1992)

45 Environmental hypersensitivity victims similarly refer to their condition as "chemical AIDS."

46 Carroll, McAfee, Riley (1992); Shorter (1992)

47 AJ Barskey and JF Borus (1999), leaders in the field of psychosomatic illness, use the term *functional somatic syndromes* to designate these sorts of illnesses. Their list of such illnesses includes environmental hypersensitivity, RSI, side effects of silicone breast implants (see chapter 17), the Gulf War syndrome, chronic whiplash, CFS, irritable bowel, and fibromyalgia. The authors provide an excellent short account of the similarity in symptoms and in the epidemiology of these conditions.

48 Braaf, Rosner (1958)

49 Ford, Bray, Swerdloff (1976)

50 Stewart, Raskin (1985)

51 Littlejohn (1989); Reilly (1995a)

52 Wessely (1990)

53 There is no evidence that the working class have fewer symptoms than the middle and classes; they just do not have the luxury of formulating their symptoms into a fashionable illness (Shorter, 1994).

54 Wessely (1990); Consumer Reports (1996) Chronic fatigue syndrome: Any closer to the answer? 60–1

55 Balla (1982)

56 States, Korn, Masengill (1970). It is often argued that because women's necks are thinner than men's they are more vulnerable to injury – an unsatisfactory explanation since children's necks are even thinner, especially when compared to the weight of their heads, yet they rarely get whiplash and then only when their parents are particularly avaricious. See Coppola (1968); Leopold, Dillon (1960)

57 Gay, Abbott (1953) Report that 35 of their 50 patients were women and most were housewives between 30 and 50 years of age. Their practice covered an industrial city surrounded by a large agricultural region; the authors specifically comment that "farmers and unskilled laborers were conspicuously absent" in their series of 50 whiplash patients. Balla (1982) in his study of 300 Australian cases of late-whiplash syndrome, found whiplash occurred most frequently in people of middle socioeconomic class, in contrast to other motor vehicle accident injuries which were much more common in people of lower socioeconomic class. Kroenke, Lucas, et al (1993). George Mendelson (1981), an Australian psychiatrist who specializes in personal injury, had more women than men in his large series of whiplash claimants. He reports that the professional, technical, and clerical workers were over-represented compared to tradesmen, production workers, and labourers. No other studies have looked at whiplash in regard to social class. It is reasonable to suppose that the aging cervical spine would be particularly vulnerable to whiplash injury but it is not the elderly who develop persistent whiplash; it is women between the ages of 20 and 40 years who do so. See Evans (1992).

58 Beard (1880)

59 Wessely (1990)

60 Bartlett (1989); Francis (1988); Wessely (1995)

61 Wessely (1995)

62 Wessely, Hotopf, Sharpe (1998)

63 Sullivan (30 Jan 1995)

64 Coutts (10 Oct 1998)

65 Manitoba doctors fined. Globe and Mail 30th January 1999 A12

66 BS. The Gifts of CFIDS. The MEssenger 12, 1955

67 Munthe (1929)
68 Shorter (1996)
69 Sullivan (30 Jan 1995) in *Chronic Fee Syndrome* examines the costs of the
treatments for chronic fatigue syndrome. He comments that single
patients have spent as much as $60,000 on dubious remedies for it.
70 Stewart (1987)
71 Stewart (1989)
72 Bell (1989); Cleland (1987); Littlejohn (1989)
73 Bell (1989)
74 Reilly (1995a); Reilly (1995b)
75 Bell (1989)
76 Littlejohn (1995) is an Australian rheumatologist.
77 Taylor (13 Mar 1993)
78 May (27 Nov 1992)
79 Springett, Johnson (29 Oct 1993)
80 Reilly (1995b); Reilly (1995a)
81 Reilly (1995b)
82 Horowitz (10 Dec 1992)
83 Jury verdict in NY product liability cases "inconsistent with scientific evidence and the law" (1996) Personal communication and press release.
84 Schrader. (1996) Personal communication
85 Grady (11 May 1996)
86 Odin: Norway Now: http://odin.dep.no/html/english/publ.html.
Updated by editors 23rd May 1996
87 Schrader. (1996) Personal communication. He is professor of clinical
neurology at the Norwegian University of Science and Technology.
88 Schrader. (1996) Personal communication
89 OECD Health Data 98: a comparative analysis of 29 countries.
90 Schrader 1997: personal communication
91 DM Fraser (1994), an alternative physician from Lewiston, New York,
writing on whiplash in the Journal of Neurology and Orthopeadic
Medicine warns: "It is mandatory to check the feet in all cases of car accident as the force comes up through the floorboards of the vehicle and
travels through the body to the neck." The author had checked 26
patients with a history of whiplash and found 25 to have subluxation of
the ankle joints. In addition, the superior tibio-fibular joint may be subluxed as well, a condition that forces the foot to turn outwards predisposing to a "Charlie Chaplin gait."
92 Intimundsøker nakkeslengskadde. Verdens Gang, 22 May 1996
93 Schrader 1997: personal communication.
94 Showalter (1997), 133
95 Haley, Kurt, Hom (1997)
96 Soetekouw, de Vries, et al (2000)

97 Macfarlane, Thomas, Cherry (2000) compared the mortality rates of all
   of UK's 53,462 Gulf war veterans with a group of similar size matched
   for age, rank, levels of fitness etc. who had not served in the war. There
   were 395 deaths among the Gulf war veterans and 378 deaths among
   the others. While the mortality from accidents was higher among the
   veterans (254 compared to 216), deaths from disease-related causes
   were lower (122 compared to 141). Deaths from accidents are higher in
   people who are stressed, angry, and demoralized, which of course these
   illness-claiming veterans had inevitably become.

98 Jaynes (May 1994)

99 France (Sep 1998)

100 Pilkington (12 Jun 1995)

101 Murrey (7 Apr 1998)

102 These suggestions include radiation from depleted Uranium used in the
    manufacture of tank-piercing shells, the effects of the nerve gas Sarin,
    the effects of pyridostigmine bromide (a drug given prophylactically to
    blunt the effects of Sarin), and the effects from the multiple vaccines
    given to protect against the possibility of germ warfare.

103 Wadman (2000): The US panel of experts based its opinion on a close
    reading of nearly 1000 papers from the scientific literature.

104 McFadyean (27 May 1995)

105 Freedland (3 Aug 1995)

106 Balla (1982)

107 Shorter (1992)

108 Koro Study Team (1969)

CHAPTER SIX

1 Livingston (1998)

2 Williams, Hadler (1983)

3 Spitzer, Skovron, et al (1995)

4 Hadler (1993); Waddell (1987)

5 Institute for Clinical Evaluative Studies in Ontario (1995)

6 Deyo, Phillips (1997); Hadler (1993)

7 Gunnar Bovim (1994) and his colleagues from the Department of
  Neurology, Tronheim University Hospital, Norway, distributed a questionnaire inquiring about neck pain to a random sample of 10,000 adult
  Norwegians. Overall, 34.4% of the respondents had experienced neck
  pain within the last year, and 13.8% reported neck pain that lasted for
  more than six months. The authors concluded that chronic neck pain is
  a frequent symptom in the general population. In Germany whiplash is
  not regarded as a chronic illness. GD Giebel, AD Bonk et al (1999)
  showed that in German patients with acute whiplash injury treated with

active neck movement had no greater neck symptoms than did controls. See also Schrader (1996) and Partheni M et al (1999)

8 Most cases both of occupational low back pain and of whiplash recover within 2 weeks, but somewhere around 15% of people with acute low back pain, and 26% of whiplash victims report symptoms lasting up to one year. Clinical Standards Advisory Group (1994); Deans, Magalliard, et al (1987); Frank, Brooker, et al (1995). See also Hogg-Johnson, Cole, et al (2000)

9 Clinical Standards Advisory Group. (1994); Deans, Magalliard, et al (1987); Frank, Brooker, et al (1995)

10 Bigos, Battié (1991) Other prospective studies on incidence of low back pain also reveal remarkably few physical factors that are predictive of future low back problems. Two studies, Heliövaara (1987); Hrubec, Nashold (1975), found tallness and greater-than-average weight (in men but not in women) to be associated with increased risk for lumbar disc problems.

11 Battié (1989)

12 Garg, Moore (1992); Hult (1954); Rowe (1983) See also Waddell (1998)

13 Cady, Bischoff, et al (1979); Gundwell, Liljeqvist, Hansson (1993)

14 Waddell (1996)

15 Waddell (1986); Waddell (1991)

16 Nachemson (1994) Waddell (1998)

17 Deyo, Cherkin, et al (1995); Galasko, Murray, et al (1993); Malleson (1994); Schutt, Dohan (1968)

18 Frank, Brooker, et al (1995); Nachemson (1994)

19 Bigos, Battié (1991); Schutt, Dohan (1968)

20 Horn (1983); Marquis Who's Who (1996)

21 Cisler (1994)

22 Harakal (1975)

23 Harriton (1988)

24 Palmer (1910). Palmer was a Canadian-born grocer from Iowa. He had practiced "magnetic healer" for eight years and then restored hearing to a man, who had lost it 17 years previously when stooping down in a mine, by realigning a painful bony prominence in the patient's back.

25 Gardner (1957), 203

26 College of Physicians and Surgeons of the Province of Quebec (Sep 1966); Hubka (1990); Lucido (1986)

27 Gatterman (1995)

28 Haas (1991), a chiropractor with the Research Department, Western States Chiropractic College, in Portland, Oregon, reviewed the studies of the reliability of chiropractic investigations and concluded: "To date, the research presented in the chiropractic literature cannot substantiate

claims concerning the reliability of any diagnostic instrumentation or palpatory procedures commonly employed by chiropractic physicians."

29 Drum (1974)

30 Office of the Inspector General (1986)

31 Kane, Olsen, et al (1974); Meade, Dyer, et al (1990)

32 Dinning (1993); Fleming (1973)

33 Frank, Brooker, et al (1995)

34 Nachemson (1994)

35 Spitzer, Bombardier, et al (1987) found these terms in the charts of patients with common low backache; often several of the terms were used in a single chart.

36 McCombe, Fairbank, et al (1989) from the Royal Orthopaedic Hospital in Birmingham, UK. Deyo (1988), the distinguished back expert from Seattle, comments: "Interobservational agreement in rating spine motion and muscle strength, even when using goniometers and dynameters, is often surprisingly poor."

37 Hayes, Solyom, et al (1993)

38 Leclaire, Esdaile, et al (1996) from Quebec enrolled 41 patients with low back pain and 46 controls matched for age and gender into their study of diagnostic reliability. Half the controls were asked to pretend they had back pain, and half the patients with back pain were asked to pretend they did not. The subjects were then sent to experienced clinicians for assessment of their low back pain. For the subjects telling the truth, the doctors got the diagnosis of back pain right 99 per cent of the time. When it came to the simulators, however, the story was different; for patients who pretended not to have low back pain when they did, and the control subjects who had no pain but pretended they did, the doctors got the diagnosis right only 22 per cent of the time. Even by using specially designed pain questionnaires it was only possible to identify 46 per cent of the simulators.

39 Leavitt (1987); Leavitt, Garron, et al (1979)

40 Awerbuch (1991)

41 A little solicitous rubbing of the injured part or its thoughtful cleaning with surgical spirit will soon bring about temperature alteration and produce a magnificently abnormal thermograph.

42 See Mahoney, McCulloch, Casma (1985); Mahoney, Wiley, McMiken (1988)

43 See Awerbuch (1991) for a list of the institutions that have condemned the use of thermography.

44 Ferrari, Russell (1998)

45 Borden, Rechtman, Gardner (1960); Gore, Sepic, Gardner (1998); Helliwell, Evans, Wright (1994)

46 Carroll, McAfee, Riley (1992)

47 Balla (1998), the Australian neurologist, in a review of 5000 whiplash cases found a poor correlation between the symptoms of headache, neck pain, neck stiffness and arm pain, and any x-ray changes. See also Ferrari, Russell (1998)

48 A damaged disc can compress nerve roots as they pass through the narrow passageways between adjacent vertebrae. In the low back, such compression causes sciatica, and in the neck it causes pain, numbness, tingling, and weakness of an arm and hand. The compression of a nerve root usually produces some signs of nerve impairment, a clinical finding that provides objective evidence that something may be physical amiss.

49 Bonica (1974); Carron, DeGood, Tait (1985)

50 Waddell (1998), 52

51 MRI = Magnetic Resonance Imaging. The result looks similar to an x-ray but the contrasting soft tissues show up in much greater detail. Nortin Hadler is professor of medicine at Chapel Hill, North Carolina, and a world authority on occupation medicine. He writes: "Since World War II, the 'ruptured disc' has hung over the American back like an imprecation." See Hadler (1993), 10.

52 Deyo, Cherkin, et al (1995)

53 Hadler (1993); Office of Health Economics (1985); Waddell (1987), 10. No equivalent statistics are available for cervical discs and neck pain, but it seems likely that the odds of the pain being caused by disc compression of the nerve root are about the same.

54 Algers, Pettersson, et al (1993); Osterweis, Kleinman, Mechanic (1996); Waddell, Kummel, et al (1979)

55 Deyo, Cherkin, et al (1995)

56 Ransohoff, Feinstein (1978)

57 Louis Teresi (1987) and his colleagues from the Department of Radiology, UCLA School of Medicine, demonstrated the presence of abnormal findings in otherwise normal necks. An MRI ordered as part of the investigation of laryngeal cancer also images the cervical discs. The radiologists took advantage of this happenstance to study the cervical discs in patients without any cervical spine symptoms. The authors found disc protrusion (herniation/bulge) was present in 20% of patients aged 45–55 and in 57% of patients older than 64 years. Furthermore, spinal impingement – a condition in which the protruding discs push into the spinal cord – was present in 16% of patients under 64, and 26% of patients over 64 years, and actual cord compression was observed in 7% of the patients. The authors concluded: "Our findings indicate that a wide variety of abnormalities may be asymptomatic and that these are seen commonly in older patients."

Scott Boden (1990), an orthopaedic surgeon, and his colleagues from the George Washington University Medical Center, used MRI scans to study 63 volunteers who had no history of neck symptoms. The scans of the volunteers were interspersed with scans from symptomatic patients and were interpreted independently by three neurologists. An abnormality was demonstrated in 19% of the healthy volunteers, 8% of whom had herniated discs. A disc was degenerated at one level or more in 25% of the healthy volunteers under 40, and in almost 60% in those over 40. The authors emphasize "the dangers of predicating operative decisions on diagnostic tests without precisely matching those findings with clinical signs and symptoms." Boden and his colleagues (1990) duplicated their MRI neck study on the lumbar spine and obtained similar results.

58 Ronnen, de Korte, et al (1996)

59 Taylor, Kakulas (1991); Taylor, Twomey (1990)

60 Aprill, Bogduk (1992); Barnsley, Lord, et al (1995); Bogduk (1996); Lord, Bogduk, Barnsley (1993); Barnsley, Lord, Bogduk (1994)

61 Jonsson, Bring, et al (1991)

62 Barnsley, Lord, Bogduk (1993)

63 Beecher (1955); Turner, Deyo, Loeser (1996)

64 Maigne (15 Jun 1997); North (1996)

65 Lord, Barnsley, et al (5 Dec 1996)

66 Drinka, Jaschob (1997): Denervated joints that develop arthritis are known as Charcot's joints.

67 Scintograms are also known as "bone scans."

68 Barton, Allen, et al (1993); Hildingsson, Hietala, Toolanen (1989)

69 Hadler (1993), 9

70 Scot Boden (1996), the orthopaedic surgeon who found all the disc lesions in healthy volunteers, also studied the efficacy of spinal manipulation. He reports that three studies suggest that one or two spinal manipulations may be useful to relieve pain and facilitate mobilization exercises within the first two to four weeks of acute back pain. He comments: "Repeated manipulations (up to 15 is the common practice in the U.S.) have not been shown to have any greater benefit than an average of one to two manipulations performed by physicians in European countries where manual medicine is performed by primary care physicians rather than chiropractors."

71 Shekelle, Adams, et al (1992)

72 Koes, Assendelft, et al (1996) from the Vrije University, Amsterdam

73 Allen, Glasziou, Del Mar (1999)

74 Waddell (1987)

75 Holm (1980); Waddell (1987)

76 Deyo, Diehl, Rosenthal (1985); Deyo, Diehl, Rosenthal (1986)

77 Bortz (1984); Nachemson (1992); Nachemson (1994)

78 Lindstrom, Ohlund, et al (1992)

79 Hall, Hadler (1995)

80 Malmivaara, Hakkinen, et al (1995)
81 Weinberger (1976)
82 National Council Against Health Fraud (1994). BR Selecki 1984, the
    Australian neurosurgeon at the Prince Henry and Prince of Wales
    Hospitals in Sydney, writes of the chiropractic treatment of whiplash:
    "Manipulation can produce frequent and unpredictable aggravation of
    underlying cervical spinal conditions, hindering the patient's convales-
    cence rather than fostering it. The average patient who did not sustain a
    cervical disc in the collision runs a risk of acquiring one with frequent
    chiropractic manipulation of the neck.
83 Horn (1983), director of an emergency department in Charlotte,
    Michigan, provided a case history of the locked-in-syndrome: "A 34-year-
    old man, previously in good health, underwent chiropractic manipula-
    tion of the cervical spine for treatment of a recent whiplash injury.
    Immediately following manipulation, the patient became unresponsive
    and was found to have sustained a brain stem infarction resulting in the
    locked-in syndrome. Ten months following the initial insult, he remained
    tetraplegic and mute but able to communicate by eye blinking and verti-
    cal eye movements." Horn references 17 further authors who have
    reported stroke after manipulation of the neck. Norris, Beletsky,
    Nadareishvili (2000), on behalf of the Canadian Stroke Consortium,
    found dissection of the cervical arteries caused by sudden movement of
    the neck to be one of the most common causes of stroke in patients
    under 45 years of age. Chiropractic manipulation was found to be a com-
    mon cause of such dissection. MVAs were an unusual cause.
84 Macnab (1966)
85 Bortz (1984)
86 Fontanna (1970)
87 Farbman (1973), an orthopaedic surgeon from Detroit, commented: "The
    prolonged encouragement or permission to wear a collar or back support
    continuously over many weeks or months is deplorable." Marshall (1976),
    an Australian surgeon, suggested the use of a "collar and short rest period
    for a very short time if necessary but mostly passive or active mobilization."
    Selecki (1984), the Australian neurosurgeon, suggested, "The collar
    should be worn during the day only and for no longer than three weeks."
    Carroll, McAfee, Riley (1992), a group of distinguished American sur-
    geons, warned that the collar should be worn "for only a short time; other-
    wise it causes atrophy of neck muscles." Carette (1994), Canada's leading
    rheumatologist from Laval University, Quebec, suggests both that a collar
    should be used only "for a few days" and that "perhaps the best way to
    make sure that this treatment will be abandoned is for governments and
    third parties to stop paying for it." Teasell, Shapiro, Maillis (1993),
    whiplash experts from Ontario, advise that the collar should not be worn

for more than two weeks. They comment about its prolonged use "leads to a variety of complications: disuse atrophy of neck muscles, soft tissue contractures, shortening of muscles, thickening of subcapsular tissues, increased dependency and enhancement of feelings of disability." Gordon Martin (1959), a consultant in rehabilitation at the Mayo Clinic, in Rochester, Minnesota, comments about whiplash that "the pain of the strain is mainly in the brain," and states that "one of the greatest problems in the treatment of prolonged and persistent pain, lasting months after whiplash injury, is due to the fact that some of the patients have been permitted or encouraged to wear the cervical spinal support continuously over a period of many weeks or months. In these patients, motion of the cervical spine may become markedly restricted and guarded in all planes, and pronounced muscle weakness and atrophy from disuse plus tenderness and hypersensitivity of the muscles may become obvious findings."

88 McKinney (1989); Mealy, Brennen, Fenelon (1986)

89 Wiley and his orthopaedic surgeon colleagues from Toronto (1986), in their assessment of 320 slow-to-recover whiplash patients, observed that 39% had continued to wear a collar for over six months after the accident. John Balla (1980), a neurologist from Melbourne, Australia, found that 60% of his 300 late (chronic) whiplash patients had worn a neck collar for six months or longer. In Sweden, Hildingsson and Toolanen (1990), in a prospective study of 93 consecutive cases of soft-tissue injury of the neck from car accidents, found 19 of the patients still sometimes used a collar at their two year follow-up appointment.

90 Kinloch (1993)

91 Legis Filius (1973)

92 Kelly (1990)

CHAPTER SEVEN

1 Trimble (1981), 27

2 Erichsen (1882)

3 Clevenger (1889)

4 Evans (1992); Russell (1863)

5 Campbell (1915), 174. He quotes Philippe Gauchet (1854–1918), the famous French physician, as the source of this statistic.

6 Campbell (1917)

7 Trimble (1981)

8 Page (1885)

9 Miller, Cartlidge (1972)

10 Fisher (1967); Shapiro (1972)

11 Bigos, Battié (1991); Frank, Brooker, et al (1995)

12 Battié (1989); Bigos, Battié (1991)

13 Frymoyer, Pope, et al (1983). Frymoyer is a professor of orthopaedics at the University of Vermont.

14 Bigos, Battié (1991); Gibb-Clark (1996); Scofield, Martin (1990); Waddell (1998)

15 Gyntelberg (1974) is from Denmark .

16 Magora (1973) from Hadassah University Hospital, Jerusalem.

17 Bigos, Battié (1991); Walsh, Dumitru (1988)

18 Bigos, Battié, et al (1989)

19 Blair, Blair, Rueckert (1994)

20 Bigos, Battié, et al (1989)

21 Crauford, Creed, Jayson (1990) from the University of Manchester, UK.

22 Graham Guest and Peter Drummond (1992): psychologists from Murdock University, Western Australia.

23 Feuerstein, Sult, Houle (1985)

24 Blair, Blair, Rueckert (1994); France, Krishnan, Trainor (1986)

25 Battié, Bigos (1991); Bigos, Battié (1991); Frank, et al (1995); Greenwood (1985); Guest, Drummond (1992); Kane, Olsen, et al (1974); Trief, Stein (1985); Waddell (1993); Walsh, Dumitru (1988)

26 Brooker, Frank, Tarasuk (1995)

27 Sarno (1991)

28 Burton, Tillotson, Troup (1989)

29 Waddell (1998)

30 Agency for Health Care Policy and Research (1992); Clinical Standards Advisory Group (1994); Frank, Brooker, et al (1995); Spitzer, Bombardier, et al (1987)

31 Bigos, Battié (1991); Wiesel, Feffer, Rothman (1984)

32 Grilli, Lomas (1992)

33 Dixon (1990)

34 Decter (2000), 25

35 Farbman (1973)

36 Livingston (1991)

37 Karlsborg, Smed, et al (1997)

38 Hadler (1993)

CHAPTER EIGHT

1 Guralnick, Kaban, Merrill (1978)

2 Costen (1934) James B Costen was an otolaryngologist from the Washington University School of Medicine

3 Marbuch (1995)

4 Some of these names are: TMJ dysfunction/disorder/syndrome, TM disorder (TMD), craniomandibular pain disorder (CMD), myofascial pain dysfunction syndrome (MPD), and many more, since experts on this

condition (and there are many) seem to like to name it themselves. See also Leonard, Dodes (1995)

5 There are eight recognized dental specialties in the U.S., TMJ disorders is not one of them, though dentists often set themselves up as TMJ experts.

6 Studies demonstrating the psychogenic aspects of TMJ disorder date from the mid-1950s. Laszlo Schwartz, a dentist from Columbia University, New York, (1955,1959), was interested in what sort of patient develops it. Instead of meticulously examining the teeth of the patients who sought care for TMJ pain, he meticulously examined their histories – 500 of them. He found more than 90% of the TMJ patients were women with a mean age of about 40 years. Besides their complaints of facial pain, they often had a history of other painful conditions and they were clearly more than averagely psychologically distressed. In contrast, their teeth and bites showed no case/control differences. Ruth Moulton (1955), a psychiatrist at Columbia University, studied 35 patients with TMJ disorder. She found that "not only [were these patients] unusually anxious, but they tended to express their anxieties in physical symptoms." Stanley Lesse (1956), a neurologist from the Presbyterian Hospital, New York, in a small series of patients (18), concluded the pain was either entirely psychogenic or a manifestation of a gross overreaction to a minor organic deficit. He found the patients generally had rigid attitudes, dominating natures, and obsessive-compulsive, perfectionist characteristics. In a methodologically excellent study, psychologist Regina Kinney and her colleagues from the University of Texas (1992), examined 50 patients who were in treatment for chronic TMD with dentists and oral surgeons in the Dallas-Fort Worth area. Using well-validated psychological instruments, Kinney and her collaborators determined the prevalence of current and past psychiatric disorders in these 50 patients and compared the results to the population norms. They found that the TMJ disorders patients had a threefold increase in the lifetime prevalence for major depression, nearly a twofold increase for a substance abuse disorder (usually alcohol or pills), and they had higher than average rates for both current and lifetime anxiety disorder. See also Haworth (23 Aug 1).

7 Newbrun (1989)

8 Schissel, Dodes (1997)

9 Kronn (1993) reports that Frankel was the first person to do so.

10 Frankel (1965)

11 Frankel writes: "In all of the patients studied there was evidence of malocclusion, usually caused by the loss of the posterior supporting teeth."

12 Roydhouse (1973)

13 Ernest (1979)

14 Ernest (1979)

15 Moses, Skoog (1986)

16 Weinberg, Lapointe (1987)

17 Kupperman (1988)

18 Mannheimer, Attanasio, et al (1989)

19 Goldberg (1990)

20 Howard, Benedict, et al (1991)

21 Heise, Laskin, Gervin (1992). Daniel Laskin is Professor and Chairman, Department of Oral and Maxillofacial Surgery, Schools of Dentistry and Medicine, Medical College of Virginia. These researchers followed up 155 whiplash patients (96 female: 59 male).

22 Pressman, Shellock, et al (1992)

23 Levandoski (1993a); Levandoski (1993b)

24 Probert, Wiesenfeld, Reade (1994)

25 Howard, Hatsell, Guzman (1995)

26 Abdel-Fattah (1993); Rogal (1987b); Teasell, Shapiro, Maillis (1993). The authors note: "Cervical traction is one of the most common modalities used in the treatment of cervical spine syndromes. Frequently, patients complain that cervical traction makes them worse. Attention is called to the possibility that they may be suffering from temporomandibular joint symptoms." Frankel's case history was of a 37-year old nurse, who had neck and shoulder pain from a non-traumatic cause. She had some back teeth missing and was treated with cervical traction. She developed TMJ disorder. See Frankel, Shore, Hoppenfeld (1964).

27 Szabo, Wellcher, et al (1994)

28 For instance, Reda Abdel-Fattah and Mervat Alatter (1984) write: "In whiplash injuries the head snaps backwards; this action occurs so quickly that the anterior cervical muscles do not have a chance to relax, forcing the mouth excessively open, the disc and the condyle travel as one functional unit down the eminence, tied together by the TMJ ligaments, the condyle, translated completely out of the TM joint, stretching and tearing the posterior ligaments, anterior ligaments, TM joint ligaments, then the condyle snaps back and slams against the anterior slope of the eminence causing the anterior belly of the pterygoid to contract and hold the disc still." Rogal uses Frankel's description in many publications about whiplash and TMJ injury. See Rogal (1982, 1984, 1986a,b, 1987a,b,). Weinberg and La Pointe presented Frankel's description as scientifically proven.

29 Pullinger, Seligman (1991)

30 Davant, et al (1993); Kircos, Ortendahl, et al (1987); Liedberg, Westesson (1988); Westesson, Erikson, Kurita (1990)

31 Major Robert Enzenauer (1989) and his army officer colleagues reviewed boxing injuries in the U.S. Forces from 1985 to 1990. They found that on average 67 army boxers were injured severely enough

each year to warrant hospital admission. Although these authors report all sorts of unpleasant injuries, injury to a TM joint was not one of them. Myer Leonard (1993), professor of oral and maxillofacial surgery at Minneapolis, with over a quarter of century of experience as a specialist in this subject, reports he has never seen TMJ disorders caused by an auto collision without the occurrence of a direct impact to the face.

32 Myers Leonard (personal communication)

33 Flyer sent by Rogal to lawyers.

34 Rugh, Solberg (1985)

35 Toufexis (25 Apr 1988)

36 Farman (1982); Juniper (1986)

37 Myodata (1996)

38 Cooper, Rabuzzi (1984)

39 Perry (1988)

40 In a deposition before a Workers' Compensation referee, Rogal had even more impressive figures, stating that 87% of people with whiplash sustained TMJ injury from which they never recover (Rogal 1986). Rogal (1987) regards "mandibular whiplash" as the common, though often unrecognized, cause of TMJ disorder.

41 Rogal (1987a), 37

42 Rugh, Solberg (1985)

43 Cooper, Rabuzzi (1984) f rom New York Medical College

44 Clarke (1982); Greene, Laskin (1983); Greene, Marbach (1982); Okeson, Hayes (1986); Cawson (1984); Juniper (1986); Eversole, Machado (1985)

45 Leonard, Dodes (1995) is professor of oral and maxillofacial surgery at Minneapolis, and John Dodes is Director, New York Chapter of National Council Against Health Fraud. Their article is a fund of interesting information about these devices. They reviewed the various studies, or lack of studies, into the reliability of these new diagnostic devices, and found nothing to support their clinical use.

46 International College of Cranio-Mandibular Orthopedics (1987)

47 Phillips (Sep 1993)

48 Lund, Lavigne, et al (1989)

49 Berry (1987)

50 Berry (1987); Leonard, Dodes (1995); Phillips (Sep 1993)

51 Rogal (1987a)

52 Journal of Craniomandibular Practice Editorial (1989)

CHAPTER NINE

1 Cherasky (1973)

2 Fry (1957)

3 Anderson, Rondeau (1954); British Medical Journal Editorial (1963); Malleson (1973); Vianna, Greenwald, Davies (1971)

4 Evans (1992); Wiesel, Fetter, Rothman (1986)

5 Frenzel lenses interfere with fixation of the gaze making the nystagmus easier to detect. Longbotham, Engelken, et al (1994)

6 Braaf, Rosner (1958)

7 Compere (1968)

8 Compere wrote: "The vestibular symptoms have a tendency to improve with time and conservative treatment (immobilization, heat, massage, traction, tranquillising, and muscle relaxing drugs)." The "decompression" was of the subclavian artery. Sometimes the surgeon decompressed the artery on one side and sometimes on both.

9 Woods (1965); Woods, Compere (1969)

10 Nine were middle-aged women whose average age was 40, and eight had been in rear-end collisions.

11 Woods, Compere (1969)

12 Toglia, Rosenberg, Ronis (1970)

13 Pang (1971)

14 Rubin (1973)

15 Hinoki, Hine, et al (1973)

16 Van de Calseyde, Ampe, Depondt (1977)

17 Hart (1979). Hart also brings out the big guns of catastrophic whiplash injury to lend added support to the fact that whiplash causes damage to the vestibular system: "Whiplash may cause contusion of the cervical muscles, damage to the vertebral ligaments, intervertebral discs, apophyseal joints, and to the spinal cord and the nerve roots ... Associated damage and dysfunction to the central nervous system may be on the basis of ischemia [decreased blood supply], thrombosis [blood clot], gross haemorrhage, or contusion [bruise] of the brain. Haemorrhage in the inner ear may also result."

18 Black, Lilly, et al (Feb 1987); Nashner, Black, Wall (May 1982) There is ongoing controversy both about the cause of these fistulas and the nature of the symptoms that such a fistula produces. Two standard textbooks of ENT surgery note that PLFS can be very varied in its symptoms and that diagnosis is often unreliable. Changes of pressure and sneezing are reported as possible causes of these fistulas, though in most cases the cause remains unknown. See Baloh (1995); Pararella, et al (1991)

19 Grimm, Hemenway, et al (1989)

20 Fitz-Ritson (1991)

21 Oosterveld, Kortschot, et al (1991)

22 Chester (1991)

23 Whiplash injuries: New hope for whiplash victims? Abstract. Executive Health Report (1991) 28, 8

24 Compere and Wood comment that "the cause of the patient's complaint is frequently overlooked or ignored by the examining physician or is summarily dismissed as due to a post-traumatic psychoneurosis or to actual malingering." Wallace reports that "prior to the utilization of the ENG most of these individuals were considered to be 'crooks' or people looking for compensation ..." Pang comments, "because the objective signs and evidences of abnormality are frequently not present to account for the severity of the subjective symptoms, some physicians are prone to attribute these symptoms to emotional factors or ulterior motives." Toglia and his colleagues say much the same: "There is a tendency even among physicians to attribute posttraumatic dizziness to psychological and emotional aetiologies unless objective evidence of otoneurologic abnormality is also available." WJ Oosterveld et al reported: "These examinations are able to add often objective substantiation, and therefore justification of the patients' complaints. In cases where legal medicine is involved, the outcome of an extensive examination can be of the utmost importance both for the doctor and the patient."

25 Shea (1992)
26 Kroenke (1995)
27 Kroenke, Lucas, et al (1993)
28 Budd, Pugh (1996); Sullivan, Katon, et al (1994)
29 Axelsson, Rosenhall, Zachau (1994)
30 Norris (1991)
31 Rubin (1973)
32 Jessner, Bol, Waldfogel (1952); Levy (1945); Pearson (1941)
33 Ministry of Health (1962)
34 Wolman (1956)
35 Bakwin (1945)
36 Fischer, Verhagen, Huygen (1997)

CHAPTER TEN

1 Hagen (1997)
2 Hadler (1993), 34
3 Swerdlow. (1998)
4 Carlow (1993); Kreeft (1993); Magnússon, Ragnarsson, Bjornsson (1996); Rogal (1986); Rogal (1987); Ziegler, Schwertfeger, Murrow (1996)
5 Cartlidge, Shaw (1981)
6 Ettlin, Kischka, et al (1992), investigators from the University Clinics in Basel, Switzerland, extensively investigated 21 unselected typical whiplash patients. Subjectively, 62% of these patients reported concentration deficits, 86% reported sleep disturbances, 43% had symptoms of depres-

sion, and 39% of the female patients reported menstrual irregularities. Psychometric testing revealed a significantly lower performance in tests related to attention and concentration compared to controls matched for sex, age, and educational status. The authors report these abnormalities to be compatible with "damage to basal frontal and upper brain stem structures." Yarnell, Rossie (1988) report on "a group of patients suffering major debility after minor whiplash head trauma," seen in one office practice, which they retrospectively studied. "Typically, acute neck and upper backaches and headache evolved into a multiple somatic, affective and cognitive dysfunction syndrome. Neuropsychological evaluations noted impairments on tests of cognitive flexibility, non-verbal reasoning, new learning/memory, psychomotor agility, and attention. However, in the subacute period, neurological examination, imaging and clinical electrophysiological studies were unable to localize, structurally or functionally, the source of the above dysfunction." Frankel (1959), a surgeon from Charlottesville, Virginia, reports: "The deceleration injury [whiplash] may, in a large number of cases (22–30%), produce concussion to the frontal and occipital areas of the brain. Torsional forces may, likewise, involve the brain stem [the part of the brain that connects to the spinal cord]. The symptoms range from loss of consciousness for a varied period to confusion, dizziness or vertigo, headache, inability to concentrate, and disorientation. Some of the symptoms have been found to last for several years." Other investigators made similar claims: Shapiro, Roth (1993); Yarnell, Rossie (1988) Di Stefano, Radanov (1993); Di Stefano, Radanov (1995); Radanov, Di Stefano, et al (1991); Radanov, Di Stefano, et al (1993); Radanov, Dvorak, Valach (1992); Radanov, Sturzenegger, et al (1994); Radanov, Sturzenegger, Di Stefano (1995); Radanov, Valach, et al (1990); Rubin (1973); Sturzenegger, Di Stefano, et al (1994); Sturzenegger, Radanov, Di Stefano (1995)

7 Berstad, Baerum, et al (1975)
8 Binder (1997a); Binder (1997b); Miller (1996); Spitzer, Skovron, et al (1995)
9 Gennarelli, Thibault, et al (1982); Ommaya, Faas, Yarnell (1968); Underharnscheidt (1983)
10 Jennett, MacMillan (1997); Jennett, Teasdale (1981)
11 Teasdale, Mathew (1996)
12 Teasdale, Mathew (1996)
13 Cook (1972); Gentilini, et al (1985); Kozol (1946); McKinlay, Brooks, Bond (1983); Stuss, Stethem, et al (1989); Young (1985)
14 Larrabee (1992)
15 Ettlin, Kischka, et al (1992); Kischka, Ettlin, et al (1991); Rothbart (1996); Stuss, Ely, et al (1985); Stuss, Stethem, et al (1989); Sweeney (1992)

16 Mandel (1992)
17 Shapiro, Torres (1960) neurologists from Minnesota Medical School
18 McMordie (1988); Pankratz, Binder (1997)
19 Gay, Abbott (1953)
20 Mayou, Bryant, Duthie (1993)
21 Gennarelli, Thibault, et al (1982)
22 Berry. Neurologist: St Michael's Hospital, University of Toronto. Unpublished work
23 Varney, Bushnell, et al (1995)
24 The exact finding were hypoperfusion in orbitofrontal, posterior temporal and basal ganglia.
25 Bench, Brown, et al (1994); Mayberg (1994); O'Connell, Van Heertum, et al (1989); Trzepac, Hertweck, et al (1992)
26 Therapeutics and Technology Assessment Subcommittee of the American Academy of Neurology (1996)
27 Bicik, Radanov, et al (1998)
28 Therapeutics and Technology Assessment Subcommittee of the American Academy of Neurology. (1989)
29 Allen, Weir-Jones, et al (1994)
30 Gouvier (1988); Lees-Haley, Brown (1993); McLean Temkin, et al (1983)
31 Trimble (1981)
32 Lewis (1942)
33 American Congress of Rehabilitation Medicine: Head Injury Interdisciplinary Special Interest group (HI-ISIG) (1993)
34 Svensson, Andersson (1989) Buchnia (1994)
35 Alina Gildiner (2001)
36 Malleson (1973a); Malleson (1973b)
37 Taylor (1997)
38 Taylor, Cox, Maillis (1994)
39 Radanov, Di Stefano, et al (1991)
40 Radanov, Dvorak, Valach (1992) NB: Radanov et al call post-concussion syndrome, cervicoencephalic syndrome. I have substituted the more familiar term.
41 Some patients "reported a short traumatic impairment of consciousness" which the investigators found "difficult to separate from dissociative reactions or very short post-traumatic amnesia."
42 Radanov, Di Stefano, et al (1994). According to the Swiss accident insurance system, a person who loses time from work because of an injury receives a proportion of his salary regardless of liability. The physician certifies disability. Some of their patients also had outstanding insurance claims.
43 Radanov, Dvorak, Valach (1992) NB: Radanov et al call post-concussion

syndrome, cervicoencephalic syndrome. I have substituted the more familiar term.

44 Bleuler (1924), 558
45 Lees-Haley, Brown (1993)
46 Sim (1992), 119; Suhr, Tranel, et al (1997)
47 For lowering of test scores in alcohol use see Mearns, Lees-Haley (1993). For scores in low IQ see Taylor, Cox, Maillis (1994). For low scores associated with somatic problems see Grigsby, Rosenberg, Busenark (1995); Olsnes (1989) . For low scores in pregnancy see Gross, Pattison (1994)
48 Suhr, Tranel, et al (1997)
49 Binder (1991); Binder (1993); Binder, Rohling (1996); Hiscock, Hiscock (1989); Pankratz, Binder (1997); Youngjohn, Burrows, Erdal (1995)
50 Pankratz, Binder (1997)
51 Bernard (1990)
52 Berry (1997) Unpublished work.
53 Hiscock, Hiscock (1989); Pankratz, Binder (1997)
54 Lees-Haley, Smith, et al (1996); Pankratz, Binder (1997)
55 Shapiro, Teasell, Steenhaus (1993)

CHAPTER ELEVEN

1 Richman (1998)
2 Dunbar (1997)
3 Sim (1992), 16
4 Kistner, Keith, et al (1994)
5 Allan, Barker, et al (1995)
6 Connolly (1981); Engel (1988)
7 Dunbar (1997); Rawson (1944)
8 Engel (1988)
9 National Safety Council: Accident Facts, 1942, Washington DC.
10 Greenwood, Woods (1919)
11 Rawson (1944)
12 Johnson (1936); O'Dowd (1988)
13 Dunbar (1942); Dunbar, Wolfe, Rioch (1936); Dunbar, Wolfe, Tauber (1939); O'Connell, Van Heertum, et al (1989)
14 Dunbar (1943)
15 Dunbar, Wolfe, Tauber (1939), 1327
16 Adler (1941)
17 Dunbar, Wolfe, Rioch (1936)
18 Angell (1996), 122
19 Collie (1917); Engel (1988)
20 Mechanic (1961); Zborowski (1952)

21 Zborowski (1952)
22 Parsons (1951); Sigerist (1960)
23 Mechanic (1961)
24 Malleson (1973)
25 Melzack, Wall (1965)
26 Sullivan, Turner, Romano (1991)
27 Florence (1981); Saunders (1990); Sullivan, Turner, Romano (1991)
28 Anderson (1991); Balint (1957)
29 International Association for the Study of Pain (1994)
30 Willis (1986), for instance, uses terms such as "victim blaming" and "in the tradition of racist medico-legal stereotypes."
31 Bell (1989)
32 Behan, Hirschfeld (1963); Hirschfeld, Behan (1963); Hirschfeld, Behan (1966)
33 Hirschfeld, Behan (1963)
34 Behan, Hirschfeld (1963)
35 Hirschfeld, Behan (1963)
36 Behan, Hirschfeld (1963)
37 Behan, Hirschfeld (1963)
38 Hodge (1971)
39 Florence (1981)
40 Florence (1981)
41 Richman (1998)
42 Loeser (Oct 1994); Loeser, Sullivan (Mar 1997)
43 Loeser, Cousins (1990)
44 Katon, Kelly, Miller (1985)
45 Kouyanou, Pither, et al (1998); and Sullivan, Turner, Romano (1991) report that psycho-social difficulties usually precede the accident and the chronic pain syndrome that is being held accountable for the difficulties. They found a high incidence of premorbid psychiatric illness – particularly of depression – and commonly a history of previous chronic pains in various locations of the body. The authors note the usefulness of the pain – since it allows time out from stressful or aversive situations (work, family, and sexual), and permits patients "to say no to demands or to ask for help when they would not usually feel so entitled." The authors emphasize the detrimental effect of medication and excess rest upon these patients.
46 Saunders (1990)
47 Weintraub (1995)
48 Hertzman, Smoller (1989)
49 Goldman (1991)
50 Saunders (1990); Waddell (1987); Waddell (1991)
51 Florence (1981)

52 Mr. Justice Hawkins: "She suffers the consequences of chronic pain syndrome." Cited in Ontario Lawyer's Weekly, 10 July 1992.

CHAPTER TWELVE

1 Hadler (1993)
2 Winfield (1997)
3 Smythe (1989)
4 See Coren (1996)
5 Moldofsky, Scarisbrick, et al (1975)
6 Carette (1995)
7 Bennett (1997). Sicca symptoms are dryness and irritation of mucus
   membranes. Raynaud's phenomenon is British Empire disease with
   hands and feet going red, white, and blue in the cold. Female urethral
   syndrome is a feeling of having to urinate all the time. Restless leg syndrome is a condition in which a leg jumps about at night.
8 Saskin, Moldofsky (1986)
9 Moldofsky, Wong, Lue (1993)
10 Wolfe, The Vancouver Fibromyalgia Consensus Group (1996)
11 Bohr (1996); Littlejohn (1989); Lorenzen (1994)
12 Bohr (1996); Brussgaard, Evensen, Bjerkedal (1993)
13 Bennett (1995); Wolfe, Ross, et al (1995)
14 Bohr (1996); Thorson (1993); Wolfe, Anderson, et al (1997); Wolfe,
   Ross, et al (1995)
15 White, Speechley, et al (1995)
16 Murrey, B. Consumer Health Service Information, Toronto Metropolitan
   Library. Personal communication 1995.
17 Wolfe (1997)
18 Shorter (1996)
19 Hirsch, Carlander, et al (1994); Jennum, Drewes, et al (1993);
   Moldofsky, Lue, Saskin (1987); Molony, MacPeek, et al (1986); Scheuler,
   Kubicki, et al (1988); Ware, Russell, Campos (1986); Russell (1995)
20 Wolfe (1994)
21 Wolfe, Smythe, et al (1990)
22 Wolfe, Smythe, et al (1990)
23 Wolfe, Smythe, et al (1990) Fibromyalgia: the Copenhagen Declaration.
   Lancet, 340, 663–4
24 Wolfe, Smythe, et al (1990)
25 Wolfe, Anderson, et al (1997)
26 Littlejohn, Granges (1993); Mikkelsson, Latikka, et al (1992); Quimby,
   Block, Gratwick (1988)
27 Bohr (1996)
28 Carette (1995); Nordstrom (1996)

29 Livingston (1995)
30 Nordstrom (1996), a physician from Colorado Springs, suggests: "An
extensive literature, often overlooked by rheumatologists, suggests that
fibromyalgia is an affective disorder such as major depression, panic disorder, vascular headache, and irritable bowel ... The view that fibromyalgia is an organic disease gives an aura of legitimacy to the pain that leads
to financial compensation and disability; it stymies treatment and crip-
ples the patient ... Patients are not well served by being declared disabled; they should be treated compassionately and urged towards health,
encouraged not entitled." Birnie, Knipping, et al (1991) from the
University Hospital, Groningen, Holland, in a well-designed study, examined the psychological characteristics of three groups of patients:
patients with acute pain, patients with chronic pain syndrome, and
patients with fibromyalgia. The patients with fibromyalgia had much in
common with the patients with chronic pain, both groups scoring high
for somatization, though the fibromyalgics had the highest scores. The
authors conclude: "Many psychological aspects of fibromyalgia can be
considered as psychological aspects of chronic pain." Bohr (1987), a
neurologist from Loma Linda University School of Medicine, California,
takes a firm stance against the uncritical acceptance of fibromyalgia as a
straightforward physical ailment. In an article entitled "Painful Questions
about Fibromyalgia," he notes the many similarities that fibromyalgia
shares with depression – sleep disorders, chronic fatigue, frequent past
histories of personal or familial depression, and positive response to antidepressants. Fibromyalgics try to avoid the "P" word. Bohr comments
that patients and insurance companies both prefer a diagnosis of
fibromyalgia to one of depression. Quimby, Block, Gratwick (1988), psychologists from the University of Maine, studied 125 patients with musculoskeletal disorders. They consigned the patients to one of three diagnostic groups: generalized non-articular rheumatism (fibromyalgia),
rheumatoid arthritis, and osteoarthritis. They found that the fibromyalgic patients, when compared to the patients in the other two groups
"demonstrated an abnormally high frequency of reporting manifold dis-
agreeable symptoms, symptoms that were likely to bring them to the
attention of various medical specialists." Forslind, Fredriksson, and Nived
(1990), rheumatologists from the University Hospital in Lund, Sweden,
question fibromyalgia's very existence. They re-examined 21 consecutive
patients (18 women and 3 men) presenting with primary fibromyalgia
over a five-year period. Six patients were found to have developed disorders other than fibromyalgia. Of the remaining 15 cases, 11 proved to
have psychiatric illness.
31 Farney, Walker (1995)
32 Thompson (1990)

33 Campbell, Clark, et al (1983); Goldenberg (1987); Livingston (1995); Wolfe (1994); Yunus, Masi, Calabro (1981)

34 Sarno (1981)

35 Kravis, Munk, et al (1993)

36 Shorter (1992)

37 Lorenzen (1994); Smythe (1989)

38 Makela, Heliovaara (1991)

39 Smythe (1989)

40 Hidding (1994) are from the University Hospital, Maastricht, Holland.

41 Patrick, Deyo (1989)

42 Russell (1995)

43 Blécourt, Knipping, et al (1993)

44 Mailis, Furlong, Taylor (2000)

45 Burton (16 Nov 1999)

46 Fitzcharles, Esdaile (1997)

47 Bohr (1996)

48 Travell, Simons (1983)

49 Bohr (1995); Bohr (1996)

50 Wolfe, Simons, et al (1992)

51 Tunks (1995)

52 Wolfe, The Vancouver Fibromyalgia Consensus Group (1996)

53 Wolfe, The Vancouver Fibromyalgia Consensus Group (1996)

54 Wolfe (1994)

55 Croft, Schollum, Silman (1994) examined the relationship between tender points, complaints of pain, and symptoms of depression, fatigue, and sleep quality. They looked for tender points in a randomly selected a sample of 250 pain respondents from two general practices. They found that women have a higher average tender point count than men (six for women and three for men). People with pain had higher counts, though most people with chronic widespread pain had fewer than eleven. Two subjects from the group of patients who reported "No present pain complaints" had eleven or more tender points. Mean symptom scores for depression, fatigue, and sleep problems increased as the tender point count rose, though these symptoms were independent of pain complaints.

56 Hadler (1993); Hadler (1997)

57 Shorter (1996)

58 These 14 consisted of 3 male, 11 female patients with a mean age of 37 years.

59 Romano (1990)

60 Boisset-Pioro, Esdaile, Fitzcharles (1995)

61 Romano (1990)

62 Greenfield, Fitzcharles, Esdaile (1992) are from Montreal

63 Weinberger (1977)
64 Wolfe, The Vancouver Fibromyalgia Consensus Group (1996)
65 Carette (1995)
66 Gunn (1995)
67 Wolfe, The Vancouver Fibromyalgia Consensus Group (1996)
68 Hadler (1997)
69 Donald (1993)

CHAPTER THIRTEEN

1 Rawlins (10 Jun 1994)
2 MMPI-2 is an upgraded version of the Minnesota Multiphasic Personality Inventory – one of the oldest screening tests for personality disorders.
3 Sprenger and Kramer: Malleus Malificarum [The Hammer of the Witches] (1487)
4 Dr Francis Skulsky, an oral and maxillofacial surgeon, testified for the defence. He believed that Dr G, the orthodontist who had diagnosed Mrs M as having TMJ disorder, had insufficient evidence to support such a diagnosis. He commented that if she had damaged the joint in the way that Dr G had suggested she would certainly have been aware of it.
5 Shorter (1996)
6 Like so many fibromyalgic patients, Mrs M consumed large amounts of non-steroidal analgesics which are ineffective in the treatment of fibromyalgia. See Wolfe, The Vancouver Fibromyalgia Consensus Group. (1996); Yunus, Masi, Aldag (1989) . However, these non-steroidal analgesics can cause a fatal gastric haemorrhage. See Champion (1993). Canada is a cold country with many wood-stoves; in consequence it has many house fires. Nevertheless three times more people die in Canada each year from gastric haemorrhage caused by non-steroidal analgesics than die in house fires. From Statistics Canada (1991) Ottawa.

CHAPTER FOURTEEN

1 Charlebois (25 Nov 1995)
2 Braaf, Rosner (1955)
3 Middleton (1956)
4 Knight (1959)
5 Dr John Gipner had reviewed in detail all the ocular symptoms of head injury, including pupillary changes and subsequent death, but only mentioned one case of head injury with loss of convergence and that was accompanied by loss of accommodation as well.
6 Horwich, Kasner (1962)
7 This observation apparently remains correct. Slamovitis, Glaser (1988).

Slamovitis and Glaser (1982) in Duane's Textbook, Clinical
Ophthalmology, suggest, "It may be impossible to separate the patient
with true post-traumatic accommodative-convergence insufficiency from
the dissembler unless objective signs are present or positive response to
therapy excludes the latter possibility.

8 Wiesinger, Guerry (1962)
9 These included a series of "31 cases of whiplash injuries that came to
   spinal fusion for the relief of symptoms."
10 Ommaya, Faas, Yarnell (1968)
11 Fite (1970)
12 Roca (1972)
13 Kelley, Hoover, George (1978)
14 Burke, Orton, et al (1992)

CHAPTER FIFTEEN

1 Lees-Haley, Dunn (1986)
2 Binder (25 Jan 1978)
3 American Psychiatric Association (1980)
4 Baskett, Henager (1983); Sim (1992)
5 American Psychiatric Association (1980)
6 Malt (1988)
7 Malt, Olafsen (1992)
8 Mayou, Bryant, Duthie (1993)
9 Kuch, Swinson, Kirby (1985)
10 Blanchard, Hickling, et al (1994)
11 Ramsay (1990)
12 van der Kolk, Herron, Hostetler (1994)
13 Platt, Husband (1989); Scrignar (1984)
14 Ward Versus Commercial Union Insurance Company (1981),
   591So.2d1286, La.Ct.App.
15 The whiplash injury victims were interviewed at home 8–54 days (mean
   25.4 days) after the accident; the other patients as soon as they were fit
   enough. The motorcyclists from 1–41 days (mean 9.5 days) after the
   accident and the car occupants from 2–26 days (mean 8.5 days).
16 Dixon, Rehling, Shiwach (1993)
17 Mendelson (1995); Shorter (1996)
18 Ramsay (1990)
19 Brent, Perper, et al (1995); McFarlane (1988); Watts (1995)
20 Blanchard, Hickling, et al (1995)
21 Paul R, Lees-Haley, and Dunn JT (1994), psychologists from California,
   tested naïve subjects, i.e., volunteers who had no reason to know more
   about PTSD symptoms than the average lay person. When these subjects

were asked to respond as if they had been psychiatrically disturbed by an accident, 86% of them satisfied the criteria in all three self-report criteria lists for the diagnosis of PTSD. The authors suggest that "through books, magazines, newspapers, television news programs, television talk shows, and radio call-in programs hosted by psychologists and psychiatrists," average laypersons are no longer naïve about such subjects. Like children with sex, people know more about these things than they are supposed to. Judith A. Lyons et al (1994), from U.S. Veterans Affairs, using the widely employed Mississippi Scale for Combat-Related PTSD, found that the scores of individuals instructed to respond "as if" they had PTSD did not differ from the scores of veterans who had it. Stephen T. Perconte and Anthony J. Goreczny (1990), from a VA Medical Center in Pittsburgh, found the MMPI failed to discriminate between Vietnam veterans seeking treatment for faked PTSD and veterans seeking treatment for other psychiatric disorders. The MMPI is a generally acclaimed psychological instrument that is used to clarify various psychiatric disturbances, but in this situation it clearly does not work.

22 Edward J. Lynn and Mark Belza (1984), VA psychiatrists, present seven cases of alleged PTSD in Vietnam veterans who were later found never to have been in combat, and in some cases, not even in Vietnam. Landy Sparr and Loren D. Pankratz (1983), also with the VA, found much the same. They report five cases of men treated in a VA Center in Oregon for symptoms of PTSD allegedly arising out of military service in Vietnam, three of whom claimed to have been prisoners of war. On investigation it was found that four of the five had never been in Vietnam, none had been prisoners of war, and two had never been in the military. The authors note: "The symptoms of PTSD can easily be simulated" and "factitious PTSD is yet another variation of the many clinical deceptions that physicians may encounter."

23 Allodi (1989); Allodi (1991); Allodi (1994)

24 Sparr, Boehnlein (1990)

25 Sparr (1995)

26 Stone (1993)

27 Daw (7 May 1998)

28 McGowan, Zigler, Peacock (1 Dec 1995); David, Leck (29 May 1997)

29 King (30 Jan 1998)

30 McGowan, Zigler, Peacock (1 Dec 1995); David, Leck (29 May 1997)

31 Daw (7 May 1998)

32 David, Leck (29 May 1997)

33 Tyndel (1974); Tyndel, Egit (1988); Tyndel, Tyndel (1984)

34 Tyndel, Tyndel (1984)

35 Dineen (1996), 15. Dineen once worked at the Toronto General Hospital but is now a psychologist in Vancouver.

36 Labi (17 May 1999)
37 Wessely, Rose, Bisson (1998)
38 Watts (1995)

  1 Ameis (1986); Binder, Rohling (1996); Bleuler (1924); Cartlidge, Shaw
      (1981); Deans (1986); Erichsen (1882); Evans (1992); Farbman (1973);
      Florence (1981); Gates, Benjamin (1967); Gorman (1979); Kennedy
      (1946); Leopold, Dillon (1960); Maguire (1993); Miller (1961a); Miller
      (1961b); Rush, Ameis (1995); States, Korn, Masengill (1970); Strub,
      Black (1988); Trimble (1981); Uomoto, Esselman (1993)
  2 Brooker, Frank, Tarasuk (1995)
  3 Hadler (1997)
  4 Erichsen (1882)
  5 Bleuler (1924), 567
  6 Kennedy (1946)
  7 Leavitt, Garron, et al (1979)
  8 Miller (1961a); Miller (1961b)
  9 Miller, Cartlidge (1972)
 10 Henry Morgentaler is a doctor who systematically challenged the abor-
      tion laws in Canadian provincial courts. He did so successfully, allowing
      Canadian women the choice to terminate a pregnancy. Unfortunately,
      antiabortionists, by murdering and threatening any doctor who provides
      this service, have managed to make "the right to choose" often a theoret-
      ic rather than a practical choice.
 11 Cartlidge, Shaw (1981), 96
 12 Guttmann (1943)
 13 Cartlidge, Shaw (1981)
 14 Uomoto, Esselman (1993), from the Department of Rehabilitation,
      University of Washington.
 15 Guy (1968)
 16 Gates, Benjamin (1967); Gates, Cento (1966)
 17 States, Korn, Masengill (1970)
 18 Champion (1992)
 19 Awerbuch (1992)
 20 Maguire (1993)
 21 Leopold, Dillon (1960)
 22 Gargan, Bannister, et al (Jul 1997)
 23 Kennedy (1946); Trimble (1981) 101
 24 Kennedy (1946)
 25 Miller, Cartlidge (1972)
 26 Gargan, Bannister, et al (Jul 1997)

27 Gargan, Bannister, et al (1997)
28 Radanov, Di Stefano, et al (1991)
29 Radanov, Sturzenegger, Di Stefano (1995)
30 Griffin (1996); O'Brien (1999); Robbins (1996)

CHAPTER SEVENTEEN

1 Berman (25 Mar 1987) 10A
2 Begley (22 Mar 1993) 62–4
3 Whelan quoted in Corcoran (24 Jun 1997)
4 Huber (1991), 2
5 Huber (1991)
6 Behan (1939), 7
7 Huber (1991), 42
8 Behan (1939), vii
9 Huber (1991), 44
10 Huber (1991); National Dairy Products Corp. v. Durham (1967), 44
11 Crane (1959)
12 Lyons (4 Feb 1991)
13 Lyons (4 Feb 1991)
14 Angell (1996a) Black (1988); The toxic tort that won't die. The Wall Street Journal, 10 July 1996; Nocera (1995a); Nocera (1995b)
15 Angell (1996b)
16 Wolf (1991)
17 Angell (1996a), 35
18 Angell (1996a), 34
19 Angell (1996b); Nocera (1995a)
20 Angell (1996a) 55
21 Angell (1996b)
22 Angell (1996a), 66
23 Angell (1996a), 69
24 Angell (1996a), 134
25 Angell (1996a), 134
26 Angell (1996a), 80
27 Angell (1996a), 80
28 Angell (1996a), 142
29 Sim (1992), 107
30 Angell (1996a), 82
31 Angell (1996a), 83
32 Angell (1996a); Nocera (1995a); Rosenbaum (6 Jun 1997).
33 Angell (1996a), 24
34 Gabriel, O'Fallon, et al (1994)
35 Nocera (1995a), 100–1

36 Hennekens, et al (1996)
37 Sanchez-Guerrero, et al (1995)
38 Nocera (1995a), 102
39 The Toxic Tort That Won't Die. (10 July 1996). The Wall Street Journal;
   Angell (1996a), 146
40 Smith (1992)
41 Angell (1996a), 145
42 Kolata (16 May 1995)
43 Angell (1996a), 146
44 Huber (1991), 207; Richards (7 Jan 1988)
45 Loevinger (1995); Winans v. New York and Erie Railroad (1858) 62 U.S.
   88,100–01.
46 American Law Institute (1997)
47 Nocera (1995a) quotation from letter, 162
48 Thomas (1998)
49 Huber (1991), 11; Calabresi (1970)
50 Glendon (1995)
51 Nocera (1995a)
52 Sugarman (1990)
53 Angell (1996b)
54 (The) Economist (1992); Sugarman (1990); Economist (2 September
   2000)
55 Epp (1992); President's Council on Competitiveness (1991)
56 Magee (1997)
57 Clarfield (30 Nov 1993)
58 Ferguson (1996)
59 Black (1988)
60 Frye v. United States, 293 F. 1013 (D.C. Cir. 1923); Freedman
   (1994)
61 Loevinger (1995)
62 Black (1988)
63 Freedman (1994)
64 Daubert vs. Merrell (1992) 509 U.S., 125 L Ed 2d 469,113 S Ct[No. 92-
   102]
65 Annas (1994)
66 Begley (22 Mar 1993); Freedman (1994)
67 Begley (22 Mar 1993)
68 Freedman (1994)
69 Freedman (1994)
70 Levy (1994)
71 Huber (1991)
72 In the U.S., 70 people have been freed from the nation's prisons –
   including 8 from death row – after DNA testing showed they had been

wrongly convicted, and this is even before the use of these tests has been widely allowed. Washington Post, 10 Sep 2000, A1 and A5.

73 Carcopino (1954)
74 Burton (1905)
75 Huxley (1880)

CHAPTER EIGHTEEN

1 Insurance Research Council Inc. (1995a), 2
2 Insurance Research Council Inc. (1994)
3 (The) Economist (27 February 1999)
4 Navin and Romilly (1989) are engineers at the University of British Columbia, who write: "It is known that during a collision, the vehicle structure deforms converting the system's kinetic energy into sound, thermal and strain energies. The rate of deformation defines the vehicle's stiffness characteristics, while the amount of recoverable deformation is a function of its elastic properties. At high impact speeds very little elastic recovery occurs and the vehicle generally behaves as plastic body. At low impact speeds, however, plastic behaviour may be absent allowing more of the total impact energy available to be recovered in elastic rebound. For the occupant, the best ride down profile occurs when the vehicle behaves as a plastic body where large deformations reduce the overall acceleration."
5 Baker (1996)
6 Insurance Research Council Inc. (1995a), 3
7 Insurance Research Council Inc. (1995a), 3
8 Insurance Research Council Inc. (1995b)
9 Insurance Research Council Inc. (1995a)
10 Insurance Research Council Inc. (1995b)
11 Insurance Research Council Inc. (1994), 4
12 Insurance Research Council Inc. (1994), 3
13 Insurance Research Council Inc. (1994), 23–5
14 Insurance Research Council Inc. (1994), 3
15 Bogduk (1996)
16 Insurance Research Council Inc. (1994), 26–7
17 Insurance Research Council Inc. (1994), 28
18 Insurance Research Council Inc. (1995a), 12
19 Insurance Research Council Inc. (1995b), 9
20 Insurance Research Council Inc. (1994), 7
21 Insurance Research Council Inc. (1994), 7
22 Insurance Research Council Inc. (1994), 49–53
23 Insurance Research Council Inc. (1994), 57, Figure 6–3
24 Insurance Research Council Inc. (1994), 61

25 Quoted by Gates, Cento (1966)
26 Cassidy, Carroll, et al (2000)
27 Van Voris (22 May 2000)
28 www.angelfire.com/nf/coalitionagainstnf/index.html
29 Back Letter Editorial (2000)
30 David Cassidy (personal communication)
31 Sim (1992)
32 Insurance Research Council Inc. (1995b), 1
33 Mitchell (1996); Rusk (1996)

CHAPTER NINETEEN

1 Caffey (1946)
2 Sim (1992) 29 and 70
3 Duffy (1992)
4 Cunnien (1997)
5 Stop Fraudulent Claims, Briefing Package: SEPTA: Fraudulent Claims Unit, 714 Market Street, Philadelphia, PA 19106.
6 McDonald (28 Sep 1988)
7 Loundsberry (31 Aug 1998)
8 Katz, E. Legal dept. SEPTA: Personal correspondence (1998)
9 Catching cheaters: an anti-fraud task force pulls in a big haul. Editorial: The Philadelphia Inquirer A18, 29 May 1992.
10 "Ghost Riders": *Eye to Eye with Connie Chung*, 18 Aug 1992. Produced by J. Martelli.
11 Kerr (18 Aug 1993); Insurance Claim Fraud. (1994); Jaffe (18 Aug 1993)
12 Rudolph (18 Aug 1993)
13 NICB Information sheets: RipOff.
14 NICB Information sheets: RipOff.
15 National Insurance Crime Bureau (1997a)
16 National Insurance Crime Bureau (1996a)
17 National Insurance Crime Bureau (1997b)
18 National Insurance Crime Bureau (1996b)
19 National Insurance Crime Bureau (1996b)
20 Ontario Legislature (1990)
21 Charlebois (25 Nov 1995)
22 Cohen (1996)
23 Lynne Cohen (1996). There is a kind of universality of problems in the delivery of healthcare. The Australian government is now bringing in laws to ensure that family doctors inform their patients of any financial interests they may have in the clinics to which they are referring them.
24 Alina Gildiner (2001) provides an excellent account of this "quagmore."

25 Daw (3 Oct 1996); Daw (7 Feb 1997)

26 Benedet (99 A.D.)

27 Daw (13 Jul 1996)

28 Gollom (7 Jun 2000)

29 DeGraaf (1995)

30 Baer (15 Jan 1925); Daw (15 Sep 1995)

31 Baer (15 Jan 1925)

32 Baer (15 Jan 1925)

33 Daw (15 Sep 1995)

34 DeGraaf (1995)

35 Such exploitation of whiplash is not confined to North America. The Japanese have "perennial problems" with gangsters who "stage-manage phoney rear-end shunts in order to collect disability pensions." The Economist (27 February 1999)

36 National Insurance Crime Bureau (1997c)

37 National Insurance Crime Bureau (1997c)

38 National Insurance Crime Bureau (1996c)

39 The Eurotunnel: Britannica: Book of the Year 1995.

40 Freud quoted by Charles Ford in Lies! Lies!!, Lies!!!: The Psychology of Deceit, 197

41 Jones, Llewellyn (1917)

42 Steinem (1994)

43 Jones (1953)

44 Perhaps novelists are a more reliable source of human behaviour than are psychiatrists. The observant eye of the novelist sees behaviour for what it is; psychiatrists see it only in terms of their discipline's belief system. Dickens writes of dishonesty: "I have known a vast quantity of nonsense talked about bad men not looking you in the face. Don't trust this idea. Dishonesty will stare honesty out of countenance any day in the week, if there is anything to be got from it."

45 Wilson (1975)

46 Darwin (1871); Morgan (1973)

47 Payne (1995); Trivers (1985) 131

48 Wiseman (1994)

49 de Waal, Lanting (1997), 35

50 National Insurance Crime Bureau (1997d)

51 Insurance Bureau of Canada (1995)

52 National Task Force on Insurance Fraud (1994)

53 Ford (1996)

54 Rogers (1997), 5

55 Sim (1992). Other authors refuse to see malingering: Teasell, McCain, Merskey, and Finestone (1991) comment: "Blaming the patients for their symptoms by labelling them 'hysterical,' 'malingerers,' or 'compensation

neurotics' only adds to the overall burden of suffering. Barnsley, Lord, and Bogduk comment (1993): "There is no real evidence, therefore, that either malingering for financial gain or pre-existing psycho-social factors contribute in any significant way to the natural history of whiplash injury. The unavoidable conclusion is that the overwhelming majority of whiplash injuries result in organic lesions." Mayou (1995) writes: "Terms such as exaggeration, simulation or malingering are rarely appropriate." Radanov, Di Stefano, Schnidrig (1993) write: "This reasonably rules out the possibility that scores of self-rated well-being were influenced by factors unrelated to injury, such as malingering." Ferrari and Russell (1997), the rheumatologists from Alberta who usually have very sensible things to say about whiplash, write: "Furthermore, we consider malingering, i.e., an attempt to deliberately mislead, to be a rare feature in whiplash patients."

56 Hirschfeld, Behan (1963)

CHAPTER TWENTY

1 Wright (1994)

2 Pinker (1997), 23

3 The association's standing committees continually review and update psychiatric diagnoses and the criteria used to make them. Every few years the American Psychiatric Association publishes a new edition of the *DSM*, the present latest edition being the *DSM-IV*.

4 Kirk, Kutchins (1992)

5 American Psychiatric Association (1994)

6 See Nadelson (1979) Theodore Nadelson, an eminent psychiatrist in charge of the consultation service at Beth Israel Hospital, Boston, sees malingering, factitious and the somatoform disorders as merging into each other. He points out that there is a continuum with psychosomatic illness (somatoform disorder) at one end and with malingering at the other end, factitious disorder being somewhere in the middle. The continuum moves from the patient's unawareness of his participation in the illness deception to his total awareness of what he is doing. Along this continuum, the conditions so blend into one another that it is impossible to know where one disorder ends and the other begins.

7 II Samuel 13

8 Grove's Dictionary of the Vulgar Tongue (1785) Trimble (1981), 57

9 Trimble (1981), 57

10 Balla (1982); Buckley (1975), 17

11 Gavin (1843)

12 Littré (1851); Skinner (1961)

13 Lasègue (1918)

14 Johnson (1849)
15 Robert T. Woolsey (1976), professor of neurology at St Louis University, reviewing the history of hysteria, stresses the prodigiously varied vicissitudes undergone by this chameleon illness. To emphasize his point Woolsey précised Kinnier Wilson's "The Approach to the Study of Hysteria" written in 1931. (S.A.K. Wilson was the eminent British neurologist after whom Wilson's disease is named.) "Possibly the outstanding feature of hysteria as revealed to us by the records of former generations is the change which its clinical syndromes have suffered. The medieval ecstatic, simulating in hands and feet the nail prints of her redeemer is long since démodée. No longer do the circus horses of the Salpetrière perform before visitors as in the palmy days of Charcot. Gone too is the 'shell shocked' young soldier of World War I who is fetched mute and amnesic from the smoking battlefield. The times have changed and we, both physician and the hysterics, have changed with them." Times had indeed changed. Two decades previously Gay and Abbott the popularity of whiplash; Wilson noted: "The contemporary hysteric has found haven in the courtroom where, equipped with neck collar and abundant x-rays, she seeks compensation for the almost unbearable and unremitting pain experienced since an automobile accident." Hysteria was reincarnated as whiplash.

Hysteria takes many forms, but one of its few constants is that in doing so it fools large numbers of doctors as to its true identity. If you are a lay reader of this book, despite your lack of an expensive medical education, you can probably now well spot hysteria in any new guise, but then you are not subjected to the financial and social presures that encourage the medical profession to keep its blind spots

Woolsey notes how difficult hysteria is to treat and suggests that the therapeutic goals should be modest. He quotes Freud's sensible dictum that much will be gained if we succeed in transforming hysterical misery into common unhappiness. But common unhappiness often seems a poor exchange for the glamour of a doctor-defeating illness and all the advantages that accrue from "sickness."
16 Freud edited by Ernest Jones (1959)
17 Trimble (1981), 45
18 Sim (1992), 71; Charcot (1889); Trimble (1981), 44
19 Mack, Semrad (1967)
20 Mott (1919)
21 Sim (1992), 70–75
22 Slater quoted by Woolsey (1976)
23 Jones, Llewellyn (1917)
24 Kennedy (1946)
25 Miller (1961)

26 Trimble (1981), 69; Rosanoff (1929)
27 Feldman, Ford (1994)
28 Spivak, Rodin, Sutherland (Jan 1994)
29 Feldman, Ford (1994), 31
30 Asher (1951)
31 Feldman, Ford (1994)
32 Feldman, Ford (1994)
33 Feldman (2000)
34 One mental hospital patient acquired enough psychiatric jargon to pass as a psychiatrist in four other mental hospitals; it is surely much easier to pass as psychiatric patient. Cooper (1974)
35 Anderson, Trethowan, Kenna (1959) Anderson Part I, 5
36 Braginsky, Braginsky, Ring (1969)
37 Earle (1973)
38 Richard Earle. Personal communication. (2000)
39 Rosenhan (1973)
40 Carlson (1973), 116
41 Szasz (1961)
42 Fink (1992)
43 Miller, Cartlidge (1972)
44 Jonas, Pope (1985)
45 Sim (1992), 117
46 Parker (1979)
47 Parker (1979)
48 Lowry (2 Mar 1994)
49 Waddell, McCulloch, et al (1980)
50 McCulloch: Personal communication 23 January 1998
51 Hartt, O'Driscoll, Rosenberg (25 Nov 1997)
52 A. Taylor, T. Hunt, G. Kumchy, J. Saint-Cyr, K. Nicholson, M. McAndrews. (1998). Letter to the OPA. The Ontario Psychologist, 30:16
53 Gorman, Winograd (1988)
54 Wright (1994), 280
55 Malcomb v. Broadhurst (1970) 3A11E.R.508at511. Hillel (1988)
56 Malleson (1990)
57 Gow (1987)

CHAPTER TWENTY-ONE

1 Fraderiks (1976); Miller, Cartlidge (1972)
2 Rigler (1879); Trimble (1981), 58
3 Sim (1992)
4 Page (1885)
5 Kretschmer quoted by Forel

6 Kamman (1951)

7 Oppenheim (1889); Page (1885); Trimble (1981); Tyndel, Tyndel (1984)

8 Buzzard, MacMillan, et al (1928)

9 Kamman (1951)

10 American Psychiatric Association (1980)

11 Goldney (1988)

12 Kennedy (1946)

13 Kennedy (1946)

14 Trimble (1981), 59

15 Sim (1992), 51

16 Awerbuch (1992)

17 Awerbuch (1992)

18 Hubbard (1982); Sim (1992), 148; Jackson (1985)

19 Bleuler (1924), 567

20 DC Turk and TE Rudy (1990) from Pittsburgh, Pennsylvania, have recently reviewed some of these studies, though they did not include all the relevant examples. The following are the studies that they did not include: John B. Cook (1972), a neurologist at the Pinderfields Hospital, Yorkshire, UK, studied 67 head-injured patients, 27 of whom had considered claims for compensation and 36 had not. The severity of these head injuries (as judged by the duration of the post traumatic amnesia), the sex ratio and the age of the patients in two groups showed no significant differences. The mean absence from work for the non-compensation group was 23.9 days and for the compensation group was 87.9 days. Cook comments about his own head injury study and those of other investigators: "Clearly, the extent of brain damage and consequent physical disability must have some influence upon recovery and return to work, but even in studies covering a wide range of severity of head injury it appears that the extent of physical brain damage is not the only factor and probably not the major factor influencing recovery."

Aaron Farbman (1973), the surgeon from Detroit who studied the factors determining recovery in 136 whiplash patients, found that 62 patients had engaged a lawyer, 48 had not, and in 26 no information was available. The median duration of symptoms was greater in the patients who had retained a lawyer, and even when the patients were categorized by estimation of severity of original injury into minor, moderate, or severe injury, this pattern still held. Whether the original injury was minor or severe, patients who consulted a lawyer took longer to recover. Farbman acknowledges the contention about the effects of litigation on whiplash symptoms, but considers his findings support the view that litigation prolongs whiplash symptoms.

CR Fee and WH Rutherford (1988), emergency physicians from

Northern Ireland, more formally demonstrated the deleterious effect of litigation – effects which persist after settlement. The authors followed up 44 consecutive concussion patients for whom a medico-legal report had been written – 22 of these patients had been involved in road traffic accidents.

The authors found that 55% had symptoms when the reports were written (mean interval from accident 12.9 months), 39% had symptoms at time of settlement (mean interval 22.1 months), and 34% had symptoms one year later. The authors compared the compensation patients to patients to other patients treated by the department. They found that the symptoms in the litigation patients one year after settlement were 2.5 times greater than comparable patients in the general series. The authors could find no organic explanation for these differences. They conclude: "It is suggested that the litigation process itself is a factor in the persistence of symptoms and this effect continues after legal settlement has been reached. Early settlement of the cases might significantly reduce morbidity."

21 Mendelson (1981); Mendelson (1982); Mendelson (1985); Mendelson (1992); Mendelson (1995) . Miller's and Mendelson's figures for rates of return to work after settlement could hardly be more different, but perhaps this difference is not so surprising. Miller collected the data for his study in the years 1955 to 1957; Mendelson published his second and larger study in 1995. Miller's figures collected over 40 years ago may well correctly reflect the rates of recovery after settlement in the UK at that time. England then was not a litigious country; Australia in the 1980s was. For other reasons also, Mendelson's findings are likely to be different.

In the 40 years between these studies, lawyers have discovered that by dragging out the litigation of their clients, the clients get sicker and sicker, the awards get bigger and bigger and lawyers get richer and richer. In the 1950s, when Miller collected his litigation data, personal injury litigation suits seldom dragged on for even a year, but many years may now elapse between the occurrence of an accident and the settlement of the injury claim. During this period, to support the cogency of his case, the injured claimant often remains off work. This lengthy process of personal injury litigation itself generates symptoms which then discourage a return to work. Litigants lose their nerve about employment, and employers, quite sensibly, knowing that litigants are often accident recidivists, are reluctant to employ them. The litigants and their families make emotional and financial adjustments to an unemployed lifestyle. The longer the litigant stays off work sick, the less are his chances of ever returning.

Even more relevant perhaps than these factors are changes in people's perceptions about recovery after settlement. In the forty or so years

since Miller published Accident Neurosis, Mendelson and his supporters
have subjected lawyers, doctors and plaintiffs to a barrage of propaganda to the effect that litigants do not recover and return to work after settlement. The enlarging numbers of litigants who fail to return to work
after settlement may just reflect the results of a self-fulfilling prophecy.
Amongst other things, the post-settlement litigant's doctor, with this
gloomy prognosis in mind, now probably does not even bother to
encourage his patient to return to work. When the settlement is too
small to provide for his patient's ongoing needs, the doctor just com-
pletes the disability forms required to obtain a state pension.

Mendelson's study (1995) serves as an excellent example of the deleterious effect of litigation upon health. Most of Mendelson's 760 personal
injury litigants only sustained minor injuries; in fact, Mendelson reports
that 28 sustained no physical injury at all. Yet almost half of his subjects
had not returned to work by the time of finalization of litigation and at
the end of the study at least 198 subjects remained unemployed, 34 of
whom were in receipt of disability support paid by the Department of
Social Security.

22 Myre Sim (1992) devotes four pages of his book to a well-researched
rebuttal of Mendelson's study, exposing its "glaring errors." Robert D.
Goldney (1988), yet another Australian psychiatrist interested in
whiplash, also meticulously re-evaluated the studies on which Mendelson
based his conclusions in Not Cured by a Verdict. Awerbuch (1992),
writes: "To assume occult injury in the absence of confirmatory medical
evidence and on the basis of persistent notionally physical symptoms
after legal settlement is at best tenuous and at worst therapeutically disastrous. Similarly, one should not assume that failure to recover from
notionally psychological symptoms necessarily reflects deep-seated psychological stress induced by the trauma of the accident."
23 Teresi, Lufkin, Reicher (1987)
24 Shapiro, Roth (1993)
25 Mayou, Radanov (1996)
26 Barnsley, Lord, Bogduk (1994)
27 Bogduk (1994)
28 Shapiro, Roth (1993)
29 Radanov, Schnidrig, et al (1992)
30 Merskey (1993)
31 Radanov, Sturzenegger (1996)
32 Barnsley, Lord, Bogduk (1993)
33 Harth, Teasell (1998)
34 Moldofsky, Wong, Lue (1993)
35 Wallis, Lord, Bogduk (1996)
36 McMurdo (1985)

CHAPTER TWENTY-TWO

1 Guinness (1997)
2 Gelernter (1997)
3 Morrow (12 Aug 1991)
4 Hughes (1993)
5 Lecky (1871) and Gage (1985) provide eye-opening information on treated of women by the church.
6 Thomas Aquinas; Freud (1961). This is another example of our capacity to muddle symbol and substance, this time not by the whiplashed but by the world's most famous psychologist. Jung's observation that the "penis is merely a phallic symbol" is certainly more realistic.
7 Craniometry is the measurement of skull size and hence brain volume. Gould (1981); Haller, Haller (1974), 48–61
8 LeBon (1879) quoted by Gould (1981)
9 Vertinsky (1990)
10 Fitch (1899)
11 Haller, Haller (1974), 174–187
12 Prendergast (1896)
13 Fitch (1899)
14 Hall (1978)
15 Vertinsky (1990). It was not only the face that suffered. Fitch (1899) writes: But do you for one moment think that a bicyclist could pose for a sculptor or an artist? Never. Behold the development of the bicyclist. The muscles of the leg, from the ankle to the knee, become enormously large, losing their symmetry and beautiful natural contour; the lower part of the thigh is disproportionately large, causing the limb to lose its beautiful shapeliness.
16 Turner (1896)
17 Rosen (1974)
18 Reich (1954)
19 Stein (1990)
20 Supreme Court of Canada (1928)
21 Showalter (1985)
22 Bly (1996)
23 Woolsey (1976)
24 Harris, Campbell (1999)
25 Well-substantiated studies confirm the psychological harm caused to a child by emotional deprivation and prolonged maternal separation. René Spitz in the late 1940s was the first scientist to demonstrate this harm. Critics savaged his work. The president of New York Psychological Association described the attacks on Spitz's reputation as "a kind of hydrogen bomb … of destructive criticism; not a paragraph is left standing for

miles around." See Hrdy (1999) for an excellent account of these deprivation studies. Jenkins (1998) provides a useful discussion on the evidence
for the harmfulness of various forms childhood compared to that of sexual
abuse.

26 Brewer (1991); Finney (1990); Fredrickson (1992); Gannon (1989);
Herman (1992); Maltz (1991)

27 Coons (1997); Ofshe, Walters (1994) 3

28 Ofshe, Walters (1994)

29 Hagen (1997)

30 Blume (1991)

31 Blume (1991)

32 See Hacking (1995)for an excellent account of this epidemic.

33 Bass, Davis (1988)

34 Ofshe, Walters (1994)

35 Ofshe, Walters (1994)

36 Bass, Davis (1988), 428–435

37 Edwards (1990); Fraser (1990); Fraser (1997); Ofshe, Walters (1994)

38 Showalter (1997), ch 12

39 Coons (1997), 179; Bottoms, Schaver, Goodman, 1993 quoted by Ofshe,
Walters (1994)

40 Ofshe, Walters (1994), 177

41 Coons (1997); Gould (1992); Putnam (1991); Showalter (1997),
174

42 van der Hart, Boon, Jansen (1997)

43 Showalter (1997)

44 Showalter (1997) ch 12

45 Horsnall, Dutta (3 Jun 1994)

46 Showalter (1997)

47 Milstone (Sep 1997)

48 La Fontaine (1998)

49 Foucault (1978)

50 American Psychiatric Association (1994)

51 Greaves (1982); Showalter (1997), ch 11. Hacking (1995) notes an epidemic of double identity around the end of the nineteenth-century
engendered by Charcot's affair with hypnotism and England's dalliance
with spiritualism.

52 Milstone (Sep 1997)

53 Hacking (1995)

54 Colin Ross quoted by Ofshe R, Watters E, in Making Monsters,: False
Memories, Psychotherapy and Sexual Hysteria (1994), 206; Showalter
(1997), 161

55 Horsnall, Dutta (3 Jun 1994); Showalter (1997), ch: 12

56 American Psychiatric Association (1994); Ross, Norton, Wozney (1989)

57 Sagan (1995); Showalter (1997), ch: 13

58 Thompson (1991)

59 Jacobs (1992)

60 Goleman (17 May 1990); Kirk, Kutchins (1992)

61 Blume (1991)

62 Dineen (1996)

63 Ofshe, Walters (1994)

64 Blackshaw, Chandarana, et al (1996)

65 Equity and Aboriginal Issues Committee (2001)

66 Showalter (1997), ch 10

67 Comfort (1967). Alex Comfort is also the comforting author of the *Joy of Sex.*

68 Biller, Trotter (1994); Friday (1996)

69 Twenty-five years ago, before the effects of childhood sexual abuse had become a fashionable condition, I acted as an expert witness for the defence of a well-known paedophile. Over the years he had kept scrupulous records of his sexual activities along with information about the fatherless boys whom he befriended. The defence lawyer managed to contact many of boys who were by then grown-up and married, and with children of their own. They all reported their relationship with the defendant in positive terms. The defendant was found guilty and remains incarcerated as a dangerous sexual offender.

70 Hacking (1995)

71 Dineen (1996)

72 Kirk, Kutchins (1992), 3

73 Feldman, Ford (1994), 26

74 Blake (1993); Field (1989); Wessely (1990); Wessely (1995)

75 Rabinbach (1982)

76 Wessely (1995)

77 Balla (1982)

78 Balint (1966); Parsons (1951); Shuval, Antonovsky, Davies (1973)

79 Eisenberg, Davis, et al (1998)

80 Office for National Statistics (1998)

81 Frankenhaeuser, Lundberg, et al (1989)

82 Reilly (1995)

83 Milstone (Sep 1997); Multiple Reckoning. The San Francisco Chronicle, (17 Feb 1997)

84 William Ernest Henley: Invictus (1875)

85 Gould (1981); Montessori (1913)

CHAPTER TWENTY-THREE

1 O'Brien (1999), 66
2 O'Brien (1999), 100
3 For instance, way back in Tudor England of 1552,in seeking to "protect the king's subjects against the hordes of quacks and impostors who preyed upon their credibility and ignorance," laws were enacted to limit medical practice to licensed practitioners. See Poynter (1971).
4 Healy (2000); Murray, Lopez (1996)
5 Hemels (2001)
6 Gardner (1957); Greenwald (23 Nov 1998); Young (1967)
7 Daly (10 Feb 2001)
8 Abbate (2000). Elizabeth Witmer, Ontario's Minister of Health estimates the cost of such fraud as somewhat lower – at between $60 million and $300 million.
9 Carlson (1975), 78
10 Webb (1910)
11 Berridge (1982); Brian (1994); Lomex (1973); Porter (1997)
12 Trall (1873). Russell T. Trall, a prominent American physician and natural hygienist, estimated that three-quarters of all medical practice was devoted to women. Trall used no medicines and claimed not to have lost a single patient.
13 Quoted by William B. Bean (1950) in Sir Wm Osler: Aphorisms, ch. 5
14 Youngson, Schott (1996)
15 Maines (1999)
16 Maines (1999)
17 Any doctor who now provided genital message would lose his licence and probably be sued by the patient for having caused psychological harm. Perhaps in the past genital message was sometimes useful. Medical authority, with its strong disapproval of female sexuality, had left some women without capacity to perceive genital sensation, and medical authority, by being permissive could sometimes bring it back again. Malleson (1942)
18 Jardine (1999), ch 7, provides an excellent account of such medical practice.
19 Gardner (1957); Hahnemann (1810)
20 Bean (1950)
21 Jardine (1999); Burnum (1986)
22 Gull (1894); Hale-White (1935)
23 Holmes, Sr. (1861)
24 Altman, Blendon (1979); Scitovsky, McCall (1976)
25 Martin, Donaldson, et al (1974)
26 Griner, Glazer (1982)

27 Lancet Editorial (1981)

28 Sandler (1979)

29 Burnum (1986)

30 Smoller, Kruskall (1986)

31 Clark (1985)

32 Mendeloff (1974)

33 Warren (1983)

34 Dunne (1993)

35 Rauws, Tytgat (1990)

36 Cassidy (1946)

37 Stallones (1980)

38 Keys, Kusukawa, et al (1958)

39 Mr. Fit Research Group (1982); WHO European Collaborative Group (1983)

40 James Le Fanu (1999), 322–55, in his book *The Rise and Fall of Modern Medicine* provides an excellent account of the politics of this epidemic.

41 'Trans' fatty acids – a major dietary risk factor of cardiovascular disease. Bruce J. Holub. Personal communication.

42 The heated vegetable oils were mixed with hydrogen in the presence of platinum. Trans fatty acid molecules are mirror images of the fat molecules found in nature.

43 Gillman, Cupples, et al (1997); Hu, Stamper, et al (1997). The trans fatty acids alter the levels of high and low-density lipoproteins in ways that probably predispose to coronary heart disease. See Holub (1991); Mensink, Katan (1990).

44 Ascherio, Willett (1997). Many manufacturers of margarine now make vegetable oils spreadable by the physical process of emulsification.

45 Black (1968)

46 Le Fanu (1999), 337, provides a graph showing the fall in coronary thrombosis rates for the U.S., Australia, New Zealand, and Canada, along with unchanged consumption of fat as percentage of energy intake.

47 Saikku, Mattila, et al (1988)

48 Shor, Kuo, Patton (1992)

49 Gupta, Leatham, et al (1997)

50 Gurfinkel, Bozovich, et al (1997)

51 Dorn, Dunn, Progulske-Fox (1999); Lip, Beevers (1997); Mendall (1998); Gupta, Camm (1979)

52 Much of the surgery for coronary heart disease is very questionable. O'Brien (1999) 128, reviews the evidence for its misuse. He quotes Dr Christian Barnard: "There is no other operation in the treatment of heart disease more misused than coronary artery surgery. You can earn a lot as a coronary artery surgeon ... I would predict that if coronary artery

surgery was made illegal in the world today, half the heart surgeons
would be out of business..."

53 Seidl, Thornton, et al (1966)
54 Schimmel (1964)
55 Hurwitz, Wade (1969)
56 Kessler (1993) see also Einarson (1993)
57 Lazarou, Pomeranz, Corey (1998)
58 (The) Economist (13 February 1999)
59 Two million hospitalized Americans acquire a nosocomial infection each
   year making these infections a major contributing factor to death in
   80,000 U.S. patients (Griffin 1996). Many nosocomial infections occur
   because, even after 150 years, doctors and hospital staff still do not follow Semmelweis's admonition to wash their hands. This failure of
   hygiene was not always by default. Oliver Wendell Holmes (of the fishes
   in the sea) introduced into the U.S. Semmelweis's insights about the
   cause of puerperal fever. Leading American obstetricians were indignant.
   Hugh Hodges wrote that physicians could never convey such a destructive illness and that "it was far more humane to keep her [the patient] in
   happy ignorance of danger." Charles D. Meigs (of ovarian tumour fame),
   accusing Holmes of "propagating a vile, demoralising superstition,"
   observed that it was impossible for doctor's hands to spread disease
   because doctors were gentlemen (O'Brien 1999, 78–9), an example of
   the assumption of the sanctity of medical intervention which cost hundreds of thousands of lives. (Griffin 1996, 78–9).
59 Vincent, Neale, Woloshynowych (2001)
60 New York Times, Dec 1978: House panel calls for more U.S. control of
   surgery, A1 27; Fineberg, Hiatt (1979)
61 Boseley (4 Nov 1998)
62 Bunker (1970)
63 (The) Economist (6 February 1999)
64 Inlander, Levin, Weiner (1988)
65 Roemer, Schwartz (1979)
66 Inlander, Levin, Weiner (1988); Preston (1981), 134–135
67 Roemer, Schwartz (1979)
68 Oswald, Priest (1965); Belleville, Frazer (1957)
69 Hartog, R (1993)
70 U.S. Bureau of Census (1971)
71 American Medical Association: Committee on Alcoholism and Addiction.
   (1965); Jackson (1976)
72 American Medical Association: Committee on Alcoholism and Addiction.
   (1965)
73 Stead AH, et al (1981)
74 Lancet Editorial (1975)

75 Stead AH, et al (1981); Charlton, Kelly, Dunnell (1993); Charlton, Kelly, Dunnell (1992)

76 James, Dean (1983)

77 Barbone, McMahon, et al (2000)

78 Doctors often seem unaware of the mayhem their prescriptions cause. In Britain in the early 1980s, Ester Rantzen in her TV show, *That's Life*, asked her viewers for feed back about problems they had had with barbiturates. The response was overwhelming. Hundreds or thousands of people were recognized as addicted to them.

79 Our Pill Epidemic. Video: Documentary Productions Ltd., Market Media Internation Corp., (1997). Centre for Addiction and Mental Health: Canadian Profile: Alcohol, Tobacco and Other Drugs, 1999. National Library of Canada.

80 Ogilvie (1952)

81 In October 2000, a Russian woman was arrested while trying to sell her grandson to an unidentified man who would take the boy to the West where his organs would be removed and sold. (The Internet)

82 George Carey, the Archbishop of Canterbury, makes the same point, although he uses the words from Abide With Me: "Change and decay in all around I see," for why people turn to their doctors for salvation. Reported by Victoria Combe, The Daily Telegraph (London) 28 Oct 2000, 1

83 Boseley, Sarah. Guardian 22 October 1998

84 Professor Richard Baker, in an audit of Dr Shipman's practice, found that Shipman had 297 more deaths than other doctors working in the Manchester area. The excess was greatest in women over 75 years of age. ("Shipman may have killed 297 report says." The Times, 10 Jan 2001)

85 Whittle, Ritchie (2000). Having injected the fatal dose of morphine, Shipman pilfered the patient's petty cash and jewellery. Seventy per cent of UK patients are cremated and the GP is paid generously for signing the cremation certificate. "Ash cash." "The more the burn the more you earn." It was the forgery of a patient's will that lead to Dr Shipman's exposure.

86 U.S. Department of Health (1973). See also Vincent, Neale, Woloshynowych (2001) for similar British findings.

87 Keeping medical mistakes hidden is certainly not good for our health. Straightforward medical errors are estimated to kill between 44,000 and 98,000 Americans each year. This compares to 43,000 deaths from car accidents. Only when such mistakes are openly acknowledged and the causes for them appropriately examined can any systemic means be found to reduce their reoccurrence. Drugs with similar sounding easily-muddled names can be given a name change; dangerous drugs that are inappropriately injected can be packaged in specially shaped and

coloured containers; and incompetent or error-prone surgeons directed to less hazardous areas of work. But, with malpractice lawyers hovering over the shoulders of doctors and overworked hospital staff, there is a strong incentive to cover up medical mishaps as quickly as possible. An airline that failed to take precautions against the inevitable human errors made by its pilots and engineers would not stay in business. Its planes would not stay in the air.

88 Medical students are now selected more on their marks than on their character. Good marks do not in anyway select for humane qualities, though they perhaps make it less likely that any disreputable behaviour will be discovered. In the past, medical school expelled students with character disorders, but as such expulsions now inevitably result in damage suits, medical schools are reluctant to put themselves at risk. The delinquent medical student becomes a delinquent doctor.

CHAPTER TWENTY-FOUR

1 Thomas (1979)
2 O'Keith (1970); Shaw, Nevel (2000)
3 Foss (2001)
4 Stone (1763)
5 Jack (1997)
6 Chalmers, Enkin, Keirse (1998); Sackett (1995)
7 Episiotomy is the cutting of the entrance of the vagina with scissors to allow easier exit of the infant's head. Additional medical intervention is then required to suture the wound.
8 Page (1996)
9 Evidence-Based Medicine Working Group (1992); Sackett, Rosenberg, et al (1996)
10 Rosser, Shafir (1998)
11 Medical Research Council (1948)
12 British Medical Journal Editorial (1998)
13 Doll (1998)
14 Craven (1950)
15 Evidence-Based Medicine Working Group (1992); Peto, Baigent (1998)
16 ISIS-2 Collaborative Group (1988)
17 Sackett (1995)
18 Rosser, Shafir (1998)
19 These cholesterol-lowering drugs are gemfibrozil, clofibrate, and colestipol. See Rosser, Shafir (1998)
20 Rosser, Shafir (1998)
21 Horsten, Wamela, et al (1997)
22 Evidence-Based Medicine Working Group (1992)

23 Chalmers (1998); Kunz, Oxman (1998)

24 BMJ Editorial (1998)

25 Hill (1966)

26 Blair (1997)

27 Maynard (1997); Page (1996); Sackett (1996); Sackett, Rosenberg, et al (1996)

28 Blair (1997)

29 Rosser, Shafir (1998), 45

30 The best-known of these huge data-bases is the Cochrane Collaboration, named after Archie Cochrane, the British epidemiologist who first sponsored it. Centred in Oxford, the Collaboration unites worldwide a large number of groups evaluating the results of RCTS.

31 Rosser, Shafir (1998)

32 Bass, Buck, Turner (1986)

33 Gracely, Dubner, et al (1985)

CHAPTER TWENTY-FIVE

1 Because Eve tempted Adam with the apple and had mankind driven out of the Garden of Eden, the church held women responsible for all the ills of the world including the crucifixion of Christ (see Gage 1985; Lecky 1871)

2 Sagan (1995); New Catholic Encyclopedia (1967)

3 Brooke (1993); Solomon (1997)

4 Even Paracelsus, the great sixteenth-century Swiss physician, seems to have thought so, for he threw all his medical works, including those of Hippocrates and Galen, into the fire, saying that he know nothing save what he had learned from the witches. See Brooke (1993); Gage (1985) 241–2; Solomon (1997)

5 Dangler (2001)

6 Bolen (1994); Stein (1988), 80

7 Estimates as to the numbers of witches burned varies greatly. Gage (1985) gives a number of nine million, while Sharpe (1996) puts the number at somewhere less than 50,000. Brooke (1993) suggests that 20 percent of women practitioners were burned.

8 Stein (1990), 84

9 Marwick (1998)

10 Boon, Kennard, et al (2000)

11 Goldbeck-Wood, Lie, et al (1996)

12 Brennan (1992); Feldenkrais (1979)

13 Morris (1971); Roemer, Schwartz (1979)

14 Smith (1976); Whitehead (1967)

15 Bucke (1901); Epstein (1995); Maslow (1968); Moore (1992);

Watts (1963); Wilber, Goleman, et al (1993); Davies (1993); Huxley (1945)

16 Delbanco (1998)

17 Eisenberg, Davis, et al (1998)

18 Eisenberg, Davis, et al (1998)

19 Greenwald (23 Nov 1998)

20 Dangler (2001), 30–1

21 Garrison (1929)

22 Economist (30 May 1998).

23 Stein (1990)

24 Levy (1996)

25 Grauds (1997); Monmaney (31 Aug 1998)

26 One unzips even a banana at one's peril! Ames, Gold (1990) found 27 natural pesticides that are rodent carcinogens to be present in virtually all the common fruits and vegetables we eat. These were just as carcinogenic as man-made pesticides but were present in about 1000 times greater amounts than were the traces of synthetic pesticides.

27 Ernst (1998)

28 Withering (1941)

29 Smith, Braunwald, Kelly (1992)

30 Mahdyoon, Battilana, et al (1990)

31 Mahdyoon, Battilana, et al (1990)

32 U.S. Newswire: Hoffman-La Roche tops list of leading corporate criminals of the decade. (3 Sep 1999) p1009245n0028 Washington.

33 Segal, D: Six vitamin firms to pay $1.1 billion: settlement would set record in antitrust case. Washington Post (7 Sep 1999)

34 Ernst (1998)

35 Tyler (1993)

36 Brevoort (1998); Ernst (2000)

37 Ang-lee, Moss, Yuan (2001)

38 Mehta (2000)

39 This excellent organization is now The National Council for Reliable Health Information. Membership Chairman, P.O. Box 1276, Loma Linda, CA 92354-1276

40 Herbert (1984)

41 The Mount Sinai School of Medicine Complete Book of Nutrition (1990) New York: St Martin's Press.

42 Herbert (1984)

43 Marwick (1998)

44 Garfinkel, Sinngal, et al (1998) in randomized single-blind control trial of treatments for carpal tunnel syndrome showed that supervised yoga and relaxation techniques are superior to the wrist splint of conventional medicine; Bensoussan, Talley, et al (1998) divided patients with irritable

bowel syndrome into three groups. The patients in one group were prescribed individualized Chinese herbal formulations, the patients in the second group were given a standard Chinese herbal formulation and those of the third group a placebo. On follow-up 14 weeks after completion of the treatment, the patients in the individualized Chinese herbal formulations group maintained improvement, while patients in the other two groups did not; Carraro, Raynaud, et al (1996) and Bach, Schmitt, Ebeling (1996) in comparing the results of herbal and conventional treatments of benign enlargement of the prostate suggest that the herbal treatments are both superior and have fewer side effects than does conventional treatment.

CHAPTER TWENTY-SIX

1 Illich (1982)
2 Poynter (1971)
3 McKeown (1979); McKeown, Lowe (1966)
4 McKeown (1971); Powles (1973)
5 Croll (2000)
6 Unwanted children are at added risk for all sorts of misfortunes; any country that reduces the number of unwanted pregnancies is likely to improve its health statistics. The accidental death rate of children in the U.S. is nearly three times higher than in Sweden where safe abortion is readily available. The U.S. has a high teenage pregnancy rate and teenagers have poor parenting skills.

Despite the essential contribution to health of smaller families, mainstream medicine was, until a few decades ago, opposed to the use of any means by which parents could limit family size. Many religious leaders still oppose all methods of family planning other than sexual abstinence. While most affluent women ignored such harsh religious sanctions and opted to do what they consider best for themselves and their families, the poor were unable to do so. Religious pressure groups, especially those in the United States, succeeded in blocking healthcare funds for family planning services to the poor and the developing countries. By having done so they bear at least partial responsibility for the continuing unnecessarily high morbidity and mortality rates in these countries.

7 Le Fanu (1999) uses this term for what he described as the apogee of medicine's success.
8 Single, Rehm, et al (2000)
9 Any person determined to kill themselves, even in a locked mental hospital ward, usually manages to do so, but once it is perceived as the psychiatrist's job to prevent suicide, the patient can keep the psychiatrist on the hop with suicide threats.

10 Bulusa, Alderson (1984)

11 Malleson (1973a); Charlton, Kelly, Dunnell (1993); Charlton, Kelly, Dunnell (1992); Bulusa, Alderson (1984); See also Hassall and Trethowan (1972)

12 Despite the fact that women complain more frequently of unhappiness, men consistently have higher suicide rates; but never before in Britain has this gender gap been so large. Perhaps men are simply handier with car exhausts and hosepipes, or perhaps women's liberation is demoralizing the English male.

13 See mortality statistic for U.S., Canada, and the U.K.

14 Lancet Editorial (2000); Bailar, Gornik (1997). See also American Cancer Society (1999) Cancer Facts and Figures.

15 Hislop (1997)

16 Thomas, Gao, et al (1997)

17 Position statement (Nov 1999).

18 Feig (1999)

19 Baines (1998)

20 Gøtzche, Olsen (2000)

21 Gøtzche, Olsen (2000); Wells (1998)

22 Miller, To, et al. (2000)

23 (The) Economist (1997)

24 Gøtzche, Olsen (2000) give the statistic that one death by breast cancer will be saved for every 1000 Swedish women screened every two years for 12 years. Black, Nease, Tosteson (1995); Bryant, Brasher (1994); Baines (2000)

25 Michaelson, Halperin, Kopans (1999); Eisenger, Geller, Holtzman (1999)

26 Baines (1998)

27 (The) Economist (5 April 1997)

28 Doll, Hill (1950)

29 WHO in World Report 1999 comments that a half of all long-term smokers will die of the habit. "If current trends continue, in the year 2030, tobacco will kill 10 million people a year – over 70% of them in developing countries where information on tobacco-related disease is often weakest." Perhaps Dr Gro Brundtland, a onetime Norwegian family physician and now the first woman director-general of the WHO, will goad her sluggish organization into exposing what she sees as "the big tobacco's worldwide campaign of deception and lies." (WHO/65 Press Release. 4 Nov 99)

30 Fenton (18 Jul 2001): The study was for the year 1999–2000.

31 Poynter (1971), 29

32 Illich (1977), 11–39; Illich (1982)

33 Barsky (1988); Dalrymple (1998); Evans, Barer, Marmor (1994)
34 Dalrymple (1998)

CHAPTER TWENTY-SEVEN

1 Carlson (1975)
2 In Evans, Barer, Marmor (1994), ch 8, 217–30
3 Beveridge (1942)
4 Poynter (1971)
5 Poynter (1971)
6 It is surprisingly difficult to find reliable information on sickness and disability rates. Waddell (Spine 1987) quotes figures supplied to him by the DHSS (UK) of 14,000 days per year per 1000 males at risk over the mid 1950s rising to 20,000 days by 1980. A comparison made 10 years after the start of the NHS of sick days lost in two similar industrial plants one in the UK and the other in Indonesia showed the English rate of 12 days a year to be more than double the Indonesian rate of 5.5 days, despite the fact that several serious and unpleasant infectious diseases remained endemic in Indonesia. See also Glyn (1970). Doctors, for instance, have become increasingly disillusioned with their choice of profession. In 1966, 14% of a cohort of UK doctors regretted entering medicine and by 1986, 58% regretted their choice. By 1996, a quarter of new English doctors had no plans to work in the National Health Service (quoted by James Le Fanu 1999).
7 Cited by Callahan in False Hopes (1998), 74
8 Dubos (1961)
9 Dubos (1961); Illich (1977); Michaelson (1970); Cochrane (1972); Powles (1973); Malleson (1973a); Malleson (1973b); McKeown (1977)
10 Carlson (1975)
11 Ezzell (2000)
12 Replacing a defective gene or even inserting the genes for a nice new tail perhaps?
13 Le Fanu (1999)
14 Actually, Le Fanu perceives "the radical ideas of social theory," – the belief that the cause of most common illnesses lies simple in people's social habits – as having also inappropriately moved in to compensate for modern medicine's doldrums. While I agree that this has happened, I disagree that these ideas should be so lightly dismissed.
15 Brook, Ware, et al (1984)
16 Organization for Economic Co-operation and Development (1998)
17 World Bank (1993)
18 Marmor, Smith (1989). Japan's increase in life expectancy is particularly

remarkable, since Japanese men smoke like old-fashioned factory chimneys.

19 WHO, World Health Report (2000)
20 OECD (1999)
21 In Evans, Barer, Marmor (1994): Is more better? 236–51
22 Simpson (16 Oct 2000)
23 O'Brien (1999)
24 O'Brien (1999), 15, 20
25 Economist (9 Oct 1999)
26 Callahan (1998).
27 Garber, Weinstein, et al (2000)
28 Carlson (1975): "Medicine has fostered a profoundly depended public which searches for cures that do not exist ... Medicine has failed to encourage the patient to assume responsibility for health; the public craves more and more services."
29 The average age, for instance, of nurses in Ontario is now 47 years. Personal communication, the Ontario College of Nurses (2000). For an excellent account of demoralised nurses and other employees of the National Health Service in the UK, see Bruggen (1997)
30 Economist (25 March 2000)
31 Economist (13 Feb 1999)
32 O'Brien (1999); Carlson (1975); Callahan (1998); Thompson (1971)
33 McKeown, Lowe (1966)
34 Charles, Whelan, Gafni (1999)
35 Decter (2000)

APPENDIX

1 White, Wolraich (1995)
2 Saravis, Schacter, et al.(1990)
3 Huber (1991); White, Wolraich (1995)
4 Gouvier (1988)
5 Guthkelch (1980); Wrightson, Gronwall (1981)
6 Binder (1997a); Binder (1997b)
7 Malleson, Eastwood, Moore (1977)
8 In developed societies tuberculosis remains a killing illness amongst the homeless.

References

Abbate Gay. 5 Nov 2000. College panel delays crackdown on fraud by MDs. Globe and Mail (Toronto) A15

Abdel-Fattah RA. 1993. Preventing Temporomandibular Joint (TMJ) and Odontostomatognathic (OSGs) Injuries in Dental Practice. Boca Raton, Florida: CRC Press

– 1996. Evaluating TMJ Injuries. New York: Wiley Law Publications

Abdel-Fattah RA, Alattar MM. 1984. Dentistry: Oral-Facial Pain: TMJ Disorders, Boca Raton, Florida: Abdel-Fattah and Alattar

Abrahamson EM, Pezet AW. 1951. Body, Mind and Sugar. New York: Holt, Rinehart and Winston

Adler A. 1941. The psychology of repeated accidents in industry. Am J Psychiatry 98, 99–101

Agency for Health Care Policy and Research. 1992. Clinical practice guideline Number 14: Acute Low Back Problems in Adults. Rockville, Maryland: Department of Health and Human Services

Algers G, Pettersson K, et al. 1993. Surgery for chronic symptoms after whiplash injury: follow-up of 20 cases. Acta Orthop Scand 64:654–6

Alker GJ, Young SO, et al. 1975. Postmortem radiology of head and neck injuries in fatal accidents. Radiology 114:611–7

Allan EL, Barker KN, et al. 1995. Dispensing errors and counselling in community practice. Am Pharm (NS35)120:25–33

Allen ME, Weir-Jones I, et al. 1994. Acceleration perturbations of daily living. A comparison to "whiplash." Spine 19:1285–90

Allen MJ, Barnes MR, Bodinah GG. 1985. The effect of seat belt legislation on injuries sustained by car occupants. Injury 16:471–6

Allen P, Glasziou P, Del Mar C. 1999. Bed rest: a potentially harmful treatment needing more careful evaluation. Lancet 354:1229–33

Allodi F. 1989. The children of victims of political persecution and torture: a psychological study of a Latin American refugee community. Int J Ment Health 18:3–15

– 1991. Assessment and treatment of torture victims. J Nerv Ment Dis 179:4–11

– 1994. PTSD in tortured Latin American refugees. Personal communication

Altman SA, Blendon R. 1979. Medical technology: the culprit behind health care costs. Washington DC: Government Printing Office, DHEW publication No:(PHS)79–3216

Ameis A. 1986. Whiplash: considerations in the rehabilitation of cervical myofascial injury. Can Fam Physician 32:1871–6

American College of Occupational and Environmental Medicine: Position Statement. 1999. Multiple chemical sensitivities: idiopathic environmental intolerance. J Occup Environ Med 4:940–2

American Congress of Rehabilitation Medicine. 1993. [HI-ISIG]. Head Injury Interdisciplinary Special Interest group: Definition of mild traumatic brain injury. J Head Trauma Rehabil 8:86–7

American Law Institute. 1997. Model Code of Evidence

American Medical Association: Committee on Alcoholism and Addiction. (1965) Dependence on barbiturates and other sedative drugs. JAMA 193:107–11

American Psychiatric Association. 1980. The Diagnostic and Statistical Manual of Mental Disorders–III (DSM-III). Washington DC: American Psychiatric Association

– 1994. The Diagnostic and Statistical Manual of Mental Disorders–IV (DSM-IV). Washington DC: American Psychiatric Association

Ames BN, Gold L. 1990. Chemical carcinogenesis: too many rodent carcinogens. Proc Nat Acad Sci 87:7772–6

Anderson EW, Trethowan WH, Kenna JC. 1959. An experimental investigation of simulation and pseudodementia. Acta Psychiatrica et Neurologica Scandinavica 34 Suppl:1–41

Anderson GW, Rondeau JC. 1954. Absence of tonsils as a factor in the development of bulbar poliomyelitis. JAMA 155:1123–30

Anderson TW. 1973. Nutritional muscular dystrophy and human myocardial infarction. Lancet 2:298–302

Anderson TP. 1991. Positive physical findings confirming chronic pain syndrome. Am J Phys Med Rehabil 70:157–8

Angell M. 1996a. Science on Trial. WW Norton & Co: London and New York

– 1996b. Shattuck Lecture: Evaluating the health risks of breast implants: the interplay of medical science, the law, and public opinion. N Engl J Med 334:1513–18

Ang-lee MK, Moss J, Yuan C-S. 2001. Herbal medicines and perioperative care. JAMA 286:208–16

Annas GJ. 1994. Scientific evidence in the courtroom: the death of the Frye Rule. N Engl J Med 330: 1018–21

Aprill C, Bogduk N. 1992. The prevalence of cervical zygapophyseal joint pain: a first approximation. Spine 17:744–7

Ariès P. 1962. Centuries of Childhood: A Social History of Family Life. New York: Alfred A Knopf

Ascherio A, Willett WC. 1997. Health effects of trans fatty acids. Am J Clin Nutr 66(4 Suppl):1006S–10S

Asher R. 1951. Munchausen's syndrome. Lancet 1: 339–41

Awerbuch MS. 1991. Thermography: its current diagnostic status in musculoskeletal medicine. Med J Aust 154:441–4

– 1991. Thermography: whither the niche? Med J Aust 154:444–7

– 1992. Whiplash in Australia: illness or injury? Med J Aust 157:193–6

Axelsson A, Rosenhall U, Zachau G. 1994. Hearing in 18-year-old Swedish males. Scand Audiol 23:129–34

Bach D, Schmitt M, Ebeling L. 1996. Phytopharmaceutical and synthetic agents in the treatment of benign prostatic hypertrophy. Phytomedicine 3:309–13

Back Letter Editorial. (2000). Half-truths, personal attacks, and innuendo cloud debate over recovery from whiplash injury. Back Letter 15(8):85

Baer N. 1997. Fraud worries insurance companies but should concern physicians too, industry says. CMAJ, 156:251–3

Bailar JC, Gornik HL. 1997. Cancer undefeated. N Engl J Med 336:1569–74

Baines C. 1998. Breast-cancer screening: will the controversy never end? Diagnosis 15:65–71

Baker LD. 1996. The Permanency of Whiplash. Eagler, Idaho: Integrity Seminars, Inc

Bakwin H. 1945. "Pseudodoxia Pediatrica." N Engl J Med 232:691–7

Balint M. 1957. The Doctor, the Patient and the Illness. New York: International Universities Press

– 1966. The Drug, Doctor. In Scott WR, Volkart EH (eds), Medical Care. New York: Wiley

Balla JI. 1980. The late whiplash syndrome. Aust N Z J Surg 50:610–4

– 1982. The late whiplash syndrome: a study of an illness in Australia and Singapore. Culture, Medicine & Psychiatry 6:191–210

– 1998. Report to the Motor Accidents Board of Victoria on whiplash injuries. 1984. In Hopkins A (ed). Headache, Problems in Diagnosis and Management. London: WB Saunders. 268–89.

Balla JI, Karnaghan J. 1987. Whiplash headache. Clinical & Experimental Neurology 23:179–82

Baloh R. 1995. Neurotology. In Joynt RJ (ed). Clinical Neurology. New York: Lippincott Raven. Vol 3, ch 42, 29

Barnsley L, Lord SM, Bogduk N. 1993b. Comparative local anaesthetic blocks in the diagnosis of cervical zygapophyseal joint pain. Pain 55:99–106

- 1993. The pathophysiology of whiplash. In Teasell RW, Shapiro AP (eds). Spine. Philadelphia: Hanley & Belfus. Vol 3(3) ch 1, 329–53

- 1994. Whiplash injury. Pain 58:283–307

Barnsley L, Lord SM, et al. 1995. The prevalence of chronic cervical zygapophyseal joint pain after whiplash. Spine 20:20–5, discussion 26

Barsky AJ.1988. Worried Sick: Our Troubled Quest for Wellness. Boston: Little, Brown and Co

Barsky AJ, Borus JF. 1999. Functional somatic syndromes. Ann Intern Med 131:910–18

Bartholomew RE, Sirois F. 2000. Occupational mass psychogenic illness: transcultural prevalence and presentation patterns. Transcultural Psychiatry 37:495–524

Bartlett J. 1989. How to survive a psychiatric interview. Interaction 2. London: ME Action Campaign

Barton D, Allen M, et al. 1993. Evaluation of whiplash injuries by technetium 99m isotope scanning. Arch Emerg Med 10:197–202

Baskett SJ, Henager J. 1983. Differentiating between post-Vietnam syndrome and preexisting psychiatric disorders. South Med J 76:988–90

Bass E, Davis L. 1988. The Courage to Heal: A Guide for Women Survivors of Child Sexual Abuse. New York: Harper and Row

Bass MJ, Buck C, Turner L. 1986. The physician's actions and outcome of illness in family practice. J Fam Practice 23:43–7

Battié MC, Bigos SJ. 1991. Industrial back pain complaints: a broader perspective. Orthop Clin North Am 22:273–82

Beard GM. 1869. Neurasthenia or nervous exhaustion. Boston Med Surg J 3:217–20

- 1880. A Practical Treatise on Nervous Exhaustion (Neurasthenia). New York: William Wood

- 1881. American Nervousness: Its Causes and Consequences. New York: GP Putnam's Sons

Beecher HK. 1955. The powerful placebo. JAMA 159:1602–6

Begley S. 22 Mar 1993. The Meaning of Junk. Newsweek

Behan RC, Hirschfeld AH. 1963. The accident process. JAMA 186:300–6

Behan RJ.1939. Relation of Trauma of New Growths: Medico-legal Aspects. Baltimore: Williams and Wilkins

Bell DS. 1989. Repetition strain injury: an iatrogenic epidemic of simulated injury. Med J Aust 151:280–4

Belleville RE, Frazer HF. 1957. Tolerance to some effects of barbiturates. J Pharm Exp Therapeut 120:469–474

Belli MM. 1970. Introduction. In Frigard LT (ed). The Whiplash Injury. Richmond Hill, NY: Richmond Hall

Bench CJ, Brown RG, et al. 1994. Neuropsychological dysfunction in depression. Psychol Med 6:849–57

Benedet J. 1991. When the Law Society is an Ass. Globe and Mail (Toronto) A17

Bennett RM. 1995. Fibromyalgia: the commonest cause of widespread pain. [Review]. Compr Ther 21:269–75

– 1997. The fibromylagia syndrome. In Kelley AB, Harris ED, Ruddy S, Sledge C. (eds). 1997. Textbook of Rheumatology. Philadelphia: WB Saunders. Ch 34, 511–19

Bensoussan A, Talley NJ, et al. 1998. Treatment of irritable bowel syndrome with Chinese herbal medicine. JAMA 280:1585–9

Berman E. 25 Mar 1987. USA Today

Bernard LC. 1990. Prospects of faking believable memory deficits on neuropsychological tests and the use of incentives in simulation research. J Clin Exp Psychol 12:715–28, 1990

Berridge V. 1998a. Opiate use in England, 1800–1926. Ann N Y Acad Sci 398:1–11

Berry JH. 1987. What can be done about dental quackery? J Am Dent Assoc 115:679–85

Berstad JR, Baerum B, et al. 1975. Whiplash: chronic organic brain syndrome without hydrocephalus ex vacuo. Acta Neurol Scand 51:268–84

Beveridge Sir W. 1942. Social Insurance and Allied Services. London: HMSO

Bicik I, Radanov BP, et al. 1998. PET with [18]fluorodeoxyglucose and hexamethylpropylene amine oxime SPECT in late whiplash syndrome. Neurology 51:345–50

Bigos SJ, Battié MC. 1991. The impact of spinal disorders in industry. In Frymoyer JW, et al (eds). The Adult Spine: Principles and Practice. New York: Raven Press. Ch 9, 147–54

Bigos SJ, Battié MC et al. 1989. A longitudinal prospective study of acute back problems. The influence of physical and non-physical factors. Abstracts. 16th Annual ISSLS Meeting (Kyoto)

Biller HB, Trotter RJ. 1994. The Father Factor: What You Need to Know to Make the Difference. New York: Pocket

Binder LM. 1978. The abuse of psychiatric disability determinations. Med Trial Tech Q (Jan):89–91

– 1991. Assessment of motivation after financially compensable minor head trauma. J Consult Clin Psychol 3:171–81

– 1993. The assessment of malingering after mild head trauma with the Portland Digit Recognition Test. J Clin Exp Psychol 15:170–82

– 1997a. A review of mild head trauma. Part l: Meta-analytical review of neuropsychological studies. J Clin Exp Psychol 19:421–31

– 1997b. A review of mild head trauma. Part ll: Clinical implications. J Clin Exp Psychol 19:432–57

Binder LM, Rohling ML. 1996. Money matters: a meta-analytic review of the effects of financial incentives on recovery after closed-head injury. Am J Psychiatry 153:7–10

Bingham R. 1968. Whiplash injuries. Med Trial Tech Q 14:69–80

Birnie DJ, Knipping AA, et al. 1991. Psychological aspects of fibromyalgia compared with chronic and nonchronic pain. J Rheumatol 18:1845–8

Bjørgen IA. 1996. Late whiplash syndrome [letter]. Lancet 348:124

Black B. 1988. Evolving legal standards for the admissibility of scientific evidence. Science 239:1508–12

Black DAK. 1968. The Logic of Medicine. London: Loiver and Boyd

Black DC, Nease RF, Tosteson ANA. 1995. Perceptions of breast cancer risk and screening effectiveness in women younger than 50 years of age. J Natl Cancer Inst 87:720–31

Black FO, Lilly DJ, et al. 1987. Quantitative diagnostic test for perilymph fistulas. Otolaryngol Head Neck Surg 96:125–34

Blackshaw S, Chandarana P, et al. 1996. Position Statement [Canadian Psychiatric Association]: Adult recovered memories of childhood sexual abuse. Can J Psychiatry 41:305–6

Blair JA, Blair RS, Rueckert P. 1994. Pre-injury emotional trauma and chronic backache. Spine 19:1144–7

Blair L. 1997. Special Report: Short on evidence. Can Fam Physician 43:427–9

Blake LS. 1993. Sick and tired. The Canadian Nurse 25–31

Blanchard EB, Hickling EJ, et al. 1995. Effects of varying scoring rules of the Clinician-Administered PTSD Scale (CAPS) for the diagnosis of post-traumatic stress disorder in motor vehicle accident victims. Behav Res Ther 33:471–5

Blanchard EB, Hickling EJ, et al. 1994. Psychological morbidity associated with motor vehicle accidents. Behav Res Ther 32:283–90

Blécourt AC, Knipping AA, et al.1993. Weather conditions and complaints in fibromyalgia. J Rheumatol 20:1932–4

Bleuler EP. 1924. Textbook of Psychiatry. Brill AA translator. New York: The Macmillan Company

Blume ES. 1991. Secret Survivors. New York: Ballantine Books

Bly Robert. 1996. The Sibling Society. Reading, Massachusetts: Addison-Wesley Publishing Co

Boden SD. 1996. Effective diagnosis and treatment for acute low back pain. Hippocrates' Lantern 4:1–3

Boden SD, Davis DO, et al. 1990. Abnormal magnetic-resonance scans of the lumbar spine in asymptomatic subjects: a prospective investigation. J Bone Joint Surg Am 72:403–8

Boden SD, McCowin PR, et al. 1990. Abnormal magnetic resonance scans of the cervical spine in asymptomatic subjects. J Bone Joint Surg Am 72:1178–84

Bogduk N. 1994. Post whiplash syndrome. Aust Fam Phys 23:2303–7

– 1996. Editorial to Scientific Monograph of the Quebec Task Force on Whiplash-Associated Disorders. Spine, 20(Suppl):8S–9S

Bohr TW. 1987. Painful questions about fibromyalgia. JAMA 258:147

– 1995. Fibromyalgia syndrome and myofascial pain syndrome. Do they exist? [Review]. Neurol Clin 13:365–84

– 1996. Problems with myofascial pain syndrome and fibromyalgia syndrome. Neurology 46:593–7

Boisset-Pioro MH, Esdaile JM, Fitzcharles MA. 1995. Sexual and physical abuse in women with fibromyalgia syndrome. Arthritis Rheum 38:235–41

Bolen JS. 1994. Crossing to Avalon. San Francisco: HarperCollins

Bonica JJ. Dec 1974. New progress against pain. US News and World Report

Boon HS, Kennard MA, et al. 2000. Use of complementary/alternative medicine by breast cancer survivors in Ontario. J Clin Oncol 8:2501–21

Borden AGB, Rechtman AM, Gardner GM. 1960. The normal cervical lordosis. Radiology 74:806–9

Bortz WM. 1984. The disuse syndrome. West J Med 141:691–4

Boseley S. 4 Nov 1998. Surgeons told operations are not always in patients' interests. Guardian (UK), Home News, 5

Bovim G, Schrader H, Sand T. 1994. Neck pain in the general population. Spine 19:1307–9

Braaf MM, Rosner S. 1955. Symptomatology and treatment of injuries of the neck. NY State J Med 55:223–42

– 1958. Whiplash injury of the neck: symptoms, diagnosis, treatment and prognosis. NY State J Med 58:1501–7

– 1966. Whiplash injury of neck – fact or fancy. Int Surg 46:176-82

Braginsky BM, Braginsky DD, Ring K. 1969. Methods of Madness. New York: Holt, Rinehart and Winston, Inc

Braun B, Schiffman EL. 1991. The validity and predictive value of four assessment instruments for evaluation of the cervical and stomatognathic systems. J Craniomandibular Dis Face Oral Pain 5:239–44

Brennan R. 1992. The Alexander Technique. Shaftesbury, Dorset: Element

Brent DA, Perper JA, et al. 1995. Post-traumatic stress disorder in peers of adolescent suicide victims: predisposing factors and phenomenology. J Am Acad Child Adolescent Psychiatry 34:209–15

Brevoort P. 1998. The booming US botanical market. Herbalgram 44:33–46

Brewer C. 1991. Escaping the Shadows: Seeking the Light. San Francisco: HarperSanFrancisco

Brian J. 1994. Opium and infant-sedation in nineteenth-century England. Health Visit 67:165–7

British Medical Journal Editorial. 1963. "Tonsils and Adenoids." Br Med J 2:698

British Medical Journal Editorial. 1998. Fifty years of randomised controlled trials. BMJ 317:1167

Brodsy CM. 1983. "Allergic to everything": a medical subculture. Psychosomatics 24:731–42

Brook RH, Ware JE, et al. 1984. The Effect of Co-insurance on the Health of Adults. Santa Monica: RAND

Brooke Elisabeth. 1993. Women Healers Through History. London: Women's Press Ltd

Brooker A-S, Frank JW, Tarasuk V. 1995. Back pain claim rates and the business cycle: Toronto: Institute of Work and Health

Bruggen P. 1997. Who Cares? True Stories of the NHS Reforms. UK: Jon Carpenter

Brussgaard D, Evensen A, Bjerkedal I. Fibromyalgia. 1993. A new cause for disability pension. Scand J Soc Med 21:116–9

Bryant HE, Brasher PMS. 1994. Risks and probabilities of breast cancer: short-term versus lifetime probabilities. CMAJ 150:211–6

Buchnia A. 1994. Rehabilitation centres owned by lawyers. Metro Morning, Canadian Broadcasting Company

Bucholz RW, Burkhead WZ, et al. 1979. Occult cervical spine injuries in fatal traffic accidents. J Trauma 19:768–71

Bucke R. 1901. Cosmic Consciousness (1961 ed). New York: EP Dutton & Co

Buckley K. 1975 Primary accumulation: a genesis of Australian capitalism. In Wheelwright EL, Buckley K (eds). Essays in Political Economy of Australian Capitalism. Melbourne: ANZ Book Co. Vol 1

Budd RJ, Pugh R. 1996. Tinnitus coping style and its relationship to tinnitus severity and emotional distress. J Psychosom Res 41:327–35

Bulusa L, Alderson M. 1984. Suicides 1950–82. Population Trends (Office of Government Statistical Service) 35:11–7

Bunker JP 1970. Surgical manpower. N Engl J Med 282:135–44

Burgess J. 1991. Symptom characteristics in TMD patients reporting blunt trauma and/or whiplash injury. J Craniomandibular Dis Face Oral Pain 5:251–7

Burke JP, Orton HO, et al. 1992. Whiplash and its effects of the visual system. Graefes Arch Clin Exp Ophthalmol 230:335–9

Burnum JF. 1986. Medical vampires. N Engl J Med 314:1250–1

Burton AK, Tillotson KM, Troup JDJ. 1989. Prediction of low-back trouble frequency in a working population. Spine 14:939–46

Burton R. 1905. Anatomy of Melancholy (1652). London: Duckworth & Co

Burton T. 16 Nov 1999. Could chronic fatigue be a bone problem? Quoted from the Wall Street Journal. Globe and Mail (Toronto) C9

Buzzard SF, MacMillan HP, et al. 1928. Discussion on traumatic neurasthenia and the litigation neurosis. J R Soc Med 21:239

Cady LD, Bischoff DP, et al. 1979. Strength and fitness and subsequent back injuries in firefighters. J Occup Med 21:269–72

Caffey J. 1946. Multiple fractures in longbones of infants suffering chronic subdural hematoma. Am J Roentgenology 56:163–73

Cain CM, Ryan GA, et al. 1989. Cervical spine injuries in road traffic accidents in South Australia. Aust NZ J Psychiatry 59:15–9

Calabresi G. 1970. The Cost of Accidents: a Legal and Economic Analysis. New Haven: Yale University Press

Caldwell IW. 1972. Seatbelts and headrests (letter). Br Med J 2:163

Callahan Daniel. 1998. False Hopes. New York: Simon & Schuster

Campbell H. 1915. Aids to Pathology (2nd ed). London: Baillière, Tindal & Cox

– 1917. Aids to Pathology (3rd ed). London: Baillière, Tindal & Cox

Campbell SM, Clark S, et al. 1983. Clinical characteristics of fibromyalgia. Arthritis Rheum 26:817–24

Capurso U, Perillo L, Ferro A. 1992. [Cervical trauma in the pathogenesis of cranio-cervico-mandibular dysfunctions] [Italian]. Minerva Stomatol 41:5–12

Carcopino J. 1954. Daily Life in Ancient Rome. London: Penguin Books

Carette S. 1994. Whiplash injury and chronic pain. N Engl J Med 330:1083–4

– 1995. Fibromyalgia 20 years later: what have we really accomplished? J Rheumatol 22:590–4

Carlow JT. 1993. Head and the eye. In Dalessio DJ, Silberstein SD (eds). Wolff's Headache and Other Head Pain. New York: Oxford University Press

Carlson RJ. 1975. The End of Medicine. New York: John Wiley & Sons

Carraro JC, Raynaud JP, et al. 1996. Comparison of phytotherapy with finasteride in the treatment of benign prostate hyperplasia. Prostate 29:231–40

Carroll C, McAfee P, Riley LH. 1992. Whiplash injuries and how to treat them. J Musculoskeletal Med (Jun) 97–113

Carron H, DeGood DE, Tait R. 1985. A comparison of low back pain patients in the United States and New Zealand: psychosocial and economic factors affecting severity of disability. Pain 21:77–89

Carson Rachel. 1962. Silent Spring. Boston: Houghton Mifflin

Cartlidge NEF, Shaw DA. 1981. Head Injury. Philadelphia: WB Saunders

Cassidy DJ, Carroll LJ, et al. 2000. Effect of eliminating compensation for pain and suffering on the outcome of insurance claims for whiplash injury. N Engl J Med 342:1179–86

Cassidy, Sir M. 1946. The Harveian Oration: Coronary Disease. Lancet 2:587–90

Castro WHM, et al. 1997. Do "Whiplash injuries" occur in low speed rear impacts? Conference Proceedings (Annual meeting). New York: North American Spine Society

Cawson RA 1984. Pain in the TM joint. Br Med J 288:1857–8

Chalmers I. 1998. Unbiased, relevant, and reliable assessments in health care. BMJ 317:1168–9

Chalmers I, Enkin M, Keirse MJNC. 1998. Effective care in pregnancy and childbirth: a synopsis for guiding practice and research. In Chalmers,

Enkin, Keirse (eds). Effective Care in Pregnancy and Childbirth. Oxford: Oxford University Press. Ch 89, 1465–75

Champion GD. 1992 Whiplash in Australia: illness or injury? Med J Aust 157:574

Champion MC. 1993. NSAID-associated mucosal damage and ulceration: incidence, etiology, prophylaxis and treatment. Can J Gastroenterology 7:427–39

Charcot JM, Trans Savill T. 1889. Clinical Lectures on Diseases of the Nervous System. London: New Sydenham Society

Charlebois MA. 1995. Why insurance fraud is everybody's problem (audeotape). In Detecting Fraud and Malingering in Disability Claims Toronto: Professional Training Seminars

Charles C, Whelan T, Gafni A. 1999. What do we mean by partnership in making decisions about treatment? BMJ 319:780–2

Charlton J, Kelly S, Dunnell K. 1992. Trends in suicide deaths in England and Wales. Population Trends (Office of Government Statistical Service) 69:10–6.

– 1993. Suicide deaths in England and Wales: trends in factors associated with suicide deaths. Population Trends (Office of Government Statistical Service) 71:34–42

Cherasky M. 1973. The Hippocratic Myth. In RJ Bulgar (ed). New York: MED-COM

Chester JB. 1991. Whiplash, postural control, and the inner ear. Spine 16:716–20

Christman OD, Gervais RF. 1962. Otologic manifestations of the cervical syndrome. Clin Orthop 24:34–9

Cisler TA. 1994. Whiplash as a total-body injury. J Am Osteopathic Assoc 94:145–8

Clarfield AM. 30 Nov 1993. Doctors take a few jabs at lawyers. Medical Post (Toronto)

Clark ML. 1985. Upper intestinal endoscopy. Lancet 1:629

Clarke NG. 1982. Occlusion and myofascial pain dysfunction: is there a relationship? J Am Dent Assoc 104:443–6

Cleland LG. 1987. RSI: a model of social iatrogenesis. Med J Aust 147:236–9

Clevenger SV. 1889. Spinal Concussion: Erichsen's Disease, as One Form of Traumatic Neurosis. Philadelphia: FA Davis

Clinical Standards Advisory Group. 1994. Epidemiology review, the epidemiology and cost of back pain. London: HMSO

Cochrane AL. 1972. Effectiveness and Efficiency. London: Nuffield Provincial Hospital Trust

Cohen L. 1996. Issue of fraud as MD self-referral comes under spotlight in Ontario. CMAJ 154:1744–6

College of Physicians and Surgeons of the Province of Quebec. Sep 1966. The Scientific Brief Against Chiropractic. New Physician

Collie J. 1917. Malingering and Feigned Sickness. London: Edward Arnold

Comfort Alex. 1967. The Anxiety Makers. London: Nelson

Compere WE. 1968. Electronystagmographic findings in patients with "whiplash" injuries. Laryngoscope 78:1226–33

Connolly J. 1981. Accident proneness. Br J Hosp Med 26:473–81

Cook JB. 1972. The post-concussion syndrome and factors influencing recovery after minor head injury admitted to hospital. Scand J Rehabil Med 4:27–30

Coons PM. 1997. Satanic ritual abuse: first research and therapeutic implications. In The Dilemma of Ritual Abuse. Washington: American Psychiatric Association Press. 105–35

Cooper BC, Rabuzzi DD. 1984. Myofascial pain dysfunction syndrome: a clinical study of asymptomatic subjects. Laryngoscope 94:68–75

Cooper D. 1974. The Gullibility Gap. London: Routledge & Kegan Paul

Corcoran T. 24 Jun 1997. World Awash in Junk Science. Globe and Mail (Toronto) B2

Coren S. 1996. Accident death and shift to daylight savings time. Perceptual and Motor Skills. 83:921–2

Costen JB. 1934. A syndrome of ear and sinus symptoms dependent upon disturbed function of the temporomandibular joint. Ann Otol Rhinol Laryngol 43:1–15

Cotteril JA. 1982. Total allergy syndrome. Lancet 1:628

Coutts J. 10 Oct 1998. Doctors scrutinized over sick notes for absent employees. Globe and Mail (Toronto) A7

Crane AR. 1959. The relationship of a single act of trauma to subsequent malignancy: single uncomplicated trauma and cancer. In Trauma and Disease, 147–58

Crauford DIO, Creed F, Jayson MLV. 1990. Life events and psychological disturbance in patients with low-back pain. Spine 15:490–4

Craven L. 1950. Acetyl salicylic acid: possible preventive of coronary thrombosis. Annals West Med Surg 4:95–9

Croft AC. 1988. Biomechanics. In Croft AC, Foreman SM (eds). Whiplash Injuries. Baltimore: Williams and Wilkins. Ch 1, 1–72

Croft AC, Foreman SM. 1988. Soft-tissue injury: long-term and short-term effects. In Foreman SM, Croft AC (eds). Whiplash Injuries: The Cervical Acceleration Deceleration Syndrome. Baltimore: Williams and Wilkins. 293

Croft P, Schollum J, Silman A. 1994. Population study of tender point counts and pain as evidence of fibromyalgia. Br Med J 309:696–9

Croll Elisabeth. 2000. Endangered Daughters: Discrimination and Development in Asia. London and New York: Routledge

Crovitz HF, Horn RW, Daniel WF. 1983. Inter-relationships among retrograde amnesia, posttraumatic amnesia, and time since injury. Cortex 19:407–12

Crowe H. 1964. A new diagnostic sign in neck injuries. California Med 100:12–3

Cumberlidge MC. 1968. The abuse of barbiturates by heroin addicts. CMAJ 98:1045–9

Cunnien AJ. 1997. Psychiatric and medical syndromes associated with deception. In Rogers R (ed). Clinical Assessment of Malingering and deception. New York: The Guilford Press. Ch 2, 23–46

Daily L. 1970. Macular and vitreal disturbances produced by traumatic vitreous rebound. South Med J 63:1197–8

Dalrymple T. 1998. Mass Listeria: The Meaning of Health Scares. London: André Deutch

Daly R. 10 Feb 2001. The peculiar practice of Albert Deep MD. Toronto Star

Dangler Jean. 2001. Mediating Fictions: Literature, Women Healers, and the Go-Between in Medieval and Early Iberia. Lewisburg: Buckness University Press

Darwin CR. 1871. The Descent of Man. London: J. Murray

Davant TS, et al. 1993. A quantitative computer assisted analysis of disc displacement in patients with internal derangement using sagittal view MRI. J Oral Maxillofac Surg 51:974–9

David T, Leck B. 29 May 1997. AG. vs. Toronto Transit Commission. Court File No.95-CU-89529: Ontario Court of Justice (General Division)

Davies P. 1993. The Mind of God. New York: Touchstone

Davis AG. 1945. Injuries to the cervical spine. JAMA 127:149–56

Davis D, Bohlman HH, et al. 1971. The pathological findings in craniospinal injuries. J Neurosurg 34:603–13

Daw J. 15 Sep 1995. Auto scam busters: MD's files seized in fraud probe. Toronto Star, B1

– 13 Jul 1996. City chiropractor denies aiding insurance scam. Toronto Star, F1 and F8

– 3 Oct 1996. Two convicted of insurer fraud: Former workers at legal firm await sentencing. Toronto Star, B3

– 7 Feb 1997. Eleven insurers sue over fraudulent accident. Toronto Star, E3

– 7 May 1998. Claimant wasn't in the TTC crash. Toronto Star

Day JH, Lees RE, et al. 1984. Respiratory response to formaldehyde and off-gas of urea formaldehyde foam insulation. CMAJ 131:1061–5

Deans GT. 1986. Incidence and duration of neck pains among patients injured in car accidents. Br Med J 292:94–5

Deans GT, Magalliard JN, et al. 1987. Neck sprain: a major cause of disability following car accidents. Injury 18:10–12

Decter M. 2000. Four Strong Winds. Toronto: Stoddart

DeGraaf Rick. 1995. How big is the problem? In Detecting Fraud and

Malingering in Disability Claims (audiotape). Toronto: Professional Training Seminars

Delbanco T. 1998. Leeches, spiders, and astrology: predilections and predictions. JAMA 280:1560–2

de Mol BA, Heijer T. 1996. Late whiplash syndrome [letter]. Lancet 348:124–5

Denny-Brown D, Russell R. 1941. Experimental cerebral concussion. Brain, 64:7–164

Departmental Committee on Telegraphists' Cramp. 1911. Report of the Departmental Committee appointed to enquire into the prevalence and causes of the disease known as telegraphists' cramp. London: HMSO

de Waal F, Lanting F. 1997. Bonobo: The Forgotten Ape. Berkeley: University of California Press.

Deyo RA. 1988. Measuring the functional status of patients with low back pain. Arch Phys Med Rehabil 69:1044–51

Deyo RA, Cherkin D, et al. 1995. Cost, controversy, crisis: low back pain and the health of the public. Annual Review of Public Health 12:141–56

Deyo RA, Diehl AK, Rosenthal M. 1985. How much bedrest for backache? A randomised clinical trial. Clin Res 33:248A

– 1986. How many days of bedrest for acute backache? N Engl J Med 315:1064–70

Deyo RA, Phillips WR. 1997. Low back pain: a primary care challenge. Spine 21:2826–32

Di Stefano G, Radanov BP. 1993. [Neuropsychological and psychosocial findings in follow-up of cervical vertebrae dislocations: a prospective clinical study] [German]. Z Unfallchir Versicherungsmed 86:97–108

– 1995. Course of attention and memory after common whiplash, a two-years perspective study with age, education, and gender pair-matched patients. Acta Neurol Scand 91:346–52

Dineen T. 1996. Manufacturing Victims. Montreal: Robert Davies Publishing

Dinning TA. 1993. Whiplash in Australia: illness or injury. Med J Aust 158:138–40

Dixon AS. 1990. The evolution of clinical policies. Med Care 28: 201–20

Dixon P, Rehling G, Shiwach R. 1993. Peripheral victims of the Herald of Free Enterprise disaster. Br J Med Psychol 66:193–202

Doggett Maeve. 1992. Marriage, Wife-Beating and the Law in Victorian England. London: Weidenfeld and Nicolson

Doll R. 1998. Controlled trials: the 1948 watershed. BMJ 317:1217–20

Doll R, Hill AB. 1950. Smoking and carcinoma of the lung. Br Med J 740–9

Donald Mr Justice. 1993. Goyer and Dorion v Stotland (B915613). Vancouver Registry, British Columbia Supreme Court

Dorn BR, Dunn WA, Progulske-Fox A. 1999. Invasion of human coronary artery cells by periodontal pathogens. Infect Immun 67:5792–8

Drinka PJ, Jaschob PT. 1997. Treatment of chronic cervical zygapophyseal joint pain. N Engl J Med 336:1530

Drum DC. 1974. The nature of the problem. JCCA 13(2):18–20

Dubos R. 1961. Mirage of Health. New York: Doubleday

Duffy JB. 1992. The red baron. N Engl J Med 327:408–11

Dukes MNG. 1980. Myler's Side Effects of Drugs. Amsterdam: Elsevier

Dunbar HF. 1942. The relationship between anxiety states and organic disease. Clinics 1:879–908

– 1943. Psychosomatic Diagnosis, with Special Reference to Cardiovascular Syndromes Including Rheumatic Disease, Diabetes and Accident Proneness. New York: Paul B. Hoeber, Inc

– 1997. Medical aspects of accidents and mistakes in the industrial army and in the armed forces. War Medicine 4:161–9

Dunbar HF, Wolfe T, Rioch J. 1936. Psychic component in fracture. Am J Psychiatry 93:649–79

Dunbar HF, Wolfe TP, Tauber ES. 1939. The psychic component of the disease process (including convalescence), in cardiac, diabetic and fracture patients. Am J Psychiatry 95:1319–41

Duncum, BH. 1947. The Development of Inhalation Anaesthesia. London: Oxford University Press

Dunn EJ, Blazar S. 1987. Soft-tissue injuries of the lower cervical spine. Instructional Course Lectures (American Academy of Orthopedic Surgeons) 36:499–512

Dunne BE. 1993. Pathogenic mechanisms in H.pylori. Gastroenterology Clin North Am 22:43–59

Durr E. 1994. [The future comes from behind] [Danish]. Sygeplejersken 94:34–6

Earle RCB. 1973. The Professional Mental Patient (unpublished doctoral Thesis), Department of Sociology, University of Toronto

Edwards LM. 1990. Differentiating between ritual assault and sexual abuse. J Child Youth Care. Special Issue 67–89

Economist. 18 Jul 1992. The legal profession: the reign of lawyers.

– 5 Apr 1997. Screening for cancer, 19

– 30 May 1998. Why rhinos recommend Viagra 76

– 6 Feb 1999. The medical profession: it hurts 30–1

– 13 Feb 1999. Health care costs on the crtical list 65–5.

– 27 Feb 1999. A pain in the neck 27

– 25 Mar 1999. A new prescription 55

– 9 Oct 1999. Politics of the week 4

– 2 Sep 2000. Hunting corporate criminals 18–20

Einarson TR. 1993. Drug-related hospital admissions. Ann Pharmacother 27:832–9

Eisenberg DM, Davis RB, et al. 1998. Trends in alternative medicine use in the United States, 1990–1997. JAMA 280:1569–75

Eisenger F, Geller G, Holtzman NA. 1999. Cultural basis for differences between US and French clinical recommendations for women at increase risk of breast and ovarian cancer. Lancet 353:919–20

Eitlinger L. 1965. Concentration camp survivors in Norway and Israel. Isr J Med Sci 1:883–95

Emzenauer RW, Montrey JS, et al. 1989. Boxing-related injuries in the US Army, 1980 through 1985. JAMA 261:1463–6

Engel HO. 1988. Accident proneness and illness proneness: a review. J R Soc Med 84:163–4

Epp CR. 1992. Do lawyers impair economic growth? Law & Soc Inquiry 17:585–624

Epstein JB. 1992. Temporomandibular disorders, facial pain and headache following motor vehicle accidents. Can J Neurol Sci 58:488–9

Epstein M. 1995. Thoughts without a Thinker: Psychotherapy from a Buddhist Perspective. New York: Basic Books

Epstein RM, Quill TE, McWinney IR. 1999. Somatization reconsidered. Arch Intern Med 159:215–22

Equity and Aboriginal Issues Committee: Report to Convocation. June 2001. Toronto: Law Society of Upper Canada

Erichsen John E. 1882. Concussion of The Spine: Nervous Shock. London: Longmans, Green and Co

Ernest EA. 1979. The orthopedic influence of the TMJ apparatus in whiplash: report of a case. Gen Dent 27:62–4

Ernst E. 1998. Harmless Herbs: a review of the recent literature. Am J Med 104:170–8

– 2000. Herbal medicines: where is the evidence? BMJ 321:395–6

Ettlin TM, Kischka U, et al. 1992. Cerebral symptoms after whiplash injury of the neck: a prospective clinical and neuropsychological study of whiplash injury. J Neurol Neurosurg Psychiatry 55:943–8

Evans RG, Barer ML, Marmor TRE (eds). 1994. Why Are Some People Healthy And Others Are Not? The Determinants Of Health Of Populations. New York: Aldine de Gruyter

Evans RW. 1992. Some observations on whiplash injury. Neurol Clin 10:976–97

– 1995. Whiplash around the world. Headache 35, 262–3

Eversole LR, Machado L. 1985. Temporomandibular joint internal derangements and associated neuromuscular disorders. J Am Dent Assoc 110:69–79

Evidence-Based Medicine Working Group. 1992. Evidence-based medicine. JAMA 268:2420–5

– 1994. Evidence-based care: 1. Setting priorities: How important is this problem? CMAJ 150:1249–53

Ezzell Carrol. 2000. The business of the human genome. Scientific American 287:48–9

Farbman AA. 1973 Neck sprain: associated factors. JAMA 223:1010–5

Farman AG. 1982. Myofascial pain dysfunction syndrome: analysis of 164 cases. Quintessence Internat 12:1–7

Farney RJ, Walker JM 1995. Office management of common sleep-wake disorders. Med Clin North Am 79:391–414

Fee CR, Rutherford WH. 1988. A study of the effect of legal settlement on post-concussion symptoms. Arch Emerg Med 5:12–17

Feig SA. 1999. Role and evaluation of mammography and other imaging methods for breast cancer detection, diagnosis and staging. Seminars in Nuclear Medicine 29:3–15

Feldenkrais M. 1979. Body and Mature Behavior. New York: International Universities Press

Feldman MD, Ford CV. 1994. Patient or Pretender: Inside the Strange World of Factitious Disorders. New York: Wiley

Feldman MD. 2000. Munchausen by Internet: detecting factitious illness and crisis on the Internet. South Med J 93:669–72

Fenton B. 18 Jul 2001. Tobacco company cites savings from early deaths of smokers. National Post (Toronto) A9

Ferguson TW. 12 Feb 1996. Tort retort. Forbes 157(3):47

Ferrari R. 1999. The Whiplash Encyclopedia: the Facts and Myths of Whiplash. Gaithersburg, Maryland: Aspen

Ferrari R, Russell AS. 1997. The whiplash syndrome: common sense revisited. J Rheumatol 24:618–23

– 1998. A minor injury: a mistaken identity. Hippocrates' Lantern 5:1–7

Feuerstein M, Sult S, Houle M. 1985. Environmental stressors and chronic low back pain: life events, family and work environment. Pain 22:295–307

Field E. 1989. Foreword to MacIntyre A. ME: Post-viral Fatigue Syndrome: How to Live with It. London: Unwin

Fineberg HV, Hiatt HH. 1979. Evaluation of medical practices. N Engl J Med 301:1086–91

Fink P. 1992. Physical complaints and symptoms of somatizing patients. J Psychosom Res 36:125–36

Finney LD. 1990. Reach for the Rainbow. New York: Putman

Fischer AJEM, Verhagen WIM, Huygen PLM. 1997. Whiplash injury: a clinical review with emphasis on neuro-otological aspects. Clin Otolaryngol 22:192–201

Fisher JL. 1967. The neglected "pain in the neck." Ind Med Surg 36: 721–30

Fitch WE. 1899. Bicycle riding: its moral effect upon young girls and its relation to diseases of women. Georgia J Med Surg IV: 154–7

Fite JD. 1970. Neuro-ophthalmologic syndromes in automobile accidents. South Med J 63:567–70

Fitzcharles M-A, Esdaile JM. 1997. Nonphysician practitioner treatments and fibromyalgia syndrome. J Rheumatol 24:937–40

Fitz-Ritson D. 1991. Assessment of cervicogenic vertigo [see comments]. J Manipulative Physio Ther 14:193–8

Fleming JFR. 1973. The neurosurgeon's responsibilities in whiplash injuries. Clin Neurol 20:242–51

Florence D. 1981. The chronic pain syndrome. Postgrad Med 70:217–28

Foletti G, Regli F. 1995. [Characteristics of chronic headaches after whiplash injury] [French]. Presse Médicale 24:1121–3

Fontanna MJ. 1970. Discussion to "The enigma of whiplash" by JD States et al. NY State. J Med 70:2977–8

Ford CV. 1996. Lies! Lies!! Lies!!!: The Psychology of Deceit. Washington, DC: American Psychiatric Press

Ford CV, Bray GA, Swerdloff RS. 1976. A psychiatric study of patients referred with a diagnosis of hypoglycemia. Am J Psychiatry 133:290–4

Forslind K, Fredriksson E, Nived O. 1990. Does fibromyalgia exist? Br J Rheum 29:368–70

Foss Krista. 1 Feb 2001. Drug firm's freebies entice doctors. Globe and Mail (Toronto) A1 and A6

Foucault M. 1978. The History of Sexuality: vol 1: An Introduction. New York: Random House

Fox EM. 1985. Urea formaldehyde foam insulation: defusing a timebomb. Am J Law Med 11:81–104

Fraderiks JAM. 1976. Changes in the higher nervous system. In Vinken PJ, Bruyn GW (eds). Handbook of Clinical Neurology. Amsterdam: North Holland Publishing Company. Vol 24 ch 27, 487–99

France D. Sep 1998. The Families Who Are Dying for Our Country. Redbook

France RD, Krishnan KR, Trainor M. 1986. Chronic pain and depression: family history study of depression and alcoholism in chronic low back pain patients. Pain 24:185–90

Francis C. 1988. A beginning. In Interaction 1. London: ME Action Campaign

Frank JW, Brooker AS, et al. 1995. Disability Due to Occupational Low Back Pain: What Do We Know about Prevention? Toronto: Institute for Work and Health

Frank JW, et al. 1995. Occupational beck pain: an unhelpful polemic. Scand J Wor Environ Health 21:3–14

Frankel CJ. 1959. Medico-legal aspects of injuries to the neck. JAMA, 169:216–23

Frankel VH. 1965. Temporomandibular joint pain syndrome following deceleration injury to the cervical spine. Bull Hosp Jt Dis 26:47–51

Frankel VH, Shore NA, Hoppenfeld S. 1964. Stress distribution in cervical traction: prevention of temporomandibular joint pain syndrome. Clin Orthop 32:114–6

Frankenhaeuser M, Lundberg U, et al. 1989. Stress on and off the job as related to sex and occupational status in white-collar workers. J Organizational Behavior 10:321–46

Fraser DM. 1994. Whiplash: a total body approach. J Neurol Orthop Med Surg 15:10–2

Fraser GA. 1990. Satanic ritual abuse: a cause of multiple personality disorder. J Child Youth care. (Special Issue):55–66

– 1997. The Dilemma of Ritual Abuse. Washington: American Psychiatric Press

Fredericks C. 1969. Low Blood Sugar and You. New York: Constellation International

Fredrickson R. 1992. Repressed Memories. New York: Simon & Schuster

Freedland J. 3 Aug 1995. Cover-up alleged as US denies Gulf war syndrome. Guardian (UK)

Freedman DH. 1994. Who's to Judge? Discover 15:78–9

Freeman MD, Croft AC. 1996. Late whiplash syndrome [letter]. Lancet 348(9020)125

Freud edited by Ernest Jones. 1959. Charcot in Collected Works of Sigmund Freud. New York: Basic Books

Freud S. 1961. Female sexuality (1931). In Institute of Psychoanalysis (ed). The Complete Psychological Works of Sigmund Freud. London: Hogarth Press. Vol 21, 223–43

Fricton JR 1993. Myofascial pain and whiplash. In Teasell RW, Shapiro AP (eds). Spine. Philadelphia: Hanley & Belfus. Vol 7(3) ch 5, 403–21

Friday N. 1996. The Power of Beauty. New York: HarperCollins

Fry J. 1957. Are all Ts and As really necessary? Br Med J 1:124

Frymoyer JW, Pope HG, Jr et al. 1983. Risk factors in low-back pain. J Bone Joint Surg 65:213–8

Gabriel SE, O'Fallon WM, et al. 1994. Risk of connective-tissue diseases and other disorders after breast implantation. N Engl J Med 330:1697–702

Gaddum JH. 1959. Pharmacology. London: Oxford University Press

Gage M. 1985. Women, Church and State (1893). Salem, New Hampshire: Ayer Company, Publishers, Inc

Gagnon NB. 1985. [Clinical observations on 76 children exposed to urea-formaldehyde insulation foam (letter)] [French]. Union Médicale du Canada 114:941–2

Galasko CS, Murray PM, et al. 1993. Neck sprains after road traffic accidents: a modern epidemic. Injury 24:155–7

Gannon JP. 1989. Soul Survivors. New York: Prentice-Hall

Garber AM, Weinstein MC, et al. 2000. Theoretical foundations of cost-effectiveness analysis. In MR Gold et al (eds). Cost-Effectiveness in Health and Medicine. New York: Oxford University Press. 25–53

Gardner M. 1957. Fads and Fallacies in the Name of Science. New York: Dover

Garfinkel MS, Sinngal A, et al. 1998. Yoga-based intervention for carpal tunnel syndrome. JAMA 280:1601–3

Garg A, Moore JS. 1992. Epidemiology of low-backpain in industry. Occup Med 7:593–603

Gargan M, Bannister G, et al. 1997. The behavioural response to whiplash injury. J Bone Joint Surg Br 79:523–6

Garrison FM. 1929. An Introduction to the History of Medicine. Philadelphia and London: WB Saunders

Gates EM, Benjamin D. 1967. Studies in cervical trauma, Part 2. Int Surg 48:368–75

Gates EM, Cento D. 1966. Studies in cervical trauma 1. The so-called "whiplash." Int Surg 46:218–22.

Gatterman MI. 1995. The articular lesion. In Gattermann MI (ed). Foundations of Chiropractic: Subluxation. Part 1, 6. St Louis: Mosby

Gavin H. 1843. On Feigned and Factitious Diseases Chiefly of Soldiers and Seamen. London: Churchill

Gay JR, Abbott KH. 1953. Common whiplash injuries to the neck. JAMA, 152:1698–704

Gelernter D. 1997. Drawing Life, Surviving the Unabomber. New York: Simon & Schuster

Gennarelli TA, Thibault LE, et al. 1982. Diffuse axonal injury and traumatic coma in the primate. Ann Neurol 12:564–74

Gentilini M, et al. 1985. Neuropsychological evaluation of mild head injury. J Neurol Neurosurg Psychiatry 48:137–9

Gérin M, Siemiatycki J, et al. 1989. Cancer risks due to occupational exposure to formaldehyde: results of a multi-site case-control study in Montreal. Int J Cancer 44:53–8

Gibb-Clark M. 1996. Employee illness: warning signs to watch. Globe and Mail (Toronto)

Gibson WJ. 1968. The eye and whiplash injuries. J Florida Med Assoc 55:917–18

Giebel GD, Bonk AD, et al. 1999. Whiplash in Germany. J Rheumatol 26:1207–10

Gildiner Alina. 2001. Ontario's Rehabilitation Sector: Understanding the Fragmentation. Toronto: Insurance Bureau of Canada

Gillman MW, Cupples LA, et al. 1997. Margarine intake and subsequent coronary heart disease in men. Epidemiology 8:144–9

Gissane W. 1966. The causes and the prevention of neck injuries to car occupants. Ann R Coll Surg Engl 39:161–3

– 1967. The causes and the prevention of car occupant neck injuries. In Selzer ML, Gikas PW, Huelke DF (eds). Proceedings of the Prevention of Highway Accidents Symposium. Ann Arbor: University of Michigan Press

Glendon MA. 1995. A Nation under Lawyers. New York: Farrar, Straus & Giroux

Glyn J. 1970. Some factors influencing the duration of morbidity in industry. J R Soc Med 63:1131

Goldbeck-Wood S, Lie LG, et al. 1996. Complementary medicine is booming worldwide. BMJ 313:131–3

Goldberg HL. 1990. Trauma and the improbable anterior displacement. J Craniomandibular Dis Face Oral Pain 4:131–4

Goldenberg DL. 1987. Fibromyalgia syndrome. JAMA 257:2782–7

Goldman B. 1991. Chronic-pain patients must cope with chronic lack of physician understanding. CMAJ 144:1492–7

Goldney RD. 1988. "Not cured by a verdict": a re-evaluation of the literature. Aust J Forensic Sci 20:295–300

Goleman D. 17 May 1990. New paths to mental health put strains on some healers. New York Times

Gollom M. 7 Jun 2000. Five doctors, paralegal charged in insurance scam. National Post (Toronto) A24

Gore DR, Sepic SB, Gardner GM. 1998. Roentgenographic findings of the cervical spine in asymptomatic patients. Spine 11:521–4

Gorman R. 1979a. Vertebral artery occlusion following manipulation of the neck. N Z Med J 89:362

Gorman WF. 1979b. "Whiplash": fictive or factual. Bull Am Acad Psychiatry Law 7:245–8

Gorman WF, Winograd M. 1988. Crossing the border from Munchausen to malingering. J Florida Med Assoc 75:147–50

Gots M. 1997. Multiple chemical sensitivities. Hippocrates' Lantern, 4:1–5

Gøtzche PC, Olsen O. 2000. Is screening for breast cancer with mammography justifiable? Lancet 355:129–37

Gould C. 1992. Diagnosis and treatment of ritually abused children. In Sakheim DK, Devine SE (eds). Out of Darkness: Exploring Satanism and Ritual Abuse. New York: Lexington Books. 207–48

Gould SJ. 1981. The Mismeasure of Man. New York: WW Norton & Co

Gouvier WD. 1988. Base rates of post-concussional symptoms. Arch Clin Neuropsychol 3:273–8

Gow Mr Justice. 1987. Price v Garcha et al. Vancouver Registry B861060.

Gracely RH, Dubner R, et al. 1985. Clinicians' expectations influence placebo response. Lancet 1:43

Grady D. 11 May 1996. The whiplash syndrome loses its validity. Globe and Mail (Toronto)

Grauds C. 1997. Botanicals: strong medicine for health and profit. The Source 3(1)

Greaves GB. 1982. Multiple personality disorder: 165 years after Mary Reynolds. J Nerv Ment Dis 168:577–96

Greene CS, Laskin DM. 1983. Long-term evaluation of treatment for myofascial pain dysfunction syndrome: a comparative analysis. J Am Dent Assoc 107:235–8

Greene CS, Marbach JJ. 1982. Epidemiological studies of mandibular dysfunction: a critical review. J Prosthet Dent 48:184–90

Greenfield S, Fitzcharles MA, Esdaile JM. 1992. Reactive fibromyalgia syndrome. Arthritis Rheum 35:678–81

Greenwald J. 23 Nov 1998. Herbal Healing. Time Magazine (Canadian Edition), 46–57

Greenwood JC. 1985. Work-related back and neck injury cases in West Virginia. Orthop Rev 14:53–61

Greenwood M, Woods HM. 1919. The incidence of industrial accidents upon individuals with special reference to multiple accidents. London: HMSO

Griffin K. 1996. They should have washed their hands. Health (Nov/Dec): 82–90

Grigsby J, Rosenberg NL, Busenark D. 1995) Chronic pain adversely affects information processing. Perceptual and Motor Skills 81:403-10

Grilli R, Lomas J. 1992. Evaluating the message: the relationship between compliance rate and the subject of a practice guideline. Hamilton, Ontario: McMaster University, Centre for Health Economics and Policy Analysis

Grimm RJ, Hemenway WG, et al. 1989. The perilymph fistula syndrome defined in mild head trauma. Acta Otolaryngol (Suppl) 464:1–40

Griner PF, Glazer RJ. 1982. Misuse of laboratory tests and diagnostic procedures. N Engl J Med 307:1336–9

Gross H, Pattison H. 1994. Cognitive failure during pregnancy. J Reproduct Infant Psychol 12:17–32

Grunsten RC, Gilbert NS, Mawn SV. 1989. The mechanical effects of impact acceleration on the unconstrained human head and neck complex. Contemp Orthop 18:199–202

Guest GH, Drummond PD. 1992. Effect of compensation on emotional state and disability in chronic back pain. Pain 48:125–30

Guinness A. 1997. My Name Escapes Me: The Diary of a Retiring Actor. London: Penguin Books

Gull Sir W. 1894. Cases of rheumatic fever treated for the most part with mint water. In A Collection of the Published Writings of Sir William Gull. Medical Papers. London: New Sydenham Society. 475–512

Gunby P. 1981. Urea formaldehyde foam insulation may be banned [news]. JAMA 245:906

Gundwell B, Liljeqvist M, Hansson TH. 1993. Primary prevention of back symptoms and absence from work: a randomized study among hospital employees. Spine 18:587–94

Gunn CG. 1995. Fibromyalgia: What have we created? Pain 60:349

Gupta S, Camm AJ. 1997. Chlamydia pneumoniae and coronary heart disease. BMJ 314:1778–9

Gupta S, Leatham EW, et al. 1997. Elevated Chlamydia pneumoniae antibodies, cardiovascular events, and azithromycin in male survivors of myocardial infarction. Circulation 96:404–7

Guralnick W, Kaban LB, Merrill RG. 1978. Temporomanibular-joint afflictions. N Engl J Med 299:123–9

Gurfinkel E, Bozovich G, et al. 1997. Randomised trial of roxithromycin in non-Q-wave coronary syndromes: ROXIS pilot study. Lancet 350: 404–7

Guthkelch AN. 1980. Posttraumatic amnesia, postconcussional symptoms and accident neurosis. Eur Neurol 19:91–102

Guttmann E. 1943. Post contusional headache. Lancet, 1:10–2

Guy JE. 1968. The whiplash: tiny impact, tremendous injury. Ind Med Surg (Sep):688–91

Gyntelberg F. 1974. One-year incidence of low back pain among male residents of Copenhagen aged 40–59. Dan Med Bull 21:30–6

Haas DC. 1991. The reliability of reliability. J Manipulative Physio Ther 14:199–208

Hacking I. 1995. Rewriting the Soul and the Science of Memory. Princeton: Princeton University Press

Haddon W, Goddard JL. 1962. An analysis of highway safety strategies. In Passenger Car Design and Highway Safety. New York: Association for the Aid of Crippled Children and Consumers Union of US

Hadler NM. 1993. Occupational Musculoskeletal Disorders. New York: Raven Press

– 1999. Occupational Musculoskeletal Disorders (2nd ed). Philadelphia: Lippincott Williams & Wilkins

– 1997. Fibromyalgia, chronic fatigue, and other iatrogenic diagnostic algorithms. Do some labels escalate illness in vulnerable patients? Postgrad Med 102:162–77

– 1997. Fibromyalgia: La maladie est morte. Vive le malade! J Rheumatol 24:1250–2

– 1999. Occupational Musculoskeletal Disorders (2nd ed). Philadelphia: Lippincott, Williams & Wilkins

Hagen MA. 1997. Whores of the Court: The Fraud of Psychiatric Testimony and the Rape of American Justice. New York: HarperCollins

Haggard HW. 1929. Devils, Drugs and Doctors. New York: Blue Ribbon Books

Hahnemann CF. 1810. Organon of Rational Medicine. Dresden

Hale-White Sir Wm. 1935. Great Doctors of the Nineteenth Century. London: Edward Arnold & Co

Haley RW, Kurt TL, Hom J. 1997. Is there a Gulf war syndrome? JAMA 277:215–22

Hall H, Hadler NM. 1995. Controversy: Low back school: Education or exercise? Spine 20:1097–8

Hall R. 1978. Dear Dr. Stopes. London: Deutsch

Harakal JH. 1975. An osteopathically integrated approach to the whiplash complex. J Am Osteopathic Assoc 74:941–56

Haller JS, Haller RM. 1974. The Physician and Sexuality in Victorian America. Chicago: University of Chicago Press

Harakal JH. 1975. An osteopathically integrated approach to the whiplash complex. J Am Osteopathic Assoc 74:941–56

Harris K, Campbell E. 1999. The plans in unplanned pregnancy: secondary gain and the partnership. Br J Med Psychol 72:105–20

Harriton MB. 1988. The Whiplash Handbook. Springfield, Il: Charles C. Thomas

Hart CW. 1979. Traumatic vestibular impairment. Med Trial Tech Q 25:301–18

Harth M, Teasell RW. 1998. Chronic whiplash revisited. J Rheumatol 25:1437

Hartog R. 1993. Barbiturate Combination: Risk Without Benefit. HAI Europe: BUKO, Pharma-Kampagn

Hartt J, O'Driscoll J, Rosenberg J. 1997. Frank Kenny vs the College of Psychologists of Ontario. File No: 19–97: Ontario Court of Justice (General Division) Divisional Court

Haslett RS, Duvall-Young J, McGalliard JN. 1994. Traumatic retinal angiopathy and seat belts: pathogenesis of whiplash injury. Eye 8:615–17

Hassall, Christine, Trethowan WH. 1972. Suicide in Birmingham. Br Med J 1:717–8

Haworth D. 23 Aug 1992. Quoted in EC fraud warning. Independent (UK)

Hayes B, Solyom CA, et al. 1993. Use of psychometric measures and nonorganic signs testing in detecting nomogenic disorders in low back pain patients. Spine 18:1254–9

Healy D. 2000. Good science or good business? Hastings Center Report 30:9–22

Heliövaara M. 1987. Body height, obesity, and risk of herniated lumbar intervertebral disc. Spine 12:469–72

Helliwell PS, Evans PF, Wright V. 1994. The straight cervical spine: Does it indicate cervical spasm? J Bone Joint Surg Br 76B:103–6

Hemels M. (Sep 2001). Rise in antidepressant use linked to advertising. Toronto: International conference on pharmacoepidemiology

Hennekens CH, et al. 1996. Self-reported breast implants and connective tissue diseases in female health professionals. JAMA 275:616–21

Hensell V. 1976. Neurologische Schaden nach Repositions – massnahmen an der Wirbelsaure. Med Welt 27:656–8

Herbert V. 1984. Snake oil nutrition: the scam of the century. In Currie MN (ed). Patient Education in Primary Care Setting, 6th Annual Conference

(Fact, Fiction and Fantasy in Health Information for Patients) Kansas City: Project for Patient Education in Family Practice, St.Mary's Hospital. 15–23, 34–36

Herman JL. 1992. Trauma and recovery. New York: Basic Books

Hertzman M, Smoller B. 1989. Early recognition. In Tollison CD (ed). The Handbook of Chronic Pain Management. Baltimore: Williams & Wilkins. Ch 44, 592–607.

Hidding A. 1994. Comparison between self-report measures and clinical observations of functional disability in ankylosing spondylitis, rheumatoid arthritis and fibromyalgia. J Rheumatol 21:818

Hildingsson C, Hietala SO, Toolanen G. 1989. Scintigraphic findings in acute whiplash injury of the cervical spine. Injury 20:265–6

Hildingsson C, Toolanen G. 1990. Outcome after soft-tissue injury of the cervical spine. Acta Orthop Scand 61:357–9

Hill Sir AB. 1966. Heberton Oration 1965: Reflections on the controlled trial. Annals Rheumatic Dis 25:107–13

Hillel D. 1988. Thin-skull claims: recovery for accident neurosis. The Advocates Society Journal 7(5):23–40

Hinoki M, Hine S, et al. 1973. Studies on ataxia of lumbar origin in cases of vertigo due to whiplash injury. Int J Equilibrium Res 3:141–52

Hirsch AE, Ommaya AK, Mahone RH. 1970. Tolerance of subhuman primate brain to cerebral concussion. In Lange WA, Patrick LM, Thomas IL (eds). Impact Injury and Crash Protection. Springfield, Il: Charles C Thomas. 352–71

Hirsch C, Nachemson AL. 1961. Clinical observation on the spine of ejected pilots. Acta Orthop Scand 31:136–45

Hirsch M, Carlander B, et al. 1994. Objective and subjective sleep disturbances in patients with rheumatoid arthritis. Arthritis Rheum 37:41–9

Hirsch SA, Hirsch PJ, et al. 1988. Whiplash syndrome: Fact or fiction? Orthop Clin North Am 19:791–5

Hirschfeld AH, Behan RC. 1963. The accident process: etiological consideration of industrial injuries. JAMA 186:193–9

– 1966. The accident process III: disability: acceptable and unacceptable. JAMA 197:125–9

Hiscock M, Hiscock CK. 1989. Refining forced-choice method for the detection of malingering. J Clin Exp Psychol 11:967–74

Hislop TG. 1997. Is breast self-examination still necessary? CMAJ 157:1225–6

Hodge JR. 1971. The whiplash neurosis. Psychosomatics 12:245–9

Hoey JR, Turcotte F, et al. 1984. Health risks in homes insulated with urea formaldehyde foam. CMAJ 130:115–7

Hogg-Johnson H, Cole D, et al. 2000. Staging treatment interventions following soft-tissue injuries. In Sullivan T (ed). Injury and the New World of Work. Vancouver: UBC Press. Ch 9

Hohl M. 1974. Soft-tissue injuries of the neck in automobile accidents: factors influencing prognosis. J Bone Joint Surg 56-A:1675–82

Holm S. 1980. Nutrition of the Intervertebral Disc: Transport and Metabolism. Göttenborg: University of Göttenborg

Holmes OW Sr. 1861. Currents and Counter-Currents in Medical Science with other Addresses and Essays. Boston: Tricknor and Field

Holub BJ. 1991. Cholesterol-free foods: Where's the trans? CMAJ 144:330

Horn SW. 1983. The "Locked-In" syndrome following chiropractic manipulation of the cervical spine. Ann Emerg Med 12:648–50

Horowitz, Janice H. 10 Dec 1992. Crippled by computers. Time Magazine (Canadian Edition) 76–8

Horsnall M, Dutta R. 3 Jun 1994. Inquiry dismisses satanic abuse as an evangelic myth. The Times (London)

Horsten M, Wamela SP, et al. 1997. Depressive symptoms, social support, and lipid profile in healthy middle-aqed women. Psychosom Med 59:521–8

Horwich H, Kasner D. 1962. The effect of whiplash injuries on the ocular functions. South Med J 55:69–71

Howard RP, Benedict JV, et al. 1991. Assessing neck extension-flexion as a basis for temporomandibular joint dysfunction. J Oral Maxillofac Surg 49:1210–3

Howard RP, Hatsell CP, Guzman HM. 1995. Temporomandibular joint injury potential imposed by the low-velocity extension-flexion manoeuver. J Oral Maxillofac Surg 53:256–62

Hrdy Sarah. 1999. Mother Nature: A History of Mothers, Infants, and Natural Selection. New York: Pantheon Books

Hrubec Z, Nashold BSJ. 1975. Epidemiology of lumbar disc lesions in the military in World War II. Am J Epidemiol 102:367–76

Hu FB, Stamper MJ, et al. 1997. Dietary fat intake and the risk of coronary heart disease in women. N Engl J Med 337:1491–9

Hubbard JH. 1982. Chronic pain of spinal origin. In Rothman RH, Simeone FA (eds). Spine. Vol 2.Philadelphia: W B.Saunders

Huber PW. 1991. Galileo's Revenge: Junk Science and the Courtroom. New York: Basic Books

Hubka MJ. 1990. Another critical look at the subluxation hypothesis. Chiropractic Technique 2:27–9

Hughes R. 1993. The Culture of Complaint: The Fraying of America. New York: Oxford University Press

Hult L. 1954. Cervical, dorsal and lumbar spine syndrome. Acta Orthop Scand 17 (Suppl)

Hurwitz N, Wade OL. 1969. Intensive hospital monitoring of adverse reactions to drugs. Br Med J 1:531–6

Huxley Aldous. 1945. The Perennial Philosophy. New York: Harper

Huxley TH. 1880. The Crayfish, an Introduction to the Study of Zoology. London: C Kegan Paul and Co

Illich Ivan. 1977. Disabling Professions. In Illich I, Zola IK, McKnigh J, et al. (eds). Disabling Professions. London: Marion Boyars

– 1982. Medical Nemesis: The Expropriation of Health. Pantheon

Inlander CB, Levin LS, Weiner E. 1988. Medicine on Trial. New York: Prentice Hall

Institute for Clinical Evaluative Sciences in Ontario. 1996. The ICES Practice Atlas: Patterns of Health Care (2nd ed). Ottawa: Ontario Medical Association

– 1995. BACK before you know it. Informed 1:2–3

Insurance Bureau of Canada. April 1995. Insurers wage war on fraud. The IBC Insurance Fraud Reporter 1-3

Insurance claim fraud: prevention and detection strategies. 1994. Toronto: Insight Press

Insurance Research Council Inc. 1994. Auto Injuries: Claiming Behavior and Its Impact on Insurance Claims. Oak Brook, Il: Insurance Research Council Inc

– 1995a. Trends in Auto Injury Claims, Part 1: Analysis of Claim Frequency (2nd ed). Wheaton, Il: Insurance Research Council Inc

– 1995b. Trends in Auto Injury Claims: Part 2: Analysis of Claim Costs (2nd ed). Wheaton, Il: Insurance Research Council Inc

International Association for the Study of Pain. 1994. Classification of Chronic Pain: Descriptions of Chronic Pain Syndromes and Definitions of Pain Terms. New York: Elsevier

International College of Cranio-Mandibular Orthopaedics. 8–9 Oct 1987. Resolution: Third Party Reimbursement. At the Las Vegas meeting.

Irvin RW. 19 Jan 1971. Iacocca, LA. As quoted in: Ford cuts back on car production. The Detroit News

ISIS2 Collaborative Group. 1988. Randomized trial of intravenous streptokinase, oral aspirin, both, or neither amongst 17,187 cases of suspected myocardial infarction. Lancet 2:349–60

Jack DB. 1997. One hundred years of aspirin. Lancet 350:437–9

Jackson CO. 1976. Before the drug culture. Barbiturate/amphetamine abuse in American society. Clio Medica 11:47–58

Jackson PR. 1985. Compensation neurosis. Med J Aust 143:176

Jackson R. 1966. Crashes cause most neck pain. AMA News

Jacobs DM. 1992. Alien Encounters: First-hand Experiences of UFO Abductions. New York: Simon & Schuster

Jacobson RR. 1995. The post-concussion syndrome: physiogenesis, psychogenesis and malingering: an integrative model. J Psychosom Res 39:721–35

Jaffe H. 18 Aug 1993. Staged bus accidents bring in rash of fake insurance claims. The Star-Ledger 1 and 13

James RTD, Dean BC. 1983. Reducing the risk: barbiturate substitution with benzodiazepine. Pharmatherapeutica 3:464–7

Janecki CJ, Lipke JM. 1978. Whiplash syndrome. Am Fam Physician 17:144–51

Janjua KJ, Goswami V, Sagar G. 1996. Whiplash injury associated with acute bilateral internal carotid arterial dissection. J Trauma 40:458

Jardine L. 1999. Ingenious Pursuits. London: Little, Brown and Co

Jaynes G. May 1994. Walking wounded. Esquire

Jenkins P. 1998. Moral Panic: Changing Concepts of the Child Molester in Modern America. New Haven: Yale University Press

Jennett B, Macmillan R. 1997. Epidemiology of head injury. Br Med J 282:101–4

Jennett B, Teasdale G. 1981. The Management of Head Injuries. Philadelphia: FA Davis

Jennum P, Drewes AM, et al. 1993. Sleep and other symptoms in primary fibromyalgia and in healthy controls. J Rheumatol 20:1756–9

Jessner L, Bol GE, Waldfogel S. 1952. Emotional implications of tonsillectomy and adenoidectomy in children. In The Psychoanalytic Study of the Child. New York: International University Press

Johnson H. 1996. Osler's Web: Inside the Labyrinth of the Chronic Fatigue Syndrome Epidemic. New York: Crown Publishers.Inc

Johnson HM. 1936. Born to Crash. Collier's

Johnson W. 1849. An Essay on the Diseases of Young Women. London: Simpkin, Marshall

Jonas JM, Pope HG. 1985. The dissimulation disorders: a single diagnostic entity? Compr Psychiatry 26:58–62

Jones BA, Llewellyn LJ. 1917. Malingering or Simulation of Disease. London: Heinemann

Jones E. 1953. Sigmund Freud: Life and Work. London: Hogarth Press

Jones Steve. 1999. Darwin's Ghost. Canada: Doubleday

Jonsson H, Bring G, et al. 1991. Hidden cervical spine injuries in traffic accident victims with skull fractures. J Spinal Disord 4:251–63

Jonsson H, Cisarini K, et al. 1995. Findings and outcome in whiplash-type neck distortions. Spine, 19:2733–43

Journal of Craniomanibular Practice Editorial. 1989. TMJ impairment: the $64,000 question. J Craniomandibular Practice 7:3

Juniper RP. 1986. Temporomandibular joint dysfunction: facts and fallacies. Nov/Dec. Dental Update, 479–90

Kamman GR. 1951. Traumatic neurosis, compensation neurosis and attitude pathosis? Arch Neurol Psychiatry 65:593

Kane RL, Olsen D, et al. 1974. Manipulating the patient: a comparison of the effectiveness of physician and chiropractic care. Lancet 1:1333–6

Karlsborg M, Smed A, et al. Feb 1997. A prospective study of 39 patients with whiplash injury. Acta Neurol Scand 95:65–72

Katano T. 1970. [Ophthalmological study of cases with whiplash injury] [Japanese]. Folia Ophthalmologica Japonica 21:525–8

Katon W, Kelly E, Miller D. 1985. Chronic pain: lifetime psychiatric diagnoses and family history. Am J Psychiatry 142:1156–60

Keaton W, Ries RK, Kleinman A. 1984. The prevalence of somatization in primary care. Compr Psychiatry 25:208–13

Kelley JS, Hoover RE, George T. 1978. Whiplash maculopathy. Arch Ophthmol 96:834–5

Kelly MC. 1990. Whiplash Syndrome. Irish Doctor (Oct):721–5

Kennedy F. 1946. The mind of the injured worker: its effects upon disability periods. Compensation Medicine 1:19

Kerr P. 18 Aug 1993. Ghost riders are target of an insurance sting. New York Times, A1

Kessel N. 1966. The respectability of self-poisoning and the fashion for survival. J Psychosom Res 10:29–36

Kessler Dea. 1993. Introducing MedWatch: a new approach to reporting medication and device adverse effects and product problems. JAMA 269:2765–8

Kewalramani L. 1982. Myelopathy following cervical spine manipulation. Am J Phys Med 61:165–75

Keys A, Kusukawa A, et al. 1958. Lessons from serum cholesterol studies in Japan, Hawaii and Los Angeles. Ann Intern Med 48:83–93

Khan H, McCormack D, et al. 1997. Incidental neck symptoms in high energy trauma victims. Ir Med J 90:143

King B. 30 Jan 1998. AG. and CO. vs Toronto Transit Commission. Court File No.95-CU-89529

Kinloch BM. 1993. Whiplash in Australia: illness or injury? Med J Aust 158:70–1

Kinney RK, Gatchel RJ, et al. 1992. Major psychological disorders in chronic TMD patients. J Am Dent Assoc 123:49–54

Kircos TL, Ortendahl DA, et al. 1987. Magnetic resonance imaging of the TMJ disc in asymptomatic volunteers. J Oral Maxillofac Surg 45 397–401

Kirk SA, Kutchins H. 1992. The Selling of DSM: The Rhetoric of Science in Psychiatry. New York: Aldine de Gruyter

Kirk WS. 1992. Whiplash as a basis for TMJ dysfunction. J Oral Maxillofac Surg 50:427–8

Kischka U, Ettlin TM, et al. 1991. Cerebral symptoms following whiplash injury. Eur Neurol 31:136–40

Kistner UA, Keith MR, et al. 1994. Accuracy of dispensing in a high-volume, hospital-based outpatient pharmacy. Am J Hosp Pharm 51:2793–7

Knight GW. 1959. Orthoptic variations. Am Orthoptic J 9:62–9

Koes BW, Assendelft WJJ, et al. 1996. Spinal manipulation for low back pain. Spine 21:2860–73

Kolata G. 16 May 1995. Legal system and science come to a differing conclusion on silicone. New York Times D6

Koro Study Team. 1969. The Koro "epidemic" in Singapore. Singapore Med J 10: 234–42

Kouyanou K, Pither CE, et al. 1998. A comparative study of iatrogenesis, medication abuse, and psychiatric morbidity in chronic pain patients with and without medically explained symptoms. Pain 76:417–26

Kozol HL. 1946. Pretraumatic personality and the psychiatric sequelae of head injury. Arch Neurol Psychiatry 53:358–64

Kraepelin E. 1902. Clinical Psychiatry. (translated by Defendorf R.) London: Macmillan

Kral VA. 1951. Psychiatric observations under severe chronic stress. Am J Psychiatry 108:185–91

Kraus JF, Nourjah P. 1988. Epidemiology of mild brain injury. J Trauma 28:1837–43

Kravis MM, Munk PL, et al. 1993. MR imaging of muscle and tender points in fibromyalgia. J Magn Imag 3:669–70

Kreeft JH. 1993. Headache following whiplash. In Teasell RW, Shapiro AP (eds). Spine. Philadelphia: Hanley and Belfus. Vol 7(3) ch 43, 391–402

Kroenke K. 1995. Dizziness in primary care. West J Med 162:73–4

Kroenke K, Lucas C, et al. 1993. Psychiatric disorders and functional impairment in patients with persistent dizziness. J Gen Intern Med 8:530–5

Kronn E. 1993. The incidence of TMJ dysfunction in patients who have suffered a cervical whiplash injury following a traffic accident. J Orofacial Pain 7:209–13

Kuch K, Cox JC, Evans RJ. 1996. Post-traumatic stress disorder and motor vehicle accidents: a multidisciplinary overview. CMAJ 41:429–34

Kuch K, Swinson RP, Kirby M. 1985. Post-traumatic stress disorder after car accidents. Can J Psychiatry 30:426–7

Kunz R, Oxman AD. 1998. The unpredictability paradox: review of empirical comparisons of randomised and non-randomised clinical trials. BMJ 317:1185–90

Kupperman A. 1988. Whiplash and disc derangement [letter]. J Oral Maxillofac Surg 46:519

La Fontaine J. 1998. The Extent and Nature of Organized Ritual Abuse. London: HMSO

La Rocca H. 1991. Cervical sprain syndrome. In JW Frymoyer, et al (eds). The Adult Spine: Principles and Practice. New York: Raven Press Ltd. Ch 50, 1051–61

Labi N. 17 May 1999. The Grief Brigade. Time Magazine (Canadian Edition) 42–3

Lancet Editorial. 1975. A two-edged sword. Lancet 2:441–2

– 1981. Reducing tests. Lancet 1:539–40

– 1991. Neck injury and the mind. Lancet 338:728–9

– 2000. Overoptimism about cancer. Lancet 157

Larder DR, Twiss MK, Mackey GM. 1985. Neck injury to occupants using seatbelts. Conference of American Association of Automedicine

Larrabee GJ. 1992. Interpretive strategies for evaluation of neuropsychological data in legal settings. Forensic Reports 5:257–64

Lasègue CE quoted by J. Babinski and J. Froment. 1918. Hysteria or Pithiatism and Reflex Nervous Disorders in the Neurology of War. London: London University Press

Lazarou J, Pomeranz BH, Corey PN. 1998. Incidence of adverse drug reactions in hospitalized patients. JAMA 279:1200–5

Leavitt F. 1987. Detection of simulation among persons instructed to exaggerate symptoms of low back pain. J Occup Med 29:229–33

Leavitt F, Garron DC, et al. 1979. Low back pain in patients with and without demonstrable organic disease. Pain 6:191–200

LeBon G. 1879. Recherches anatomiques et mathématiques sur les lois des variations du volume du cerveau et sur leurs relations avec l'intelligence. Revue d'Anthropologique, 2nd series. Vol 2, 27–104

Lecky WEH. 1871. The History of European Morals. New York: Appleton

Leclaire R, Esdaile JM, et al. 1996. Diagnostic accuracy of technologies used in low back pain assessment. Spine 21:1325–31

Lees-Haley PR, Brown RS. 1993. Neurological complaint base rates of 170 personal injury claimants. Arch Clin Neuropsychol 8:202–9

Lees-Haley PR, Dunn JT. 1994. The ability of naive subjects to report symptoms of mild brain injury, post-traumatic stress disorder, major depression, and generalized anxiety disorder. J Clin Psychol 50:252–6

Lees-Haley PR, Dunn RS. 1986. Pseudoposttraumatic stress disorder. Trial Diplomacy, Winter, 17–20

Lees-Haley PR, Smith HH, et al. 1996. Forensic neuropsychological test usage: an empirical study. Arch Clin Neuropsychol 2:45–51

Le Fanu J. 1999. The Rise and fall of Modern Medicine. London: Little, Brown & Co

Legis Filius. 1973. Whiplash injury, or homage to Minerva. Med J Aust 2:1028

Leighton AH, Hughes CC, et al. 1963. The Stirling County Study of Psychiatric Disorder and Socio-cultural Environment. New York: Basic Books

Leonard M. 1993. On TMD. Personal communication.

Leonard M, Dodes JE. 1995. TMJ: Unnecessary diagnostic devices. Hippocrates' Lantern 3:7–11

Leopold RL, Dillon H. 1960. Psychiatric considerations in whiplash injuries of the neck. Pennsylvania Med J 63:385–9

Lesse S. 1956. Atypical facial pain syndromes of psychogenic origin. J Nerv Ment Dis 124:543–6

Levack BP. 1993. The Witch-Hunt in Early Modern Europe. London: Longman

Levandoski RR. 1993a. Mandibular whiplash. Part II. An extension flexion injury of the temporomandibular joints. Functional Orthodontist, 10: 45–51

– 1993b. Mandibular whiplash. Part I: An extension flexion injury of the temporomandibular joints. Functional Orthodontist 10:26–9

Levy DM. 1945. Psychic trauma of operations in children. Am J Dis Child 69:7

Levy G quoted in DH Freedman. 1994. Who's to Judge? Discover 15:78–9

Levy S. 1996. The Antibiotic Paradox: How Miracle Drugs are Destroying the Miracle. New York: Pelnum Press

Lewis A. 1942. Discussion on the differential diagnosis and treatment of post-concussional states. J R Soc Med 35:607–14

Liedberg J, Westesson P-L. 1988. Sideways position of the temporomandibular joint disc: coronal cryosectioning of fresh autopsy specimens. Oral Surg Oral Med Oral Pathol 66:644

Linde K, Ramirez G, et al. 1996. St John's Wort for Depression: an overview and meta-analysis of randomised clinical trials. BMJ 313:253–8

Lindstrom I, Ohlund C, et al. 1992. The effect of graded activity on patients with subacute low back pain. Phys Ther 72:291–3

Lip GYH, Beevers DG. 1997. Can we treat coronary disease with antibiotics? Lancet 350:378–9

Littlejohn GO 1989. Fibrositis/fibromyalgia syndrome in the workplace. Rheum Dis Clin North Am 15:45–60

– 1995. Key issues in repetitive strain injury. J Musculoskeletal Pain 3:25–33

Littlejohn GO, Granges C. 1993. Pressure pain threshold in pain-free subjects, in patients with chronic regional pain syndromes, and in patients with fibromyalgia syndrome. Arthritis Rheum 36:642–50

Littré E. 1851. Oeuvres Complètes d'Hippocrate. Paris: Baillière

Livingston M. 1991. Neck and back sprains from MVAs: a retrospective study. B C Med J 33:654–6

– 1991. Whiplash (Letter). Lancet 338:1207–8

– 1992. Whiplash injury: misconceptions and remedies. Aust Fam Phys 21:1642–7

– 1995. Fibromyalgia, fibrositis and myofascial pain syndrome: a preliminary report. B C Med J 37:690–3

– 1998. Common Whiplash Injury: A Modern Epidemic. Springfield, Il: Charles C Thomas

– 1999a. Report on World Whiplash Congress. B C Med J 41:281–3

– 1999b. Letter to the Editor. Spine 24:99–101

Loeser JD. Oct 1994. John J. Bonica 1917–1994. Pain 59:1–3

Loeser JD, Cousins MJ. 1990. Contemporary pain management. Med J Aust 153:208–12

Loeser JD, Sullivan MD. Mar 1997. Doctors, diagnosis, and disability: a disastrous diversion. Clin Orthop 336:61–6

Loevinger L. 1995. Science as evidence. Jurimetrics J, 153–90

Lomex E. 1973. The uses and abuses of opiate in nineteenth-century England. Bull Hist Med 47:167–76

Longbotham HG, Engelken E, et al. 1994. Nonlinear approaches for separation of slow and fast phase nystagmus signals. Biomed Sci Instrum 30:99–104

Lord SM, Barnsley L, et al. 1994. Third occipital nerve headache: a prevalence study. J Neurol Neurosurg Psychiatry 57:1187–90

Lord SM, Barnsley L, et al. 5 Dec 1996. Percutaneous radio-frequency neurotomy for chronic cervical zygapophyseal-joint pain. N Engl J Med 335:1721–6

Lord SM, Bogduk N, Barnsley L. 1993. Cervical zygapophyseal joint pain in whiplash. In Teasell RW, Shapiro AP (eds). Spine. Philadelphia: Hanley & Belfus. Vol 7(3) ch 2, 355–71

Lorenzen I, 1994. Fibromyalgia: a clinical challenge [Review]. J Intern Med 235:199–203

Loundsberry E. 31 Aug 1998. Doctor 73, lauded as charitable, caring, gets jail for mail fraud. Philadelphia Inquirer

Lowry The Honourable Mr Justice. 2 Mar 1994. Spencer vs Soans. Supreme Court of British Columbia: Vancouver Registry, No B901809, B901810, B922884

Lucido VP. 1986. The dilemma of "subluxation." J Chiropractic 23:5–10

Lund JP, Lavigne G, et al. 1989. The use of electronic devices in the diagnosis and treatment of temporomandibular disorders. J Can Dent Assoc 55:749–50

Lynn EJ, Belza M. 1984. Factitious PTSD: the veteran who never got to Vietnam. Hosp Community Psychiatry 35:697–701

Lyons J. 4 Feb 1991. It's not a wonderful situation. Forbes 90–1

Lyons JA, Caddell JM, et al. 1994. The potential for faking on the Mississippi Scale for Combat-related PTSD. J Traumatic Stress 7:441–5

Macfarlane GJ, Morris S, et al. 1999. Chronic widespread pain in the community: the influence of psychological symptoms and mental disorder on healthcare seeking behavior. J Rheumatol 26:413–19

Macfarlane GJ, Hunt IM, Silman A. 2000. Role of mechanical and psychosocial factors in the onset of forearm pain: prospective population study. BMJ 321:676–84

Mack JE. 1994. Alien Encounters: Human Encounters with Aliens. New York: Simon & Schuster

Mack JE, Semrad EV. 1967. Classical Psychoanalysis. In Freedman AM, Kaplan HI (eds). Comprehensive Textbook of Psychiatry. Baltimore: Williams and Wilkins

Macnab I. 1966. Whiplash injuries of the neck. Manitoba Med Review 46:172–4.

– 1971a. The "whiplash syndrome." Orthop Clin North Am 2:, 389–403

– 1971b. Acceleration injuries of the cervical spine. J Bone Joint Surg 2:389–403

– 1973. The whiplash syndrome. Clin Neurosurg 20:232–41

– 1982. Acceleration extension injuries of the cervical spine. In The Spine. Philadelphia: Saunders. Vol 1 ch 10, 647–660

Magee SP. 1997. The optimum number of lawyers: a reply to Epp. Law & Soc Inquiry 17:667–94

Magnússon T. 1994. Extracervical symptoms after whiplash trauma. Cephalalgia 14:223–7, discussion 181–2

Magnússon T, Ragnarsson T, Bjornsson A. 1996. Occipital nerve release in patients with whiplash trauma and occipital neuralgia. Headache, 36:32–6

Magora A. 1973. Investigation of the relation between low back pain and occupation. V. Psychological aspects. Scand J Rehabil Med 5:191

Maguire WB 1993. Whiplash in Australia: illness or injury. Med J Aust 158:138

Mahdyoon H, Battilana G, et al. 1990. The evolving pattern for digoxin intoxication: observations at a large urban hospital from 1980 to 1988. Am Heart J 120:1189–94

Mahoney L, McCulloch JA, Casma A. 1985. Thermography as a diagnostic aid in sciatica. Thermology 1:43–50

Mahoney L, Wiley M, McMiken D. 1988. Thermography in whiplash injuries of the neck. Advocates' Quarterly 10:1–10

Maigne R. 1972. A New Approach to Vertebral Manipulations (translated by WT Liberson). Springfield, Il: Charles C Thomas

Mailis A, Furlong W, Taylor AE. 2000. Chronic pain in a family of six in the context of litigation. J Rheumatol 27:1315–7

Maines RP. 1999. The Technology of Orgasm. Baltimore: The Johns Hopkins University Press

Makela M, Heliovaara M. 1991. Prevalence of fibromyalgia in the Finnish population. Br Med J 303:216–9

Malleson AG. 1973a. Need Your Doctor Be So Useless? London: George Allen & Unwin

– 1973b. The Medical Runaround. New York City: Hart Publishing Co

– 1973c. Suicide prevention: a myth or a mandate? Br J Psychiatry 123: 612–3

– 1990. Whiplash, folly and fakery. Humane Med 6:193–6

– 1994. Chronic whiplash syndrome: a psychosocial epidemic. Can Fam Physician 40:1906–9

– 1996. Chronic whiplash: How long a pain in the neck? Hippocrates' Lantern 4:11–5

Malleson AG, Eastwood R, Moore S. 1977. Overvaluation of health care. CMAJ 116:11

Malleson Joan. 1942. Vaginismus: its management and psychogenesis. Brit Med J 2:213–6

Malleson Kate. 1999. The New Judiciary: the Effects and Expansion and Activism. Aldershot, UK: Dartmouth

Malmivaara A, Hakkinen U, et al. 1995. The treatment of acute low back pain: bed rest, exercises, or ordinary activity? N Engl J Med 332, 351–5

Malt UF. 1988. The long-term psychiatric consequences of accidental injury. Br J Psychiatry, 153:810–8

Malt UF, Olafsen OL. 1992. Psychological appraisal and emotional responses to physical injury. Psychiatric Medicine 10:117–33

Maltz W. 1991. The Sexual Healing Journey. New York: HarperCollins

Mandel S. 1992. Minor head injury may not be "minor." Postgrad Med 85:213–7

Mannheimer J, Attanasio R, et al. 1989. Cervical strain and mandibular whiplash: effects upon the craniomandibular apparatus. Clin Prev Dent 11:29–32

Marbuch JJ. 1995. Is myofascial face pain a regional expression of fibromyalgia? J Musculoskeletal Pain 3:93–7

Marco GJ. 1987. Silent Spring Revisited. Washington DC: American Chemical Society

Marmor TR, Smith GD. 1989. Why are the Japanese living longer? Br Med J 299:1547–51

Marquis Who's Who. 1996. The Official ABMS Directory of Board Certified Medical Specialists (28th ed). New Providence, NJ: Reed Reference Publishing Co

Marshall LL. 1976. The "whiplash" injury. Med J Aust 2:26–7

Martin GM. 1959. Sprains, strains and whiplash injuries of the neck. Physical Therapy Review 39:808–18

Martin SP, Donaldson MC, et al. 1974. Inputs into coronary care during thirty years: a cost-effectiveness study. Ann Intern Med 81:289–93

Martinez JL, Wickstrom JK, Barcelo BT. 1965. The whiplash: a study of head-neck action and injuries in animals. Am Soc Mech Engin Paper 65–WA/HUF-6, 1–8

Marwick C. 1998. Alterations are ahead at the Office of Alternative Medicine. JAMA 280:1553–4

Marx Karl quoted by FH Garrison. 1928. Bull N Y Acad Med 4:1001

Maslow A. 1968. Towards a Psychology of Being. New York: van Nostrand

Maudsley H. 1868. Illustrations of a variety of insanity. J Ment Sci 14:149

May M. 27 Nov 1992. Screens of protest over rules. The Times (London)

Mayberg HS. 1994. Frontal lobe dysfunction in secondary depression. J Neuropsychiatry Clin Neurosci 6:428–42

Maynard A. 1997. Evidence-based medicine: an incomplete method for informing treatment choices. Lancet 349:126–8

Mayou RA. 1995. Medico-legal aspects of road traffic accidents. J Psychosom Res 39:789–98

Mayou RA, Bryant B. 1994. Effects of road traffic accidents on travel. Injury 25:457–60

Mayou RA, Bryant B, Duthie R. 1993. Psychiatric consequences of road traffic accidents. BMJ 307:647–51

Mayou RA, Radanov BP. 1996. Whiplash neck injury. J Psychosom Res 40:461–74

McCain GA. 1993a. Diagnosis and treatment of fibromyalgia. In Teasell RW, Shapiro AP (eds). Spine. Philadelphia: Hanley & Belfus. Vol 7(3) ch 6, 423–441

– 1993b. Clinical picture of whiplash injuries. In Teasell RW, Shapiro AP (eds). Spine. Philadelphia: Hanley & Belfus. Vol 7(3) ch 373–90

McCombe PF, Fairbank JCT, et al. 1989. Reproducibility of physical signs in low-back pain. Volvo award in clinical sciences. Spine 14:908–18

McConnell WE, Howard PR, et al. 1993. Analysis of human test subject kinematic responses to low velocity rear end impacts. In Vehicle and Occupant Kinetics: Simulation and Modelling. Warrendale PA: Society for Automotive Engineers. 21–9

McDonald M. 28 Sep 1988. SEPTA does its math homework. Philadelphia Daily News

McFadyean M. 27 May 1995. Soldier on. Guardian (UK) Weekend 25ff

McFarlane AC. 1988. The longitudinal course of posttraumatic morbidity. The range of outcomes and their predictors. J Nerv Ment Dis 176:30–9

Macfarlane GJ, Thomas E, Cherry N. 2000. Mortality among UK Gulf war veterans. Lancet 356:17–21

McGowan M, Zigler R, Peacock GD. 1 Dec.1995. AG. vs Toronto Transit Commission. Court File No.95-CU-89529: Ontario Court of Justice (General Division)

McIntire RT. 1956. Opening remarks of conference on whiplash. International Record of Medicine and General Practice Clinics 169:2

McKenzie JA, Williams JF. 1971. The dynamic behaviour of the head and cervical spine during "whiplash." J Biomech 4:477–90

McKeown Thomas. 1971. Medical History and Medical Care. London: Oxford University Press

– 1977. The Role of Medicine: Dream, Mirage or Nemesis. Princeton: Princeton University Press

– 1979. The Role of Medicine. Oxford: Basil Blackwell

McKeown T, Lowe CR. 1966. An Introduction to Social Medicine. Oxford: Blackwell Scientific Publications

McKinlay WW, Brooks DV, Bond MR. 1983. Post-concussional symptoms, financial compensation and outcome of severe blunt head injury. J Neurol Neurosurg Psychiatry 46:1084–91

McKinney LA. 1989. Early mobilisation and outcome of acute sprains of neck. Br Med J 229:1006–8

McKinney MB. 1994. Treatment of dislocations of the cervical vertebrae in so-called "whiplash injuries" [German]. Orthopäde 23:287–90

McLaren L. 29 Apr 2000. Non-scents. Globe and Mail (Toronto) R1 and R6

McLean A, Temkin NR, et al. 1983. The behavioral sequelae of head injury. J Clin Neuropsychol 5:361–76

McMordie RW. 1988. Twenty-year follow-up of the prevailing opinion on the posttraumatic or postconcussional syndrome. Clin Neuropsychol 2:198–212

McMurdo R. 1985. Compensation neurosis. Med J Aust 143:324

McWinney IR, Epstein RJ, Freeman TR. 1997. Rethinking somatization. Ann Intern Med 126:747–50

Meade TW, Dyer S, et al. 1990. Low back pain of mechanical origin: randomised comparison of chiropractic and hospital outpatient treatment. BMJ 300:1431–7

Mealy K, Brennen H, Fenelon GCC. 1986. Early mobilisation of acute whiplash injuries. Br Med J 292:656–7

Mearns J, Lees-Haley PR. 1993. Discriminating neuropsychological sequelae of head injury from alcohol-abuse-induced deficits: a review and analysis. J Clin Psychol 49:714–20

Mechanic D. 1961. The concept of illness behaviour. J Chron Dis 15:189–94

Medical Research Council. 1948. Streptomycin treatment of pulmonary tuberculosis. Br Med J 2:769–82

Mehta U. 2000. Potentially serious drug interactions between St John's Wort and other medicines. S Afr Med J 90:698

Melville PH. 1963. "Research" in car crashing. CMAJ 89:275

Melzack R, Wall PD. 1965. Pain mechanisms: a new theory. Science 150:971–9

Mendall MA. 1998. Inflammatory responses and coronary heart disease. BMJ 316:953–4

Mendeloff A. 1974. What has been happening to duodenal ulcers? Gastroenterology 67:1020–2

Mendelson D. 1995b. Legal and medical aspects of liability for negligently occasioned nervous shock: a current perspective. J Psychosom Res 39:721–35

Mendelson G. 1981. Persistent work disability following settlement of compensation claims. Law Institute J 55:342–5

– 1982. Not cured by a verdict: the effect of legal settlement on compensation claims. Med J Aust 2:132–4

– 1985. "Compensation neurosis": an invalid diagnosis. Med J Aust 142:561–4

– 1992. Compensation and chronic pain. Pain 48:121–3

– 1995. "Compensation neurosis" revisited: outcome studies of the effects of litigation. J Psychosom Res 39:696–706

Mensink RP, Katan MB. 1990. Effect of dietary fatty acids on high-density and low-density lipoprotein cholesterol levels in healthy subjects. N Engl J Med 323:439–45

Merskey H. 1984. Psychiatry and the cervical syndrome. CMAJ 130:1119–21

– 1986. The importance of hysteria. Br J Psychiatry 149:23–8

– 1993. Psychological consequences of whiplash. In Teasell RW, Shapiro AP (eds) Spine. Philadelphia: Hanley & Belfus. Vol 7(3) ch 9, 471–9

– 1997. Whiplash in Lithuania. Pain Res Management 2:13

Mertz HJ, Patrick LM. 1967a. Investigation of the kinematics and kinetics of whiplash. SAE, Paper 670919

– 1967 b. Investigation of the kinematics and kinetics of whiplash. Paper presented at the 11th Stapp Car Crash Conference

Michaelson JS, Halperin E, Kopans DB. 1999. Breast cancer: computer simulation method for estimating optimal intervals for screening. Radiology 212:551–60

Michaelson MM. 1970. The failure of American medicine. The American Scholar 39(4)

Middleton JM. 1956. Ophthalmic aspects of whiplash injuries. Int Record Med and Gen Pract Clinics 19–20

Mikkelsson M, Latikka P, et al. 1992. Muscle and bone pressure pain threshold and pain tolerance in fibromyalgia. Pain 73:814–8

Milicic A, Jovanovic A, et al. 1994. [Evaluation of long-term prognosis in patients with whiplash syndrome] [SerboCroatian]. Med Pregl 47:341–3

Miller AB, To T, et al. 2000. Canadian National Breast Screening Study-2: 13-year results of a randomized trial in women. J Natl Cancer Inst 92:1490–9

Miller H. 1961a. Accident neurosis, Part 1. Br Med J 5230:920–5

– 1961b. Accident neurosis, Part 2. Br Med J 5231:992–8

Miller H, Cartlidge NEF. 1972. Simulation and malingering after injuries to the brain and spinal cord. Lancet 1:580–5

Miller L. 1996. Neuropsychology and pathophysiology of mild head injury and the postconcussion syndrome: clinical and forensic considerations. J Cogn Rehabil (Jan/Feb): 8–23

Mills H, Horne G. 1986. Whiplash: manmade disease? N Z Med J 99:373–4

Milstone Carol. Sep 1997. Sybil minds. Saturday Night, 35–42

Ministry of Health. 1962. Deaths from tonsillectomy. In Report on Hospital In-Patient Inquiry for the Year 1961. London: HMSO

Mitchell B. 1996. Drivers with no insurance face new plan. Toronto Star, A10

Moldofsky H, Lue FA, Saskin P. 1987. Sleep and morning pain in primary osteoarthritis. J Rheumatol 14:124–8

Moldofsky H, Scarisbrick P, et al. 1975. Musculoskeletal symptoms and non-REM sleep disturbance in patients with "fibrositis syndrome" and healthy subjects. Psychosom Med 37:341–51

Moldofsky H, Wong MT, Lue FA. 1993. Litigation, sleep, symptoms and disabilities in postaccident pain (fibromyalgia). J Rheumatol 20:1935–40

Molony RR, MacPeek DM, et al. 1986. Sleep, sleep apnoea and fibromyalgia syndrome. J Rheumatol 13:797–800

Monmaney T. 31 Aug 1998. Labels' potency claims often inaccurate, analysis finds. Los Angeles Times A10

– 31 Aug 1998. Remedy's US sales zoom, but quality control lags. Los Angeles Times A1

Montessori M. 1913. Pedagogical Anthropology (English Edition). New York: FA Stokes and Co

Moore T. 1992. Care of the Soul. New York: HarperCollins

Morgan E, 1973. The Descent of Woman. London: Souvenir Press Ltd

Morris D. 1971. Intimate Behavior. New York: Random House

Morrow L. 12 Aug 1991. A Nation of Finger Pointers. Time Magazine (Canadian Edition) 30–4

Moses AJ, Skoog GS. 1986. Cervical whiplash and TMJ. Trial (Mar):63–6

– 1986. Cervical whiplash and TMJ. Basic Facts 8:61–3

Mott FW. 1919. War Neuroses and Shell Shock. London. Oxford University Press

Moulton RE. 1955. Oral and dental manifestations of anxiety. Psychiatry 18:261–73

Mr Fit Research Group. 1982. Multiple-risk factor intervention trial. JAMA 248:1465–77

Munthe A. 1929. The Story of San Michele. London: Murray

Murray C, Lopez A. 1996. The Global Burden of Disease. Cambridge, Mass: Harvard University Press

Murrey J. 7 Apr 1998. Is burning semen newest Gulf war complication? Medical Post (Toronto) 34:1 and 82

Myodata. 1996. Catalogue. PO Box 803394, Dallas, Texas 75380: TMJ & Stress Center

Nachemson AL. 1992. Newest knowledge of low back pain. Clin Orthop 279:8–20

– 1994. Chronic pain: the end of the welfare state? Qual Life Res 3:S11–S17

Nadelson T. 1979. Munchausen syndrome: borderline character features. Gen Hosp Psychiatry 2:11–7

Naf E. 1978. Post-traumatic Horner's syndrome [German]. Klin Monatsbl Augenheilkd 172:517–20

Nashner LM, Black FO, Wall C. May 1982. Adaptation to altered support and visual conditions during stance: patients with vestibular deficits. J Neurosci 2:536–44

National Council Against Health Fraud. 1994. Position Paper on Chiropractic. Loma Linda, California: NCAHF

National Dairy Products Corp. vs Durham. 1967. Georgia Court of Appeals (quoted by Peter Huber [1991] in Galileo's Revenge: Junk Science and the Courtroom. New York: Basic Books)

National Highway Traffic Safety Administration. 1998. Traffic Safety Facts 1996 (Motor vehicle crash data from FARS and GES), Washington

National Insurance Crime Bureau: 1996a. Operation "Paper Accidents." Spotlight on Insurance Crime. Fall/Winter 17

– 1996b. Quacks, Crooks and Con Artists. Spotlight on Insurance Crime. Spring/Summer 9

– 1996c. Insurance fraud: the quiet catastrophe. Spotlight on Insurance Crime. Fall/Winter 18–19

– 1997a. Team Operation Backbone Scores Big. Spotlight on Insurance Crime IV:8–9

– 1997b. Operation Sideswipe. Spotlight on Insurance Crime, II:2–3

– 1997c. Crack down on soft-tissue injury. Spotlight on Insurance Crime I:6–7

– 1997d. Ripoff: Information Pamphlets. NICB Corporate Communications

National Library of Medicine. 1997. MedLine. Bethesda, MD

National Task Force on Insurance Fraud. 1994. Insurance Fraud in Canada. Toronto: Insurance Bureau of Canada

Navin FPD, Romilly DP. 1989. An investigation into vehicle and occupant response subjected to low-speed rear impacts. In Proceedings of the Multidisciplinary Road Safety Conference VI. Fredericton, New Brunswick: University of New Brunswick. 48–58

Nemiah JC. 1975. Neurasthenic neurosis. In Freedman AM, Kaplan HI, Sadock BJ. (eds). Comprehensive Textbook of Psychiatry. Baltimore: Williams and Wilkins. Vol II, Ch 21. 7, 1664.

Newbrun E. 1989. Effectiveness of water fluoridation. J Public Health Dent 49 (5 Special Issue), 279–88

New Catholic Encyclopedia. 1967. Philippines: Catholic University of America

Newcombe F, Rabbitt P, Briggs M. 1994. Minor head injury: Pathophysiological or iatrogenic sequelae? J Neurol Neurosurg Psychiatry 57:709–16

New Jersey Insurance Department, Fraud Division. 1993

Nice CM. 1908. Neurasthenia. South Med J 1:104–12

Nixon PGF. 1982. "Total allergy syndrome." Lancet 1:404

Nocera J. 1995a. O'Quinn's personal wealth cited in "Fatal Litigation." Part 1. Fortune 138, 60–82

– 1995b. O'Quinn's average out–of–court settlement cited in "Dow Corning Succumbs." Part 2. Fortune 138, 137–58

Nordstrom D. 1996. Disabling fibromyalgia: appearance vs reality. J Rheumatol 21:1776

Norman GR. 1986. Science, public policy and media disease. CMAJ 134:719–20

Norman GR, Newhouse MT. 1986. Health effects of urea formaldehyde foam insulation: evidence of causation. CMAJ 134:733–8

Norman GR, Pengelly LD, et al. 1986. Respiratory function of children in homes insulated with urea formaldehyde foam insulation. CMAJ 134:1135–8

Norris JW, Beletsky V, Nadareishvili ZG. 2000. Sudden neck movement and cervical artery dissection. CMAJ 163:38–40

Norris JW. 1991. Whiplash. Lancet 338:1207–8

North RB. 1996. Treatment of spinal pain syndromes. N Engl J Med 335:1763–4

Nygren A. 1984. Injuries to car occupants: some aspects of interior safety of cars. Acta Otolaryngol 395(Suppl):1–164

O'Brien LJ. 1999. Bad Medicine. Amherst, New York: Prometheus Books

O'Connell RA, Van Heertum RL, et al. 1989. Single photon emission tomography (SPECT) with [123] IMP in the differential diagnosis of psychiatric disorders. J Neuropsychiatry Clin Neurosci 1:145–53

O'Dowd T. 1988. Five years of heartsink. Br Med J 297:528

O'Neill B, Haddon W, et al. 1972. Automobile head restraints: frequency of neck injury claims in relation to the presence of head restraints. Am J Public Health 62:399–406

Obelieniene D, Schrader H, et al. 1999. Pain after whiplash: a prospective controlled inception cohort study. J Neurol Neurosurg Psychiatry 66:279–83

Office for National Statistics. 1998. Social Focus on Men and Women. London: Stationery Office.

Office of Health Economics. 1985. Back Pain. London

Office of the Inspector General. 1986. Inspection of chiropractic services under Medicare. Washington: Dept of H&HS

Ofshe R, Walters E. 1994. Making Monsters: False Memories, Psychotherapy, and Sexual Hysteria. New York: Scribners

Ogilvie WH. 1952. Whither medicine? Lancet 2:820

Okeson JP, Hayes DK. 1986. Long-term results of treatment for temporomandibular disorders: an evaluation by patients. J Am Dent Assoc 112:473–8

Olin M. 1990. Components of complex TM disorders. J Craniomandibular Dis Face Oral Pain 4:193–6

Olney DB, Marsden AK. 1986. The effect of head restraints and seat belts on the incidence of neck injury in car accidents. Injury 17:365–7

Olsen JH, Dossing M. 1982. Formaldehyde-induced symptoms in daycare centers. Am Ind Hyg Assoc J 43:366–70

Olsnes BT. 1989. Neurobehavioral findings in whiplash patients with long-lasting symptoms. Acta Neurol Scand 80:584–8

Ommaya AK, Faas F, Yarnell PR. 1968. Whiplash injury and brain damage. JAMA 204:285–9

Ontario Legislature. 1990. Bill 68, C2, SO1990

Oosterveld WJ, Kortschot HW, et al. 1991. ENG findings following cervical whiplash injuries. Acta otolaryngol 111:201–5

Oppenheim H. 1889. Die traümische Neurosen. Berlin: Hershwald

Organization for Economic Co-operation and Development. 1998. Better Health at Lower Cost? Paris: OECD

–1999. Health Data Package 98. Paris: OECD

Osselton MD. 1984. Poisoning-associated deaths for England and Wales between 1973 and 1980. Human Toxicology 3:201–21

Osterweis M, Kleinman A, Mechanic D. 1996. Pain and Disability: Clinical, Behavioral and Public Policy Perspectives. Washington, DC: National Academic Press

Oswald I, Priest RE. 1965. Five weeks to escape the sleeping pill habit. Br Med J 2:1093–5

Pabst R. 1987. Exposure to formaldehyde in anatomy: an occupational health hazard? Annat Rec 219:109–12

Page HW. 1885. Injuries of the Spine and Spinal Cord without Apparent Mechanical Lesions, and Nervous Shock in their Surgical and Medico-legal Aspects (2nd ed). London, UK: J & A Churchill

Page L. 1996. The backlash against evidence-based care. Birth 23:191–2

Palmer DD. 1910. The Science, Art and Philosophy of Chiropractic. Portland, Oregon: Portland Printing House

Pang LQ. 1971. The otological aspects of whiplash injuries. Laryngoscope 81:1381–7

Pankratz LD, Binder LM. 1997. Malingering on intellectual and neuropsychological measures. In Rogers R (ed). Clinical Assessment of Malingering and Deception. New York: Guilford Press. Ch 11, 223–36

Paparella MM, et al. 1991. Menière's disease and other labyrinthine diseases. In Paparella MM, et al (eds). Otolaryngology, 49. Philadelphia: Saunders Co

Pappworth MH. 1966. Human Guinea Pigs. London: Routledge & Kegan Paul

Parker N. 1979. Malingering: a dangerous diagnosis. Med J Aust 2:318–22

Parmar HV, Raymakers R. 1993. Neck injuries from rear-impact road traffic accidents: prognosis in persons seeking compensation. Injury 24:75–8

Parsons T. 1951. The Social System. Glencoe, Il: Free Press

Partheni M, et al. 1997. Whiplash injury following car accident. In New York: Annual Meeting of the North American Spine Society

Partheni M, Miliaris G, et al. 1999. Whiplash injury. J Rheumatol 26: 1206–7

Patrick DL, Deyo RA. 1989. Generic and disease-specific measures in assessing health status and quality of life. Med Care 27(3 Suppl): S217–32

Payne Roger. 1995. Among Whales. New York: Scribner

Peabody FW. 1927. The care of the patient. JAMA 88:877–82

Pearce JMS. 1989. Whiplash injury: a reappraisal. J Neurol Neurosurg Psychiatry 52:1329–31

– 1994. Polemics of chronic whiplash injury. Neurology 44:1993–7

Pearson GHJ. 1941. Effects of operative procedures on the emotional life of children. Am J Dis Child 69:716

Peck SM. 1978. The Road Less Traveled. New York: Simon & Schuster

Pennie BH, Agambar LJ. 1991. Patterns of injury and recovery in whiplash. Injury 22:57–9

Perconte ST, Goreczny AJ. 1990. Failure to detect fabricated posttraumatic stress disorder with the use of the MMPI in a clinical population. Am J Psychiatry 147:1057–60

Percy JS. 1994. Whiplash syndrome: a doctor's dilemma. CMAJ 6:63–8

Perry HT. 1988. Above all else, do no harm. J Am Dent Assoc 117:662

Peto R, Baigent C. 1998. Trials: the next 50 years. BMJ 317:1170

Peveler R. 1998. Understanding medically unexplained physical symptoms: faster progress in the next century than this? Psychosomatics 45:93–7

Phillips DJ. Sep 1993. Transcript of testimony. Geraldine Heffinger vs. Rosalie Wilson. (The Circuit Court of the 15th Judicial Circuit, Palm Beach, Florida). Honorable Edward Fine. CL-90-13342-AN

Pilkington E. 12 Jun 1995. Gulf war veterans fear for their families. Guardian (UK)

Pinker Steven. 1997. How the Mind Works. New York: WW Norton & Co

Platt JJ, Husband SD. 1989. Post-traumatic stress disorder in forensic practice. Am J Forensic Psychol 4:29–56

Porter KM. 1989. Neck sprains after car accidents: a common cause of long-term disability. Br Med J 298:973–4

Porter R. 1997. The Greatest Benefit to Mankind. London: HarperCollins

Powles J. 1973. On the limitations of modern medicine. Science, Medicine & Man 1:1–30

Poynter N. 1971. Medicine and Man. London: CA Watts & Co

Prendergast JF. 1896. The bicycle for women. Am J Obstet 14:245–53

President's Council on Competitiveness. 1991. Agenda for Civil Justice Reform. Washington DC: Government Printing Offices

Pressman BD, Shellock FG, et al. 1992. MR imaging of temporomandibular joint abnormalities associated with cervical hyperextension/hyperflexion (whiplash) injuries. J Magn Imag 2:569–74

Preston T. 1981. The Clay Pedestal. Seattle: Madrona

Probert TC, Wiesenfeld D, Reade PC. 1994. Temporomandibular pain dysfunction disorder resulting from road traffic accidents: an Australian study. Int J Oral Maxillofac Surg 23:338–41

Pullinger AG, Seligman DA. 1991. Trauma history in diagnosis groups of temporomandibular disorders. J Oral Surg Med Pathol 71:529–34

Putnam FW 1991. The satanic ritual abuse controversy. Child Abuse Negl 15:175–9

Quill TE. 1985. Somatic disorder, one of medicine's blind spots. JAMA 254:3075–9

Quimby LG, Block SR, Gratwick GM. 1988. Fibromyalgia: generalized pain intolerance and manifold symptom reporting. J Rheumatol 15:1264–70

Rabinbach A. 1982. The body without fatigue: a nineteenth century Utopia. In Drescher S, Sabean D, Sharlin A (eds). Political Symbolism in Modern

Europe: Essays in Honour of George Mosse. London: Transaction Books. 42–62

Radanov BP. 1997. Common whiplash: research findings revisited. J Rheumatol 24:624–5

Radanov BP, Begre S, et al. 1996. Course of psychological variables in whiplash injury: a two-year follow-up with age, gender and education pair-matched patients. Pain 64:429–34

Radanov BP, Di Stefano G, Schnidrig A. 1993. Cognitive functioning after common whiplash. Arch Neurol 50:87–91

Radanov BP, Di Stefano G, et al. 1991a. Role of psychosocial stress in recovery from common whiplash. Lancet 338:712–5

– 1991b. Role of psychosocial stress, cognitive performance and disability after common whiplash. Lancet 338:712–5

Radanov BP, Di Stefano G, et al. 1993. Psychological stress, cognitive performance and disability after common whiplash. J Psychosom Res 37:1–10

– 1994. Common whiplash: psychosomatic or somatopsychic? J Neurol Neurosurg Psychiatry 57:486–90

Radanov BP, Dvorak J, Valach L. 1989. [Psychological changes following whiplash injury of the cervical vertebrae] [German]. Schweiz Med Wochenschr 119:536–43

– 1992. Cognitive deficits in patients after soft-tissue injury of the cervical spine. Spine 17:127–31

Radanov BP, Schnidrig A, et al. 1992. Illness behaviour after common whiplash. Lancet 339:749–50

Radanov BP, Sturzenegger M, Di Stefano G. 1994. [Prediction of recovery from dislocation of the cervical vertebrae (whiplash injury of the cervical vertebrae) with initial assessment of psychosocial variables] [German]. Orthopäde 23:282–6

– 1995. Long-term outcome after whiplash injury: a two-year follow-up considering features of injury mechanism and somatic, radiologic, and psychosocial findings. Medicine 74:281–97

Radanov BP, Sturzenegger M, et al. 1993a. [Results of a 1-year follow-up study of whiplash injury] [German]. Schweiz Med Wochenschr 123:1545–52

– 1993b. Factors influencing recovery from headache after common whiplash. BMJ 307:652–5

– 1996. Predicting recovery from common whiplash. Eur Neurol 36:48–51

– 1994. Relationship between early somatic, radiological, cognitive and psychosocial findings and outcome during a one-year follow-up in 117 patients suffering from common whiplash. Br J Rheum 33:442–8

Radanov BP, Valach L, et al. 1990. [Neuropsychological findings following whiplash injury of the cervical spine] [German]. Schweiz Med Wochenschr 120:704–8

Raffle PAB. 1963. Automation and repetitive work: their effect on health. Lancet 1:733–7

Ramsay R. 1990. Invited review: post-traumatic stress disorder: a new clinical entity? J Psychosom Res 34:355–65

Ransohoff DF, Feinstein AR. 1978. Problems of selection and bias in evaluating the efficacy of diagnostic tests. N Engl J Med 299:926–30

Ratliff AH. 1997. Whiplash injuries. J Bone Joint Surg Br 79:517–9

Rauws EAJ, Tytgat GNJ. 1990. Cure of duodenal ulcers associated with eradication of H. pylori. Lancet 335:1233–5

Rawlins Mme Justice. 1994. Mackie vs Wolfe. Alberta Court of Queen's Bench No.9201-12776

Rawson AJ. 1944. Accident proneness. Psychosom Med 6:88–94

Reich A. 1953. Narcissistic object choice in women. J Am Psychoanal Assoc 1:22–44

Reilly PA. 1995a. "Repetitive strain injury": from Australia to the UK. J Psychosom Res 39:783–8

– 1995b. Approaches to RSI in the United Kingdom. J Musculoskeletal Pain 3:123–5

Rembold CM. 1998. Number needed to screen: development of a statistic for disease screening. Br Med J 317:307–12

Richards B. 7 Jan 1988. Doctors seek crackdown on colleagues paid-for testimony in malpractice suits. Wall Street Journal, sect 2, 1

Richman J. 1998. Manufacturing disability. Canadian Insurance, 28–34

Rigler CTJ. 1879. Über die Folgen der Verletzungem auf Eisenbahnen. Berlin: Reimer

Robbins J. 1996. Reclaiming our Health. Tiburton, Ca: HJ Kramer

Roca PD. 1972. Ocular manifestations of whiplash injuries. Ann Ophthalmol 4:63–73

Roemer MI, Schwartz JL. 1979. Doctor slowdown: effects on the population of the Los Angeles County. Soc Sci Med 13C: 213–8

Rogal OJ. 1982. The Medical Legal Aspects of Whiplash and TMJ. Lawyer's Digest (Feb)

– 1984. Mandibular Whiplash. Published by author

– 1986. Successful treatment for Head, Facial and Neck Pain. Philadelphia: The TMJ Dental Trauma Center for Head, Facial & Neck Pain

– 1986. The Medical-Legal Aspects of Whiplash and TMJ Injuries. Philadelphia: The TMJ Dental Trauma Center for Head, Facial & Neck Pain

– 1987a. Mandibular Whiplash: Medical-Legal Aspects of Whiplash and TMJ Injuries (video recording). Philadelphia: The TMJ Dental Trauma Center for Head, Facial & Neck Pain

– 1987b. Mandibular Whiplash: Medical-Legal Aspects of Whiplash and TMJ Injuries. Published by the author

– 1986. Court Testimony, Robert Barley vs Boekel Industries before Walter

M Leonard. Commonwealth of Pennsyivania Department of Labor and Industry Workers' Compensation Referees: No.181-42-0485

Rogers R. 1997. Introduction. In Rogers R (ed). Clinical Assessment of Malingering and Deception. New York: The Guilford Press. 1–19

Romano TJ. 1990. Clinical experiences with post-traumatic fibromyalgia syndrome. W V Med J 86:198–202

Ronnen HR, de Korte PJ, et al. 1996. Acute whiplash injury: is there a role for MR imaging? A prospective study of 100 patients. Radiology 201:93–6

Rosanoff AJ. 1929. Traumatic hysteria versus malingering. California State J Med 30:197

Rosen A. 1974. Lydia Becker quoted in: Rise up Women! The Militant Campaign of the Women's Social and Political Union, 1903–1914. Routledge and Kegan Paul, 8

Rosenbaum JT. 1997. Lessons from litigation over silicone breast implants: a call for activism by scientists. Science 276:1524–5

Rosenhan DL. 1973. On being sane in insane places. Science 179:250–8

Ross CA, Norton GR, Wozney K. 1989. Multiple personality disorder: an analysis of 236 cases. Can J Psychiatry 34:413–18

Ross SE. 1999. "Memes" as infectious agents in psychosomatic illness. Ann Intern Med 131:867–71

Rosser WW, Shafir MS. 1998. Evidence-Based Family Medicine. Hamilton, Canada: BC Decker Inc

Rothbart PJ. Oct 1996. Snapping back at whiplash. Can J Diagnosis 91–104

Rowe ML 1983. Backache at Work. Fairport, NY: Perington Press

Roydhouse RH. 1973. Whiplash and temporomandibular dysfunction. Lancet 1:1394–5

– 1985. Torquing of neck and jaw due to belt restraint in whiplash-type accidents. Lancet 1:1341

Rubin W. 1973. Whiplash with vestibular involvement. Arch Otolaryngol 97:85–7

Rudolph R. 18 Aug 1993. Two Newark police officers, East Orange doctor charged for insurance fraud. The Star-Ledger, 13

Rugh JD, Solberg WK. 1985. Oral health status in United States: temporomandibular disorders. J Dent Educ 49:398–405

Rush PJ, Ameis A. 1995. Trauma and fibromyalgia: does the punishment fit the crime? J Rheumatol 22:372–4

Rusk J. 1996. Uninsured drivers, false claims face crackdown. Globe and Mail (Toronto) A5

Russell AS. 1995. Fibromyalgia: a historical perspective. J Musculoskeletal Pain 3:43–7

Russell J. 1863. Cases illustrating the influence of exhaustion of the spinal cord in inducing paraplegials. Medical Times Gazette (London) 2:456

Sackett DL. 1995. The need for evidence-based medicine. J R Soc Med 88:620–4

–1996. The Doctor's (Ethical and Economic) Dilemma. London: Office of Health Economics

Sackett DL, Rosenberg WMC, et al. 1996. Evidence-based medicine: what it is and what it isn't. BMJ 312:71–2

Sagan C. 1995. The Demon-haunted World: Science as a Candle in the Dark. New York: Random House

Saikku P, Mattila K, et al. 1988. Serological evidence of an association of novel Chlamydia, TWAR, with chronic coronary heart disease and acute myocardial infarction. Lancet 2:983–5

Sanchez-Guerrero J, et al. 1995. Nurses' Health Study. N Engl J Med 332:1666–70

Sandler G. 1979. Costs of unnecessary tests. Br Med J 2:21–4

Saravis S, Schacter R, et al. 1990. Aspartame: effects on learning, behavior and mood. Pediatrics 86:75–83

Sarno JE. 1981. The etiology of neck and back pain: an autonomic myoneuralgia? J Nerv Ment Dis 169:55–9

– 1991. Healing Back Pain: The Mind-Body Connection. New York: Warner Books

Saskin P, Moldofsky H. 1986. Sleep and post-traumatic rheumatic pain modulation disorder (fibrositis syndrome). Psychosom Med 48:319–23

Saunders HD. 1990. Defining chronic pain and the chronic pain syndrome. Can J Diagnosis (Nov): 95–112

Schaefer JH. 1986. Importance of whiplash injury. Basic Facts 8:62

Scheuler W, Kubicki S, et al. 1988. The alpha-sleep pattern: quantitative analysis and functional aspects. In Koella WP, Obal F, Schultz H, Visser P (eds). Sleep. Stuttgart: Fischer

Schimmel EG. 1964. The hazards of hospitalization. Ann Intern Med 60:100

Schissel MJ, Dodes JE. 1997. "Wellness" and quackery. NY State Dent J 52:7

Schneider K, Zernicke RF, Clark G. 1989. Modelling of jaw-head-neck dynamics during whiplash. J Dent Res 68:1360–5

Schrader H, Obelieniene D, et al. 1996. Natural evolution of late whiplash syndrome outside the medicolegal context. Lancet 347:1207–11

Schutt CH, Dohan C. 1968. Neck injury to women in auto accidents: a Metropolitan plague. JAMA 206:2689–92

Schwartz LL. 1956. A temporomandibular joint pain-dysfunction syndrome. J Chron Dis 284–93

– 1959. Disorders of the Temporomandibular Joint. Philadelphia: WB Saunders

Schwartzmann LC, Teasell RW, et al. 1996. The effects of litigation status on adjustment to whiplash injury. Spine 21:53–8

Scitovsky AA, McCall N. 1976. Changes in the costs of treatment of selected illnesses, 1951-1964-1971. Washington DC: Government Printing Office (DHEW publication No:(HRA)77-3161)

Scofield ME, Martin W. 1990. Development of the AT&T Health Audit for measuring organizational health. Occup Med 5:755–70

Scrignar CB. 1984. Post-traumatic Stress Disorder: Diagnosis, Treatment and Legal Issues. New York: Praeger

Seidl LG, Thornton GF, et al. 1966. Studies on the epidemiology of adverse drug reactions. 3. Reactions in patients on a general medical service. Bull Hopkin's Hosp 119:299

Selecki BR. 1984. Whiplash: a specialist's view. Aust Fam Phys 13:243–7

Seletz E. 1958. Whiplash injuries. JAMA 168:1750–5

Severy DM, Mathewson JH, Bechtol CD. 1955. Controlled automobile rear-end collisions: an investigation of related engineering and medical phenomena. Can Serv Med J (Nov): 727–53

Shapiro AP, Teasell RW, Steenhaus R. 1993. Mild traumatic brain injury following whiplash. In Teasell RW, Shapiro AP (eds). Spine. 7(3) ch 8, 455–70

Shapiro AP, Roth RS. 1993. The effects of litigation on recovery from whiplash. In Teasell RW, Shapiro AP (eds). Spine. 7(3) ch 13, 531–55

Shapiro SK, Torres F. 1960. Brain injury complicating whiplash injuries. Minnesota Med 43:473–6

Shapiro SL. 1972. The otologic symptoms of cervical whiplash injuries. Eye, Ear, Nose & Throat Monthly 51:259–63

Sharpe J, 1996. Instruments of Darkness. London: Hamish Hamilton Ltd

Shaw DL, Nevel JP. 2000. The information value of medical science news. Journalism Q 44:548

Shea JJ. 1992. The myth of spontaneous perilymph fistula. Otolaryngol Head Neck Surg 107:613–6

Shekelle P, Adams AH, et al. 1992. Spinal manipulation for low-back pain. Ann Intern Med 117:590

Shepherd M, Cooper B, et al. 1966. Psychiatric illness and General Practice. London: Oxford University Press

Shor A, Kuo CC, Patton DL. 1992. Detection of Chlamydia pneumonia in coronary arterial fatty streaks and atheromatous plaques. S Afr Med J 82:158–61

Shorter E. 1992. From Paralysis to Fatigue: A History of Psychosomatic Illness in the Modern Era. Canada: Maxwell Macmillan

– 1994. From the Mind into the Body: The Cultural Origins of Psychosomatic Symptoms. New York: Free Press

– 1996. The role of hysteria in pseudo-diseases. Hippocrates' Lantern 4:1–5

Showalter E. 1985. The Female Malady: Women, Madness and English Culture. New York: Pantheon Books

– 1997. Hystories: Hysterical Epidemics and Modern Culture. New York: Columbia University Press

Shuval JT, Antonovsky A, Davies AM. 1973. Illness: a mechanism for dealing with failure. Soc Sci Med 7:259–65

Sim M. 1992. Insurance, Legal and Medical Aspects. Victoria, BC: Emmes

Simmons K, et al. 1982. Trauma to vertebral artery related to neck manipulation. Med J Aust 1:187–8

Simpson, Jeffrey. 16 Oct 2000. Nothing like tossing moolah at health care. Globe and Mail (Toronto) A15

Single E, Rehm J, et al. 2000. The relative risks and etiologic fractions of different causes of death and disease attributable to alcohol, tobacco, and illicit drug use in Canada. CMAJ 162:1669–75

Skinner HA. 1961. The Origin of Medical Terms. Baltimore: Williams and Wilkins

Slamovitis TL, Glaser JS. 1988. The pupils and accommodation. In Duane's Clinical Ophthalmology. Philadelphia: JB Lippincott. Ch 15, 23

Slater Elliot. 1965. Hysteria. Br Med J 1:1395–9

Smith H. 1976. The Forgotten Truth. New York: Harper & Row

Smith T. 1992. Against lawyers. BMJ 305:837

Smith TW, Butler VP, et al. 1982. Treatment of life-threatening digitalis intoxication with digoxin-specific Fab antibody fragments. N Engl J Med 307:1357–66

Smoller BR, Kruskall MS. 1986. Phlebotomy for diagnostic laboratory tests in adults. N Engl J Med 314:1233–5

Smythe H. 1989. Nonarticular rheumatism and psychogenic musculoskeletal syndromes. In Daniel McCarthy (ed). Arthritis and Allied Conditions. Philadelphia: Lea and Febger. 1241–54

Soetekouw PM, de Vries M, et al. 2000. Somatic hypotheses of war syndromes. Europ J Clin Invest 30:566–9

Solomon M. 1997. Women healers and the power to disease in late medieval Spain. In Lilian R Furst (ed). Women's Healers and Physicians: Climbing a Long Hill. Lexington: University of Kentucky. Ch 4, 79–92

Sparr LF. 1995. PTSD. Does it exist? Neurol Clin 13:413–29

Sparr LF, Boehnlein JK. 1990. PTSD in tort actions: forensic minefield. [Review]. Bull Am Acad Psychiatry Law 18:283–302

Sparr LF, Pankratz LD. 1983. Factitious PTSD. Am J Psychiatry 140:1016–9

Spender D. 1982. Women of Ideas. London: Pandora

Spitzer WO, Bombardier C, et al. 1987. Scientific approach to the assessment and management of activity-related spinal disorders. Spine 12(7S): S1–S42

Spitzer WO, Skovron ML, et al. 1995. Scientific monograph of the Quebec Task Force on Whiplash-associated disorders: redefining "whiplash" and its management. Spine 20(Suppl): 2S–68S

Spivak H, Rodin G, Sutherland AJ. 1994. The psychology of factitious disorders: a reconsideration. Psychosomatics 35:25–34

Springett P, Johnson A. 29 Oct 1993. RSI ruling may only delay claims avalanche. Guardian (UK) 3

Stallones RE. 1980. The rise and fall of ischemic heart disease. Scientific American 243:43–9

Starhawk, 1988. Dreaming the Dark: Magic, Sex and Politics. Boston: Beacon Press

States JD, Korn MW, Masengill JB. 1970. The enigma of whiplash injury. N Y State J Med 70: 2971–8

Stead AH, Allan AR, Ardrey RE, et al. 1981. Drug misuse: the barbiturate problem. J Forensic Sci Soc 21:41–53

Stein D. 1988. The Women's Book of Healing. St Paul, Minnesota: Llewellyn Publications

– 1990. All Women are Healers: A Comprehensive Guide to Natural Healing. Freedom, California: The Crossing Press

Steincrohn PJ. 1972. Low Blood Sugar. Chicago: Henry Regnery Co

Steinem G. 1994. What if Freud were Phyllis? In Moving Beyond Words. New York: Simon & Schuster

Stewart DE. 1989. The changing faces of somatization. Psychosomatics, 31:53–8

Stewart DE, Raskin J. 1985. Psychiatric assessment of patients with "20th-century disease." CMAJ 133:1001–5

Stone AA. 1993. PTSD and the law: critical review of the new frontier. Bull Am Acad Psychiatry Law 21:23–36

Stone E. 1763. An account of of the success of the bark of the willow in the cure of agues. Philosoph Trans 53:195

Stovner LJ. 1996. The nosological status of the whiplash syndrome: a critical review based on a methodological approach. Spine 21:2735–45

Strauss I, Savitsky N. 1934. Head injury: neurologic and psychiatric aspects. Arch Neurol Psychiatry. 31:893–955

Strole L, Langer TS, et al. 1962. Mental Health in the Metropolis: The Midtown Manhattan Study. New York: McGraw-Hill

Strother CE, James MB. 1987. Evaluation of seat back strength and seat belt effectiveness in rear end impacts. SAE Technical Paper Series: 872214, 369–77

Strub RL, Black FW. 1988. In Neurobehavioral Disorders: a Clinical Approach. Ch 9, 313–48. Philadelphia: FA Davis

Sturzenegger M, Di Stefano G, et al. 1994. Presenting symptoms and signs after whiplash injury: the influence of accident mechanisms. Neurology 44:688-93

Sturzenegger M, Radanov BP, Di Stefano G. 1995. The effect of accident mechanisms and initial findings on the long-term course of whiplash injury. J Neurol 242:443–9

Stuss DT, Ely P, et al. 1985. Subtle neuropsychological deficits in patients with good recovery after closed head injury. Neurosurgery, 17:41–6

Stuss DT, Stethem LL, et al. 1989. Reaction time after head injury: fatigue, divided and focused attention, and consistency of performance. J Neurol Neurosurg Psychiatry 52:742–8

Sugarman SD. 1990. The need to reform personal injury law: leaving scientific disputes to scientists. Science 248:823–7

Suhr J, Tranel D, et al. 1997. Memory performance after head injury: contributions of malingering, litigation status, psychological factors, and medication use. J Clin Exp Psychol 19:500–14

Sullivan MD, Katon W, et al. 1994. Coping and marital support as correlates of tinnitus disability. Gen Hosp Psychiatry 16:259–66

Sullivan MD, Turner JA, Romano TJ. 1991. Chronic pain in primary care: identification and management of psychosocial factors. J Fam Practice 32:193–9

Sullivan RL. 30 Jan 1995. Chronic fee syndrome. Forbes 114

Sun M. 1986. Formaldehyde poses little risk, study says [news]. Science 231:1365

Supreme Court of Canada. 1928. Meaning of the word "persons" under section 24 of the British North American Act. Supreme Court Reports 276–304

Svensson H-O, Andersson GBJ. 1989. The relationship of low back pain, work history, work environment, and stress. Spine 14:517–22

Sweeney JE. 1992. Non-impact brain injury: grounds for clinical study of neuropsychological effects of acceleration forces. Clin Neuropsychol 6:443–7

Swerdlow B. 1998. Whiplash and Related Headaches. Boca Raton: CRC Press

Szabo TJ, Wellcher JB, et al. 1994. Human occupation kinematic response to low speed rear-end impacts. SAE Technical Paper Series: 940532

Szasz T. 1961. The Myth of Mental Illness. New York: Dell

– 1996. A brief history of medicine's war on responsibility. J Clin Epidemiol 49:609–13

Talaga T. 24 Aug 1995. TTC facing $55 million crash lawsuit. Toronto Star

Taylor AE. 1997. Mild traumatic brain injury: an author responds. Arch Phys Med Rehabil 78:334–5

Taylor AE, Cox CA, Maillis A. 1994. Persistent neuropsychological deficits following whiplash: evidence for mild traumatic brain injury? Arch Phys Med Rehabil 77:529–35

Taylor JR, Kakulas BA. 1991. Neck injury. Lancet 338:1343

Taylor JR, Twomey LT. 1990. Disc injuries in cervical trauma. Lancet 338:1318

Taylor P. 13 Mar 1993. Danger at the keyboard. Globe and Mail (Toronto) A1 and A4

Teasdale G, Mathew P. 1996. Mechanisms of cerebral concussion, contusion, and other effects of head injury. In Youmans JR (ed). Neurological Surgery. Philadelphia: WB Saunders. Ch 66, 1533

Teasell RW. 1993. Clinical picture of whiplash injuries. In Teasell RW, Shapiro AP (eds). Spine. Philadelphia: Hanley & Belfus. Vol 7(3) ch 3, 373–89

Teasell RW, McCain GA. 1992. Painful Cervical Trauma. Baltimore: Williams and Wilkins

Teasell RW, McCain GA, et al. 1991. Cervical strain of whiplash injury. Humane Med 7:183–7

Teasell RW, Shapiro A, Maillis A. 1993. Medical management of whiplash injuries. In Teasell RW, Shapiro AP (eds). Spine. Philadelphia: Hanley & Belfus. Vol 7(3) ch 10, 481–99

Teasell RW, Shapiro AP. 1993. Preface.In Teasell RW, Shapiro AP. (eds). Spine. Philadelphia: Hanley & Belfus. Vol 7(3) Preface xi–xii

Teife A, Degrief J, et al. 1993. Der Sicherheitsgurt: Auswirkungen auf das Verletzungsmuster von Autoinsassen. Rofo fortschr Geb Rontgenstr Neuen Bildgeb Verfahr 159:278–83

Teresi LM, Lufkin RB, Reicher MA. 1987. Asymptomatic degenerative disc disease and spondylosis of the cervical spine: MR imaging. Radiology, 164:83–8

Terr AI. 1986. Environmental illness: a clinical review of 50 cases. Arch Intern Med 146:145–9

Therapeutics and Technology Assessment Subcommittee of the American Academy of Neurology. 1996. Assessment of brain SPECT. Neurology 46:278–85

– 1989. Assessment: EEG brain mapping. Neurology 39:1100–1

THM. 1982. The dump that wasn't there. Science 215:645

Thomas DB, Gao DL, et al. 1997. Randomized trial of breast self-examination in Shanghai: methodology and preliminary results. J Natl Cancer Inst 89:355–65

Thomas DJ, Ewing CL, Majewski PL. 1979. Clinical medical effects of head and neck response during biodynamic stress experiments. In (AGARD) Conference Proceedings at Lisbon. Advisory Group for Aerospace Research and Development, ch 15, 1–15

Thomas R. 8 Nov 1998. Woolf pounces on experts' fees. Observer News 5

Thompson JM. 1990. Tension myalgia as a diagnosis at the Mayo Clinic and its relationship to fibrositis, fibromyalgia and myofascial pain syndrome. Mayo Clin Proc 65:1237–48

Thompson K. 1991. Angels and Aliens: UFOs and the Mythic Imagination. New York: Random House

Thompson WI. 1971. Planetary Vistas. Harpers 243:73

Thorson K. 1993. Fibromylagia Network: newsletter for fibromyalgia/fibrositis/CFS support groups

Toglia JU. 1972. Vestibular and medico-legal aspects of closed cranio-cervical trauma. Scand J Rehabil Med 4:126–32

– 1976. Acute flexion-extension injury of the neck. Electronystagmographic study of 309 patients. Neurology 26:808–14

Toglia JU, Rosenberg PE, Ronis ML. 1969. Vestibular and audiological aspects of whiplash injury and head trauma. J Forensic Sci 14:219–26

–1970. Posttraumatic dizziness: vestibular, audiologic, and medicolegal aspects. Arch Otolaryngol 92(S5):485–92

Torres F, Shapiro SK. 1961. Electroencephalograms in whiplash injury. Arch Neurol 5:40–7

Toufexis A. 25 Apr 1988. Treating an "In" Malady. Time Magazine (Canadian Edition) 102

Tounge DJ, O'Reilly MJ, et al. 1972. Traffic crash fatalities: injury patterns and other factors. Med J Aust 2:5–17

Trall RT. 1873. The Health and Diseases of Women. Battle Creek, Michigan: Health Reformer

Travell J, Simons DG. 1983. Myofascial Pain and Dysfunction: The Trigger Point Manual. Baltimore: Williams & Wilkins

Trief P, Stein N. 1985. Pending litigation and rehabilitation outcome of chronic back pain. Arch Med Rehabil 66:95–9

Trimble MR. 1981. Post-traumatic Neurosis: From Railway Spine to Whiplash. Chichester UK: John Wiley & Sons

Trivers RL. 1985. Social Evolution, Menlo Park, CA: Benjamin/Cummings Publishing Co

Trzepac PT, Hertweck M, et al. 1992. The relationship of SPECT Scans to behavioral dysfunction in neuropsychiatric patients. Psychosomatics 33:62–71

Tunks E. 1995. Comparing fibromyalgia, myofascial pain and control groups. J Musculoskeletal Pain 3:81–5

Turk DC, Rudy TE. 1990. Neglected factors in chronic pain treatment outcome studies: referral patterns, failure to enter treatment and attrition. Pain 43:7–25

Turner EB. 1896. A report on cycling in health and disease. Br Med J 1158

Turner JA, Deyo RA, Loeser JD. 1996. The importance of placebo effects in pain treatment. JAMA 271:1609–14

Twomey LT, Taylor JR, Taylor MM. 1989. Unsuspected damage to lumbar zygapophyseal (facet) joints after motor-vehicle accidents. Med J Aust 151:210–7

Tyler VE. 1993. The Honest Herbal: A Sensible Guide to the Use of Herbs and Related Remedies (3rd ed). New York: Pharmaceutical Products Press

Tyndel M. 1974. Offenders without victims? In Drapkin I, Viano E (eds). Victimology: A New Focus. Lexington: DC Heath

Tyndel M, Egit M. 1988. Concept of nomogenic disorders. Med Law 7:167–76

Tyndel M, Tyndel FJ. 1984. Post-traumatic stress disorder: a nomogenic disease. Emotional First Aid 1:5–10

Tyrer S. 1994. Repetitive strain injury. J Psychosom Res 38:493–8

Underharnscheidt F. 1983. Traumatic alterations in the Rhesus monkey undergoing –GX accelerations. Neurotraumatology 6:151–67

Uomoto JM, Esselman PC 1993. Traumatic brain injury and chronic pain: differential types and rates by head injury severity. Arch Phys Med Rehabil 74:61–4

US Bureau of Census. 1971. Statistical Abstract of the USA. Washington DC: US Government Printing Office

US Department of Health, Education and Welfare. 1973. Report of the Secretary's Commission on Medical Malpractice. Washington DC: Government Printing Office

Van de Calseyde P, Ampe W, Depondt M. 1977. ENG and the cervical syndrome neck torsion nystagmus. Adv Otorhinolaryngol 22:119–24

Van der Hart O, Boon S, Jansen OH. 1997. Ritual abuse in European countries: a clinician's perspective. In Fraser GA (ed). The Dilemma of Ritual Abuse, 137–63. Washington: American Psychiatric Association Press

Van der Kolk BA, Herron N, Hostetler A. 1994. The history of trauma in psychiatry. Psychiatric Clin North Am 17:583–600

Van Voris B. 22 May 2000. No gain, no pain? National Law Journal, 1

Varney NR, Bushnell DL, et al. 1995. NeuroSPECT correlates of disabling mild head injury: preliminary findings. J Head Trauma Rehabil 10:18–28

Vertinsky PA. 1990. The Eternally Wounded Woman. Manchester and New York: Manchester University Press

Vianna NJ, Greenwald P, Davies JNP. 1971. Tonsillectomy and Hodgkin's Disease: The lymph barrier. Lancet 1:431

Vincent C, Neale G, Woloshynowych M. 2001. Adverse events in British hospitals: preliminary retrospective record review. Br Med J 322:517–9

von Korff M, Ormel J, et al. 1992. Disability and depression among high utilizers of health care, a longitudinal analysis. Arch Gen Psychiatry 49:91–100

Waddell GA. 1986. Provision of orthopaedic services for backache in Oman. Report to the Minister of Health, Muscate Sultanate of Oman

– 1987. A new clinical model for the treatment of low-back pain. Volvo Award in Clinical Sciences. Spine 12:632–44

– 1991. Low back disability. A syndrome of Western civilization. Neurosurg Clin North Am 2:719–38

– 1993. Simple low back pain: rest or active exercise. Ann Rheum Dis 52:17–9

– 1996. Low back pain: a twentieth-century health problem. Spine 21:2820–5

– 1998. The Back Pain Revolution. Edinburgh: Churchill Livingstone

Waddell GA, Kummel EG, et al. 1979. Failed lumbar disc surgery and repeat surgery following industrial injury. J Bone Joint Surg 61A: 201–7

Waddell GA, McCulloch JA, et al. 1980. Non-organic physical signs in low back pain. Spine 5:117–25

Wadman M. 2000. US panel draws blank on Gulf war symptoms. Nature 407:121

Wallis BJ, Lord SM, Barnsley L. 1996. Pain and psychological symptoms of Australian patients with whiplash. Spine 21:804–10

Walsh NE, Dumitru D. 1988. The influence of compensation on the recovery from low back pain. Occup Med 3:109–21

Walz F. 1987. [Whiplash trauma of the cervical vertebrae in traffic: biomechanical and expert-opinion aspects] [German]. Schweiz Med Wochenschr 117:619–23

– 1994. [Biomechanical aspects of injuries of the cervical vertebrae] [German]. Orthopäde 23:262–7

Ware JC, Russell J, Campos E. 1986. Alpha intrusions into sleep of depressed and fibromyalgic syndrome (fibrositis) patients. Sleep Research 15:210

Warren JR. 1983. Unidentified curved bacilli in gastric epithelium in active chronic gastritis. Lancet 1:1273–5

Watts A. 1963. The Wisdom of Insecurity. New York: Random House

Watts R. 1995. Post-traumatic stress disorder after a bus accident. Aust NZ J Psychiatry 29:75–83.

Webb, S.and W. 1910. The State and the Doctor. London: Longmans

Weinberg S, La Pointe H. 1987. Cervical extension-flexion injury (whiplash) and internal derangement of the temporomandibular joint. J Oral Maxillofac Surg 45:653–6

Weinberger LM. 1976. Trauma or treatment? The role of intermittent traction in the treatment of cervical soft-tissue injuries. J Trauma, 16:377–82

– 1977. Traumatic fibrositis. West J Med 127:99–103

Weintraub MI. 1995. Chronic pain in litigation. Neurol Clin 13:341–9

Weiss HD, Stern BJ, Goldberg J. 1991. Post-traumatic migraine: chronic migraine precipitated by minor head or neck trauma. Headache 31: 451–6

Wells Jane. 1998. Mammography and the politics of randomised controlled trials. BMJ 317: 1224–7

Wessely S. 1990. Old wine in new bottles: neurasthenia and "ME". Psychol Med 20:35–53

– 1995. Social and cultural aspects of chronic fatigue syndrome. J Musculoskeletal Pain 3:111–22

– 1997. Chronic fatigue syndrome: a twentieth-century illness? Scand J Wor Environ Health 23 (Suppl 3):17–34

Wessely S, Hotopf M, Sharpe M. 1998. Chronic Fatigue and its Syndromes. London: Oxford University Press

Wessely S, Rose S, Bisson J. 1998. Psychological "debriefing": a systemic review of the brief psychological interventions for the treatment of immediate trauma related symptoms and the prevention of PTSD. The Cochrane Library (4)

West DH, Gough JP, Harper GTK. 1993. Low speed rear-end collision testing using human subjects. Accid Reconstruct J 5:22–6

Westesson P-L, Erikson L, Kurita K. 1990. TMJ: variation of normal arthrographic anatomy. Oral Surg Oral Med Oral Pathol 69:514–9

White JW, Wolraich M. 1995. Effect of sugar on behavior and mental performance. Am J Clin Nutr 62(suppl):242S–9S

White KP, Speechley M, et al. 1995. Fibromyalgia in rheumatology practice: a survey of Canadian rheumatologists. J Rheumatol 22:722–6

Whitehead AN. 1967. Science and the Modern World. New York: Macmillan

Whittle B, Ritchie J. 2000. Prescription for Murder: The True Story of the Mass Murderer Harold Frederick Shipman. London: Warner

WHO European Collaborative Group. 1983. Multi-factorial trial in prevention of heart disease incidence and mortality results. European Heart J 4:141–7

Wickstrom JK, Martinez JL, Rodriguez R. 1967. Cervical sprain syndrome: experimental acceleration injuries of the head and neck. In Selzer ML, Gikas PW, Huelke DF (eds). Proceedings of the Prevention of Highway Accidents Symposium. Ann Arbor: University of Michigan Press. 182–7

Wickstrom JK, Martinez JL, et al. 1970. Hyperextension and hyperflexion injuries to the head and neck of primates. In Gurdjian ES, Thomas LM (eds). Neckache and Backache. Springfield, IL: Charles C Thomas. 108–19

Wiesel SW, Feffer HL, Rothman RH. 1984. Industrial low back pain. A prospective evaluation of a standardized diagnostic and treatment protocol. Spine 12:199–203

Wiesel SW, Fetter HL, Rothman RH. 1986. Neck Pain. Charlottesville: The Michie Co

Wiesinger H, Guerry D. 1962. The ocular aspects of whiplash. Virginia Med Monthly 89:165–8

Wilber K, Goleman D, et al. 1993. Paths Beyond Ego. New York: CP Putnam

Wiley AM, Lloyd GJ, et al. 1986. Musculo-skeletal sequelae of whiplash injuries. Advocates' Quarterly 7:65–78

Williams JF, McKenzie JA. 1975. The effect of collision severity on the motion of the head and neck during "whiplash." J Biomech 8:257–9

Williams ME, Hadler NM. 1983. The illness as focus of geriatric medicine. N Engl J Med 308:1357–60

Willis E. 1986. RSI as a social process. Community Health Studies 10:210–9

Wilson Edward O. 1975. Sociobiology: a Modern Synthesis. Cambridge, Mass: Harvard University Press.

Wilson SAK. 1931. The approach to the study of hysteria. J Neurol Psychopathol 11:193–206

Winfield JB. 1997. Fibromyalgia: What's next? Arthritis Care & Research 10:219–21

Wiseman R. 1994. Megalab. Daily Telegraph (UK)

Withering W. 1941. An account of the foxglove and some of its medical uses: with practical remarks on dropsy and other diseases (1785). In Willius FA, Key TE.(eds). Classics in Cardiology. New York: Henry Schuman. 231–52

Wolf N. 1991. The Beauty Myth: How Images of Beauty are Used against Women. New York: William Morrow

Wolfe F. 1994. When to diagnose fibromyalgia. Rheum Dis Clin North Am 20:485–500

– 1997. The fibromyalgia problem. J Rheumatol 24:1247–9

Wolfe F, Anderson J, et al. 1997. The work and disability status of persons with fibromyalgia. J Rheumatol 24:1171–8

Wolfe F, Ross K, et al. 1995. The prevalence and characteristics of fibromyalgia in the general population. Arthritis Rheum 38:19–28

Wolfe F, Simons DG, et al. 1992. The fibromyalgia and myofascial pain syndromes: a preliminary study of tender points and trigger points in persons with fibromyalgia, myofascial pain syndrome and no disease. J Rheumatol 19:944–51

Wolfe F, Smythe H, et al. 1990. The American College of Rheumatology 1990 criteria for the classification of fibromyalgia. Arthritis Rheum 33:160–72

Wolfe F and the Vancouver Fibromyalgia Consensus Group. 1996. The fibromyalgia syndrome: a consensus report of fibromylagia and disability. J Rheumatol 23:534–9

Wolman IJ. 1956. Tonsillectomy and adenoidectomy: an analysis of a nationwide inquiry into prevailing practices. Q Rev Pediatr 2:109

Woods WW. 1965. Personal experiences with the surgical treatment of 250 cases of cervicobrachial neurovascular compression syndrome. Arch Emerg Med 5:12–7

Woods WW, Compere WE. 1969. Electronystagmography in cervical injuries. Int Surg 51:251–8

Wool CA, Barsky AJ. 1994. Do women somatize more than men? Psychosomatics 35:445–51

Woolsey RM. 1976. Hysteria: 1875 to 1975. Diseases of the Nervous System 37:379–86

World Bank. 1993. World Development Report 1993: Investing in Health. Washington DC: World Bank

Wright Robert. 1994. The Moral Animal. New York: Pantheon Books

Wrightson P, Gronwall D. 1981. Time off work and symptoms after minor head injury. Injury 12:445–54

Yarnell PR, Rossie GV. 1988. Minor whiplash head injury with major debilitation. Injury 2:255–8

Young, B. 1985. Sequelae of head injury. In Wilkins RH, Rengachary S (eds). Neurosurgery. New York: McGraw-Hill Book Co. Ch 209, 1691.

Young JH. 1967. A Social History of Health Quackery in Twentieth-Century America. Princeton: Princeton University Press

Youngjohn JR, Burrows L, Erdal K. 1995. Brain damage or compensation neurosis? The controversial post-concussion syndrome. Clin Neuropsychol 9:112–23

Youngson R, Schott I. 1996. Medical Blunders. New York: New York University Press

Yunus MB, Masi AT, Calabro JJ. 1981. Primary fibromyalgia (fibrositis): clinical study of 50 patients with matched controls. Semin Arthritis Rheum 11:151–71

Yunus MB, Masi AT, Aldag JC. 1989. Short-term effects of ibuprofen in primary fibromyalgia syndrome: a double blind placebo controlled study. J Rheumatol 16:527–32

Zborowski M. 1952. Cultural components in response to pain. J Soc Issues 8:17–30

Figure Credits & Permissions

FIGURE CREDITS

Fig. 1–1   Carroll, McAfee, Riley (1992) 99b
Fig. 2–1   Gay, Abott (1953) 152:1694
Fig. 2–2   Ommaya, Fass, Yarnell (1968) 204, 285–9
Fig. 3–1   National Highway Traffic Safety Administration (1998)
Fig. 4–1   Lees-Haley, Brown (1993) 8:202–9
Fig. 6–1   Waddell (1996) 2821. Based on statistics supplied by the Department of Social Security, U.K.
Fig. 8–1   Courtesy of Hippocrates' Lantern
Fig. 8–2   Courtesy of Hippocrates' Lantern
Fig. 10–1   Adapted from Radanov, Dvorak, Valach (1992)
Fig. 12–1   Wolfe, Smythe, et al (1990)
Fig. 15–1   Adapted from Mayou, Bryant, Duffie (1998)
Fig. 19–1   Insurance Research Council Inc. (1994)
Fig. 19–2   Adapted from Insurance Research Council Inc. (1994) 61
Fig. 20–1   New Jersey Insurance Department, Fraud Division (1993)
Fig. 21–1   British Columbia Insurance Commission
Fig. 22–1   George Cruikshank (1833)
Fig. 23–1   Kessel (1966)
Fig. 26–1   Malleson, Eastwood, Moore (1977)
Fig. 26–2   Registrar General's Report and National Statistics U.K.
Fig. 26–3   Mortality Statistics for U.S., Canada, and the U.K.

PERMISSIONS

The author and publisher would like to thank the following organizations and journals for kindly granting permission to reprint previously published material:

American Medical Association: Illustrations "Action of Whiplash," Gay and Abbott, *JAMA* (1953) 152: 1693–704, and "Simulated Whiplash," *JAMA* (1968) 204: 75–9. Quotation from Timothy Quill, *JAMA* (1985) 254: 3075–9.

Archives of Clinical Neurology: "The neurological base rates of 170 personal injury litigants." P.R. Lees-Haley and R.S. Brown (1993) 8:202–9.

Journal of Musculoskeletal Medicine and Teri J. McDermott: Illustration: "The Mechanism of Whiplash," C. Carroll, M. McAlfee, and L.H. Riley (June 1993): 97–113.

The American College of Rheumatology: "The Three Graces." F. Wolfe, H. Smythe, H.B. Yunus et al, *Arthritis & Rheumatism* (1990) 33:160–72.

Index

Abbott, Kenneth. *See* Gay and Abbott
abortion, 226n10, 371
acceleration, 13–14, 17, 138–9; and brain damage, 19, 135–6; and whiplash, 124
accident neurosis, 224–6
accident proneness, 152–3, 158; as psycho-social disorder, 158–9
accidents: as cause of whiplash, 13–14; causes of, 151, 348; deliberate, 158, 271; effect of compensation on, 309–10; railway, 304–5; simulated, 267–8, 270, 274; subway, 38–42; useful, 153. *See also* accident proneness; motor vehicle accidents
accommodation (optical), 200–2, 205–7
acting out, 152–3
acupuncture, 183, 361
Adams, Jim, 274
addiction, 346, 348
adenoids, 117

Adler, Alfred, 153
Agambar, Lindsay, 25, 36–7
Agency for Health Care Policy and Research (AHCPR), 99
AIDS, 60
alien abduction, 327
Allen, Murrey E., 138–9
allergies. *See* environmental hypersensitivity
Allodi, Federico, 217
alternative healthcare, 80, 335, 338–9, 362; and fibromyalgia, 174; and the media, 363, 367–8; as reaction to patriarchal healthcare system, 360–1, 385; regulation of, 363. *See also specific healthcare treatments and providers;* complementary healthcare
American Academy of Neurology, 137–8
American Academy of TMJ Orthopedics, 115
American Association of

Orthoptic Technicians, 199–200
American Child Health Association, 127
American College of Rehabilitation Medicine, 140
American College of Rheumatology, 169, 176–7, 189
American Dental Association, 115–16
American Law Institute, 245
American Psychiatric Association, 212, 309. *See also DSM*
anaesthetists, 188–9
analgesics, 155, 156, 193n6
Anderson, Terry, 343
Angell, Marsha, 241, 245, 252
anger: about court awards, 261–2; as factor in psycho-social disorders, 52, 160, 289, 305–6; as factor in whiplash, 98, 194, 227, 230; in